The Gourmet's Companion™
Italian
Menu Guide
&
Translator

Other Titles by Bernard Rivkin

The Gourmet's Companion: French Menu Guide & Translator

The Gourmet's Companion: German Menu Guide & Translator

The Gourmet's Companion: Spanish Menu Guide & Translator

The Author wishes to express appreciation to the Italian government tourist office for their cooperation and assistance, and the supply of some of the information used in the preparation of this book.

The Gourmet's Companion™
Italian
Menu Guide
&
Translator

Bernard Rivkin

John Wiley & Sons, Inc.

New York • Chichester • Brisbane • Toronto • Singapore

This book is dedicated to my associate, Myrna Childs Rivkin, without whose patience, effort, and efficiency the project could not have been completed. Thank you! Dear wife.

In recognition of the importance of preserving what has been written, it is a policy of John Wiley & Sons, Inc. to have books of enduring value published in the United States printed on acid-free paper, and we exert our best efforts to that end.

Reproduction or translation of any part of this work beyond that permitted by section 107 or 108 of the 1976 United States Copyright Act without the permission of the copyright owner is unlawful. Requests for permission or further information should be addressed to the Permission Department, John Wiley & Sons, Inc.

Copyright © 1991 by Bernard Rivkin of Bellaire Publishing
Published by John Wiley & Sons, Inc.
All rights reserved. Published simultaneously in Canada.

This publication is designed to provide accurate and authoritative information in regard to the subject matter covered. It is sold with the understanding that the publisher is not engaged in rendering legal, accounting, or other professional service. If legal advice or other expert assistance is required, the services of a competent professional person should be sought. FROM A DECLARATION OF PRINCIPLES JOINTLY ADOPTED BY A COMMITTEE OF THE AMERICAN BAR ASSOCIATION AND A COMMITTEE OF PUBLISHERS.

Library of Congress Cataloging-in-Publication Data

Rivkin, Bernard.
    The gourmet's companion: Italian menu guide and
      translator / Bernard Rivkin.
      p. cm.
    Includes bibliographical references.
    ISBN 0-471-52515-4
    1. Food—Dictionaries. 2. Cookery, Italian—Dictionaries.
3. Cookery—Italy. I. Title.
TX349.R495   1991
641.5945'03—dc20   90-40994

Printed in the United States of America

91 92 10 9 8 7 6 5 4 3 2 1

Contents

**Section 1   Food and Wine in Italy:
A Regional Overview   1**

Restaurants   1
  Suggestions on Tipping   1
Piedmont Cuisine   2
Lombardy Cuisine   3
Trentino-Alto (Upper) Adige Cuisine   4
Liguria Cuisine   4
Emilia-Romagna Cuisine   4
Tuscany Cuisine   5
The Marches Cuisine   5
Umbrian Cuisine   6
Latium Cuisine   6
The Abruzzi and Molise Cuisine   6
Campania Cuisine   7
Apulian Cuisine   7
Basilicata (Lucania)   8
Calabrian Cuisine   8
Sicilian Cuisine   8
Sardinian Cuisine   9
Roman Cuisine   9
  Fettucine   11
  Lasagne   11
  Ravioli with Ricotta   11
  Spaghetti   12
  Soups   12

**Section 2   How to Say It:
English to Italian   13**

Numbers   13
Words and Phrases   15

Foods and Beverages   22
In the Restaurant: To Order or Make Requests   31
Problems   38
To Pay   40
Doctor/Dentist/Emergency   41
Telephone   42

Section 3   How to Understand It:
Italian to English   45

Appetizers   45
Beverages   57
Bread   58
Cakes and Pastries   60
Cheese and Butters   65
Desserts, Fruits, Nuts   68
Dumplings, Polenta   79
Eggs   81
Fritters, Pancakes, Croquettes   85
Game   86
Meat   92
Pasta   122
Pizza, Calzone   136
Poultry   138
Rice   148
Salads   152
Sauces   155
Seafood   162
Soup   176
Spices, Condiments, Herbs   182
Vegetables   183
Wines, Beer, Liquor   197

Section 4   What It Means: A Complete
Alphabetical Dictionary of
Italian Food and Drink   205

Food and Wine in Italy: A Regional Overview

Restaurants

Italy has many restaurants of international renown as well as an infinite number of *trattorie* and *rosticcerie*, where excellent meals are offered at very moderate prices. Many *pizzerie* serve a variety of foods in addition to the popular pizza and are usually open later than other eating establishments.

Restaurants in most deluxe, first class, and second class hotels serve international as well as local cuisine. You will also find restaurants in many third and fourth class hotels and in pensions

Main meals are served between noon and 3 p.m. and between 8 and 11 p.m., but may also be available at other hours.

Most Italian restaurants and hotel dining rooms offer both fixed-price meals and a la carte menus. Fixed-price meals usually include two courses, dessert, taxes, and service charges.

Bars in Italy are open from early morning to late at night and usually serve drinks, refreshments, and a variety of snacks at reasonable prices. There is an extra charge if you want food and drinks served at your table.

Suggestions on Tipping

Restaurants: A service charge of approximately 15 percent is added to all restaurant bills. It is customary, however, to leave the waiter a small tip (five to ten percent) for good service.

Cafes and Bars: Leave a 15 percent tip if you are at a table and if your bill does not already include a service charge. Leave 200 lire (change) if you are at a counter or bar drinking an espresso, cappuccino, etc.; and 500 lire or more if you are at a counter or bar having cocktails or other alcoholic beverages, sandwiches, pastries, and desserts.

Credit cards: The following major credit cards are honored in Italy: American Express, Carte Blanche, Diners Club, MasterCard, and Visa.

There is so much to see and do in Italy—her cities and villages, ruins and landscapes, the waters of her seas, woodland paths, and monuments and galleries. But no visit to Italy would be complete without experiencing the variety of her local dishes and wines. Imagine the tasty dishes prepared with spices and aromatic herbs in Genoa, Queen of the Orient Seas; or the Abruzzi shepherd's *cottura*, which takes its name from the tightly sealed pot he has used for centuries to stew his lamb, with only salt and water added.

Too often, visitors fail to take the opportunity to taste and get to know the wonderful variety of excellent wines that Italy has to offer. Some tourists stick closely to the three or four types of wine most commonly in use: Chianti, Barolo, Barbera, Soave, and Valpolicella. These are certainly excellent wines and worthy of their fame, but you haven't really been to Sardinia if you have not tasted Vernaccia or Malvasia. Similarly, you cannot boast of knowing Campania unless you have tasted Gragnano. Nor should you leave Sicily without trying its Faro and Calatafimi. Regional wines provide a wonderful way to experience the areas of Italy you visit.

Piedmont Cuisine

Piedmontese and Aostan cooking evolved as responses to the appetites of strong, hungry men, accustomed to the cold and to hard work. Highly seasoned dishes are popular, as are the first-rate roasts and the plentiful use of garlic in sauces and stews. France is not far, however, as you will discover when you taste certain subtle combinations of cream cheese, cream, and butter.

Alba produces fragrant white truffles, which can be slivered into fine flakes and sprinkled over a risotto or sliced turkey breasts; there is firm yellow polenta, spread out on freshly scoured boards, and eaten with a substantial sauce; steaming hot boiled beef or veal—whose shining streaks impart an air of gelatinous tenderness—dressed with a spicy green sauce; real partridges, pheasants, and thrushes; haunches of venison roasted over hot coals; beans baked in the oven and brought to the table in all the glory of their native aroma; gorgeous yellow peaches; and chestnuts coated in crystallized sugar, the very ones that Pietro Aretino called *marroni confetti* (chestnut sweetmeats). Coffees, biscuits, and two excellent local cheeses—Robiola and Fontina d'Asti— are renowned in Piedmont.

Lombardy Cuisine

The cuisine of Lombardy is a tasty, refined, and aromatic affair that takes advantage of excellent local products, such as rice, smoked meats, dairy products, and beef. These are prepared to suit the tastes of modern, demanding people who belong, even when at the table, to one of the most important cities of Europe.

You can prepare your palate for a real holiday in Lombardy, whether you eat in a crowded fashionable restaurant, a quiet suburban trattoria, the railway station buffet, or with a family. After a long day's work in the office, even the busiest Lombard business person relaxes at the table in order to enjoy the delights of good cooking.

Among the specialties of the Lombard cuisine: a curious tripe dish called *busecca*; the world-famous Milanese cutlet; the no less famous *risotto*; marrow bones, stew, and *polenta*; tasty sausage; stuffed turkey; Carthusian risotto; salami from Brianza; rich, nourishing broths; whipped cream; delicious fruit pickles and nougat from Cremona; and last but not least, the famous, classic, and inimitable Milanese *panettone*, an airy synthesis of all that is best in the art of the pastry chef. Local cheeses include Mascarpone, Gorgonzola, Robiola, Stracchino, Toleggio, Bel Paese, and Groviera.

Trentino-Alto (Upper) Adige Cuisine

Trentino-Alto (Upper) Adige Cuisine is naturally influenced by German and Austrian traditions, although certain types of sauces have been forgotten and have been replaced by others of a more Mediterranean cast. For example, you will find wurstel and strudel, side by side with excellent gnocchi, ravioli, stuffed meat roasts, and potatoes—baked rather than roasted—and delicious fish brought from alpine lakes, with all the aroma of the genuine fresh-water article.

Liguria Cuisine

The gastronomic specialties of Liguria certainly do not lag behind its excellent wines. The most famous specialty is pesto, a sauce made of oil, basil, cheese, garlic, and walnuts, which is used to dress several local dishes. Also try the *buridda* (fish soup), the *cappon magro* (Russian salad). You will find wonderful mussel soups and other seafood, Genoiese buns, pesto broth, San Remo tangerines, noodles, figs, and a delicious cake called the *Pasqualina*.

Emilia-Romagna Cuisine

The immortal Pellegrino Artusi, in his famous *La scienza in cucina* (The Science of Cooking) writes: "When you hear mention made of Bolognese cooking, drop a little curtsy, for it deserves it. It is a rather heavy cuisine, if you like, because the climate requires it; but how succulent it is, and what good taste it displays! It is wholesome too and, in fact, octogenarians and nonagenarians abound there as nowhere else."

The cuisine of Emilia-Romagna, and particularly that of Bologna, is a hymn to the taste, a triumph of the palate, and a sublimation of the best that anyone has been able to achieve in the field of gastronomy. Bologna is a real school of cooking and enumerates, among its many glories, the following dishes: *tagliatelle, tortellini,* and *capelletti* (all varieties of "macaroni"); *zampone* (pig's foot), *cotechino* (a highly spiced pork sausage); fillets of turkey; rice with duck; mortadella (a type of bologna); prosciutto (ham); Parmesan cheese; Bolognese cutlets; *passatelli* (spinach balls); eel; *lasagne al forno* (alternate layers of macaroni dough and meat sauce baked in the oven); *involtini* (stuffed veal rolls); and an endless list of fragrant smoked meats.

Tuscany Cuisine

Tuscany has succeeded in conferring refinement and subtlety on the most obvious and persistently "ordinary" dishes. Living in the midst of beauty and history has kept the Tuscan on the straight and narrow path in the aesthetics of cooking. Basic cooking materials are incomparable olive oil, the tenderest of meat, and excellent wine.

Fagioli all'uccelletto, with its reminder of game in both name and flavor, cooked with sage, garlic, and tomato is "once tasted, and never forgotten." And *fagioli al fiasco*? What genius of the kitchen perfected that system of boiling beans in a flask so that none of their substance might be lost, and then dressing them with uncooked olive oil, salt, and pepper. *Baccalà alla Livornese*! And try such famous sweets as Siennese *panforte* and *ricciarelli*!

The Marches Cuisine

The lovely region of the Marches, as elsewhere in Italy, has both local country dishes and those inspired by the fish that comes from the numerous ports and harbors along the coast. There are delicious fish stews, huge pastries, aromatic roast piglet, and veal stewed in wonderful sauce. The Marches produces very good wines, better known for their quality than their quantity, which is somewhat restricted. The best of these is undoubtedly the *Verdicchio dei Castelli di Jesi*, and that becomes still better after aging.

Umbrian Cuisine

The best culinary offerings of Umbria are the black truffles from Norcia (with a different and stronger flavor than those from Alba, in Piedmont; Perugian suckling-pig; pigeon; fish caught in Lake Trasimeno; sausages dried along with hams; and tartlets flavored with pine seeds.

Latium Cuisine

Rome is one of the most important tourist centers of the world, and as the meeting point for millions of Italians and foreigners, offers its guests the gastronomic specialties of every large city in their own countries. The local eating habits of Latium, and of Rome in particular, include healthy portions of well-seasoned, tasty and even somewhat vigorous dishes. Garlic, aromatic herbs, spices, wines, vinegar, goat, and every other kind of meat are all summoned to dress the table for meals that delight the palate, even if they are somewhat hard on the digestive organs and the liver.

Unless you have sat down to eat in a small *osteria* (lit. "hostelry") and have ordered the simplest of its dishes, it is difficult to appreciate how important this way of cooking can be—catering, as it does, to the taste of the landlord and his plump and smiling wife rather than to that of the customer.

The Abruzzi and Molise Cuisine

Abruzzi and Molise form two distinct regions: one is bounded by the rivers Tronto, Velino, Salto, part of the Liri and the Sangro, and by the Trigno and the Adriatic Sea; the other lies between the Trigno, part of the Volturno, and of course, the Adriatic Sea.

The types of food prepared along the coastal strip differ considerably from those of the interior. Coastal cuisine, with its *brodetto* (fish soup) and *scapece* (fried fish in vinegar), have fish as their basis, while cuisine from the interior takes its base from the pig—although there are delicious macaroni dishes (*alla chitarra*, for example), sweets, and vegetable stews, as well.

Campania Cuisine

The Campanian cuisine has given rise to many legends and anecdotes, both sad and merry. It revolves around the famous spaghetti, which, as a nineteenth-century writer put it, "God has provided as a basis for an entire meal." Many a slanderous word concerning macaroni, and their widespread use throughout the country, has been put forward by their detractors.

The fact is that, notwithstanding early prejudices concerning the social and digestive acceptability of the dish, this is the one Italian specialty that has conquered the world, and forced itself on the attention of the gourmet, in spite of its humble origins.

But this region has other culinary boasts: Neapolitan pizza, the tastily filled *calzoni* (pastries), cutlets *alla pizzaiola* (a highly spiced sauce), golden-brown fish fries, spaghetti with mussels, Neapolitan sausages, and the smoked meats of Secondigliano. There are also such sweets as the *sfogliatella*, the *pastiera*, and a host of delicious table fruits.

Apulian Cuisine

Apulian cooking, with its strong and tasty dishes, is an admirable accompaniment to the serving of generous wines. Its specialties include the fish soup or stew; macaroni baked in the oven; *capocollo*, a strongly flavored seasoned sausage; roast lamb; stuffed eggplant; seafood in general; and oysters and mussels, which at Taranto are especially magnificent.

The roasts, too, which are prepared with great care in this region, are admirably suited to the local production of red wine. Do not forget to try the Apulian *provole*, a mild but tasty cheese, sometimes smoked; the *ricotta* (cottage cheese); *pan pepato* (a dry cake, made of almonds, raisins and candied fruit); the juicy, juicy figs from Taranto; and the aromatic melon (*popone*) from Brindisi, to be eaten chilled.

Basilicata (Lucania)

Some of the best products of the Basilicata Lucania kitchens include vegetable soups; smoked meats, or meat preserved in oil, which are the *soppressate* (sausages kept in oil); strong cheeses; artichokes; and jugged hare.

You will find the pungent aroma of ginger (which is simply called "strong" by the local population) present in every dish—from the humble fried egg to the "jugging" sauces—and always ready to promote thirst!

Among the cheeses, you should try *caciocavallo*, hard and fairly mild; *provolone*, which is quite strong; the buttery cream cheeses; the *casiddi*, little hard cheeses; cottage cheese, sweet, salt, fresh or dried, but always delicious.

Calabrian Cuisine

Calabrian cooking has some pleasant surprises for the gourmet, among them being macaroni with *ricotta* (cottage cheese); roast pork; trout from the Sila; the highly seasoned smoked sausages—such as the *capocollo* (end of neck), the *soppressata* (pressed pork), and Lucanian sausage—which leave a pleasant memory of their fragrance and seasoning.

Sicilian Cuisine

Sicilian cooking is in no way inferior to the wines that accompany it. The cuisine tends to be rather strong, and in its choice of ingredients reflects the optimistic and rugged character of the Sicilians themselves. Complicated and aromatic sauces are used for the macaroni. You will also find stews and fries of seafood (the best in Italy), delicious sweetmeats, stuffed olives, ice cream, and fresh and preserved fruit.

Sardinian Cuisine

Sardinia takes its place among the most typical of Italy's gastronomical regions. Its wines alone are second to none— whether strong, mild, liquerish, or perfumed—and all have poetic names: Canonau, Monica, Malvasia del Campidano, Oliena, to name a few. The Vernaccia, clear and transparent, is a pale yellow soul-mate to the delights of a Sardinian fish dish. All of these wines synthesize centuries of human experience. They are elaborated and refined, and yet fundamentally simple and pure in the tastes they reveal.

The Sardinian cuisine is of a lineage as ancient as the wines, and is intended for people of discriminating taste. The fine, fat fish that appear on Sardinian tables are a triumph. So is the game—from the partridge to the grive (thrush), from the quail to the black wild boar. There are also the *porceddi* (suckling pigs roasted the same now as they were 2,000 years ago), *malloreddus, taccula, corda, cassola,* and a host of others whose names defy ready translation. There is the special, thin bread eaten by the herdsmen and called "music paper." And there are magnificent mussels, eels, lobster, and tuna fish, and a wide variety of fruits.

Roman Cuisine

Perhaps the most outstanding characteristic of the universally recognized excellence of Roman cuisine is the fact that, in Rome, you can eat very well everywhere. This is as true of luxurious restaurants as it is of the simplest downtown *osteria*, as well as of out-of-town or even provincial eating places. Your choice of eating establishment is limited only by the size of your wallet—and not, certainly, by the quality of the cooking. The quality is guaranteed, regardless of whether you dine *a la carte* or *a prezzo fisso*. (In fact, a great many restaurants have welcomed the proposal made by the Region of Latium—Offices of the Assessor for Tourism and for Commerce and Industry, and offer selections on the "all included" formula.

The first course is a plate of pasta. The *antipasto* course, or hors d'oeuvres, is not a Romanesque tradition.

Only in country inns, or *trattorias*, or in the Castelli Romani, is it usual to anticipate the first course with a large tray of red, hand-cut *prosciutto*, various salamis, some *lonza* (salted pork loin) and, in a separate dish, some Gaeta olives, served with a mixture of chopped garlic and hot pepper, oregano, fennel seeds, anise, celery slices, a little oil, and lemon slices. This genuine betrayal is extremely difficult to resist.

A place must be set aside for *bruschetta*—an accompaniment for the entire meal that is neither a dish on its own nor does it appear on the menu. Offered by the house, it is a tidbit made of slices of home-style bread toasted over a fire or on the grill, rubbed with a garlic clove, and sprinkled with oil, a pinch of salt and another of freshly ground pepper.

In the *trattorias* along the coast, the owner might slip a little seafood salad beneath your nose before you have a chance to consider the menu: small shrimp, clams, mussels and prawns, boiled and shelled, pieces of boned, boiled mullet and cod, all seasoned with a sauce made of olive oil, capers, anchovies, parsley, celery, lemon, salt, and pepper.

The real test of a cook's ability is his/her treatment of fettucine, spaghetti, bucatini, and all the various types of pasta, freshly made with egg, and dried. If he/she doesn't pass this test, then it's time to change *osteria*. But it would be hard to find an *osteria*, *trattoria*, or restaurant in Rome where you can't get a really good plate of pasta.

Fettucine

Fettucine should immediately bring to mind homemade (or at least hand-made) pasta of durum wheat flour, eggs (one per person), salt, and olive oil. Once the dough has been well kneaded, a thin—very thin—layer is rolled out and long, narrow strips are cut, no wider than a centimeter: The fettucine is made. It is then boiled in well-salted water, strained when it is *al dente*, or a little hard, and served with various sauces—with meat sauce (lean beef, onion, carrot, celery, parsley, cloves, red wine, tinned or strained tomatoes, salt, pepper and olive oil, which has taken the place of the original lard); or with chicken livers (giblets, various edible innards, livers browned in olive oil with onion, a good sprinkling of white wine, salt, and pepper); or with pecorino cheese; or tomato sauce with basil leaves, butter, and grated Parmesan cheese; or even a little sauce based on melted butter and anchovy fillets crushed in a mortar.

In the appropriate season, fettucine is served with a sauce of meat, peas, and *prosciutto*, or tossed in a frying pan with grated pecorino or parmesan cheese, together with thin slices of artichokes cooked in a mixture of butter and oil.

Lasagne

Lasagna is like fettucine, but wider and thicker; it can be served with stewed pork sauce, ricotta cheese, and grated Parmesan, or baked with meat sauce, chicken livers, chopped veal, mushrooms, mozzarella cheese, and grated Parmesan cheese. The mozzarella cheese can be substituted with bechamel, and the chopped veal with meatballs.

Ravioli with Ricotta

Alone or bonded to spinach, ricotta cheese is an exquisite filling for ravioli, and Latium abounds in excellent ricotta cheese. Ravioli filled with ricotta by itself, or together with spinach, is served with either meat sauce or melted butter and grated Parmesan cheese.

Spaghetti

Spaghetti has become an international favorite, with its numerous sauces. The most typical and the best known ways of serving spaghetti are *alla matriciana* and then *alla carbonara*.

Soups

In the sacred texts of Roman and Romanesque cuisine, the chapter dealing with soups is no less important than the one about pasta. A good, hearty dish of pasta and lentils, or pasta and chick-peas, or pasta and potatoes, is certainly no less important than a plate of spaghetti with tomato sauce. And the same can be said of pasta and broccoli, pasta and broad beans, or pasta and peas.

A typical Roman soup, not much called for today, is one made with the so-called *battuto*, which the elderly remember with nostalgia today. This soup belongs to their youth, to that *Italietta* when meat and even macaroni was eaten only once a week. The *battuto* is made with the fat pieces and then water. When the water boils, in goes the spaghetti, broken into pieces, however. Salt, pepper and grated Pecorino complete the offering.

In tradition-minded families, soups are a must for holiday celebrations. Easter calls for *brodetto* (made with stale bread, beef and lamb broth and egg yolks beaten with grated cheese, salt, marjoram, and lemon juice); for Christmas, instead, *cappelletti in brodo* (beef and chicken broth, together with Roman cappelletti stuffed with a mixture of pork, mortadella, prosciutto, chicken, brains, grated cheese, nutmeg, egg, Marsala wine, salt and pepper).

How to Say It:
English to Italian

Numbers

0	nought, zero	zero
1	one	uno, una
2	two	due
3	three	tre
4	four	quattro
5	five	cinque
6	six	sei
7	seven	sette
8	eight	otto
9	nine	nove
10	ten	dieci
11	eleven	undici
12	twelve	dodici
13	thirteen	tredici
14	fourteen	quattordici
15	fifteen	quindici
16	sixteen	sedici
17	seventeen	diciassette
18	eighteen	diciotto
19	nineteen	dicannove
20	twenty	venti
21	twenty-one	ventuno
22	twenty-two	ventidue
23	twenty-three	ventitrè

24	twenty-four	ventiquattro
25	twenty-five	venticinque
26	twenty-six	ventisei
27	twenty-seven	ventisette
28	twenty-eight	ventotto
29	twenty-nine	ventinove
30	thirty	trenta
31	thirty-one	trentuno
32	thirty-two	trentadue
40	forty	quaranta
50	fifty	cinquanta
60	sixty	sessanta
70	seventy	settanta
80	eighty	ottanta
90	ninety	novanta
100	one hundred	cento
101	one hundred and one	centouno
105	one hundred and five	centocinque
150	one hundred and fifty	centocinquanta
200	two hundred	duecento
300	three hundred	trecento
400	four hundred	quattrocento
500	five hundred	cinquecento
600	six hundred	seicento
700	seven hundred	settecento
800	eight hundred	ottocento
900	nine hundred	novecento
1,000	one thousand	mille
1,001	one thousand and one	milleuno
1,002	one thousand and two	milledue
1,100	one thousand one hundred	millecento
1,150	one thousand one hundred and fifty	millecento-cinquanta
1,200	one thousand two hundred *or* twelve hundred	milleduecento
1,900	one thousand nine hundred *or* nineteen hundred	millenovecento

2,000	two thousand	duemila
3,000	three thousand	tremila
10,000	ten thousand	diecimila
1,000,000	one million	un milione

Words and Phrases

ACCOMMODATE, TO accomodare
ACCOMPANY, TO accompagnare
AFTER dopo
AGAIN ancora
ALL tutto
ALL RIGHT benissimo
ASH TRAY il portacenere
ASSORTED CHEESES i formaggi assortiti
AT a, ad, da, in
BAD male, cattivo
BAKED al forno
BAKED IN PARCHMENT al cartoccio
BATHROOM il bagno
BEFORE prima
BITTER amaro
BOILED lesso
BOTTLE la bottiglia
BRAISED brasato
BREAKFAST la colazione
CALL AN AMBULANCE Chiamate un'ambulanza
CAN YOU RECOMMEND A GOOD DENTIST? Può
  raccomandarmi un buon dentista?
CASHIER il cassiere
CHAIR la sedia
CHANGE il cambio
CHEF'S SPECIALTY la specialità della casa
CLOSED chiuso
COAT il soprabito, il cappotto
COLD DISHES i piatti freddi
COLD freddo

COME IN   Avanti
CONTENT, HAPPY   contento
COURSE (OF A DINNER)   la pietanza
CUP   la tazza
CURED   salato
DELICIOUS   delizioso
DENTIST   il dentista
DENTIST, JUST FIX IT TEMPORARILY   Dentista, faccia
  una medicazione provvisoria
DESIRE, TO   volere
DESSERT   il dolce
DIET   la dieta
DINING ROOM   la sala da pranzo
DINNER   il pranzo
DO YOU SPEAK ENGLISH?   Parla inglese?
DO YOU UNDERSTAND?   Capisce?
DOCTOR WHO SPEAKS ENGLISH, A   un dottore che
  parla inglese
DOCTOR, IT HURTS HERE   Dottore, fa male qui
DOES ANYONE SPEAK ENGLISH?   Qualcuno parla
  inglese?
DOES NOT INCLUDE THE TIP   Il servizio non è
  compreso
DOWN   giù
EARLY   di buon'ora
EAT, TO   mangiare
EMERGENCY   l'emergenza
END   la fine
ENOUGH   abbastanza
EVENING   la sera
EVERYTHING INCLUDED   tutto completo
EXCELLENT   eccellente
EXCUSE ME!   Mi scusi!
EXPENSIVE   caro
EYEGLASSES   gli occhiali
FEW, SOME   alcuni
FIRE   il fuoco

FIXED PRICE   il prezzo fisso
FOOD   il cibo
FORBIDDEN   proibito
FORK   la forchetta
FROM   da
GLASS   il bicchiere
GOOD   buono
GOOD AFTERNOON   buon giorno
GOOD DAY   buon giorno
GOOD EVENING   buona sera
GOOD MORNING   buon giorno
GOOD NIGHT   buona notte
GOOD-BYE   arrivederci, addio
GRILLED   ai ferri
HARD   duro
HAT   il cappello
HAVE YOU ANY...?   Avete del (della, dello)...?
HEADWAITER   il capocameriere
HEART ATTACK   l'attacco cardiaco
HELLO   ciao
HELP   aiuto
HERE IS   ecco
HERE   quá
HOSPITAL   l'ospedale
HOT   caldo
HOT DISHES   i piatti caldi
HOT FIRST COURSES   i primi piatti caldi
HOT MAIN COURSES   i secondi piatti caldi
HOW ARE YOU?   Come sta?
HOW   come
HOW DO YOU DO?   Come sta?
HOW FAR?   Quanto è lontano?
HOW LONG WILL IT TAKE?   Quanto tempo ci vorrà?
HOW MANY?   quanti?
HOW MUCH IS THAT?   Quanto costa?
HOW MUCH?   Quanto?
HUNGRY, TO BE   avere fame

HURRY   la fretta
I AM A VEGETARIAN   Sono vegetariano(a)
I AM COLD   Ho freddo
I AM HOT   Ho caldo
I AM HUNGRY   Io ho fame
I AM SORRY   Mi dispiace
I AM WAITING FOR SOMEONE   Aspetto qualcuno
I AM WARM   Ho caldo
I ASKED FOR...   Avevo chiesto...
I CAN, I MAY, I AM ABLE TO   io posso
I DON'T UNDERSTAND   Non capisco
I DRINK   Io bevo
I HAVE HAD ENOUGH, THANKS   Nient'altro, grazie
I HAVE LOST MY COAT   Ho perduto il cappotto
I HAVE LOST MY MONEY   Ho perduto il denaro
I HAVE LOST MY PASSPORT   Ho perduto il passaporto
I MUST, I HAVE TO   Io devo
I SPEAK ONLY ENGLISH   Parlo solo inglese
I UNDERSTAND   Capisco
I WANT TO GO TO THE HOTEL   Desidero andare
    all'albergo
I'LL TAKE THIS   Prenderò questo
I'M HUNGRY   Ho fame
ICE CUBES   il ghiaccio
IF YOU PLEASE   prego
IMMEDIATELY   subito
INCLUDES TIP   Il servizio è compreso (*or* incluso)
INSTEAD   invece
KNIFE   il coltello
KOSHER   kosher
LADIES'   per signore
LARGE SPOON   il cucchiaio grande
LATE   tardi
LAVATORY   la toilette
LEAN   magro
LIGHT   leggero
LITTLE   piccolo

LITTLE SUPPER, A   la cenetta
LOOK FOR, TRY, TO   cercare
LUNCH   la colazione del mezzogiorno
MAIN MEALS SERVED COLD   i piatti freddi
MARINATED   marinato
MASHED   il puré
MATCH   il fiammifero
MAY I HAVE OUR HATS AND COATS PLEASE?   Mi dia
   i cappelli e le giacche, per favore
MAY I HAVE THE MENU?   La lista, per favore
MAY I HAVE THE WINE LIST?   La lista dei vini, per
   favore
MAY I HAVE THIS?   Vorrei questo
MAYBE   forse
MEAL   il pasto
MEALS SERVED QUICKLY   i piatti pronti
MEDIUM   non troppo cotto
MEN'S   per signori
MENU   la lista delle vivande
MID MORNING SNACK   lo spuntino
MORE   più
MUCH   molto
MY   mio
NAPKIN   il tovagliolo
NEED   la necessità
NO   no
NO SMOKING   Vietato fumare
NOTHING MORE, THANKS   Nient'altro, grazie
NOTHING   niente
NOW   adesso
OCCUPIED   occupato
OF COURSE   certo
OF EXCELLENT QUALITY   di ottima qualità
ON THE CONTRARY   al contrario
OPEN, TO   aprire
ORDINARILY   generalmente
OVERCOAT   il soprabito

PARDON ME   Scusatemi
PASTRY CART   il carrello della pasticceria
PEN   la penna
PENCIL   la matita
PEPPER MILL   il macinapepe
PIECE   il pezzo
PITCHER   la caraffa
PLACE SETTING   il coperto
PLATE   il piatto
PLATES PREPARED TO ORDER   i piatti da farsi
PLEASE CALL THE HEADWAITER   Per favore (piacere),
   chiami il capocameriere
PLEASE   prego
PLEASE SERVE US QUICKLY   Per favore, ci serva in
   fretta
PLEASE TELEPHONE FOR A TAXI   Per favore, telefoni
   per un tassì
POACHED   affogato
PORTION   la porzione
PREFER, TO   preferire
PREPARED AT THE TABLE   preparato al tavolo
PREPARED FAST SERVICE MEALS   i piatti pronti
PRICE   il prezzo
PURSE   la borsa
QUESTION   la domanda
QUICKLY   subito
RARE   al sangue *or* poco cotto
RAW   crudo
READY   pronto
RED   rosso
REQUEST   la domanda
RESTAURANT   il ristorante
ROAST   l'arrosto
ROASTED   arrostito
SALTY   salato
SALTY, THIS IS TOO   Questo è troppo salato
SANDWICH   il panino imbottito

SAUTÉED   fritto in padella
SEASONING   il condimento
SELL, TO   vendere
SERVICE INCLUDED   il servizio compreso
SERVICE NOT INCLUDED   il servizio non compreso
SICKNESS   la malattia
SMALL BOTTLE OF   una mezza bottiglia di
SMALL   piccolo
SMOKED   affumicato
SOFT   soffice
SOME MORE   ancora
SOUP SPOON   il cucchiaio da minestra
SOUR   agro
SPARKLING   spumante
SPOON   il cucchiaio
STOP   la fermata
STRONG   forte
SUPPER   la cena
SURE   certo
SWEET   il dolce
TABLE   la tavola
TABLESPOON   il cucchiaio da tavola
TAXI   il tassì
TEASPOON   il cucchiaino
THANK YOU   grazie
THANK YOU VERY MUCH   grazie mille
THANK YOU, THIS IS FOR YOU   Grazie, questo è per
   Lei
THAT WAS A VERY GOOD MEAL   È stato un pasto
   molto buono
THAT'S ALL   finito
THE MENU, PLEASE   La lista, per favore
THERE ARE   ci sono
THERE HAS BEEN AN ACCIDENT   C'è stato un incidente
THERE IS   c'è
THIRSTY, TO BE   avere sete
TO   a

TOASTED   tostato
TODAY   oggi
TOILET FOR LADIES   la toilette per signore
TOILET FOR MEN   la toilette per signori
TOILET   il gabinetto
TOMORROW   domani
TONIGHT   stasera
TOOTHPICK   uno stuzzicadenti
UMBRELLA   l'ombrello
UP   su
URGENT   urgente
VARIED   diverso
VERY DRY   molto secco
VERY GOOD   ottimo
WAITER   il cameriere
WAITRESS   la cameriera
WALLET   il portafoglio
WASH, TO   lavare
WE ENJOYED IT, THANK YOU   Ci è piaciuto, grazie
WELL   bene
WELL-DONE   abbastanza cotto *or* ben cotto
WET   bagnato
WHEN CAN THE DOCTOR COME?   Quando può venire
   il dottore?
WINE GLASS   il bicchiere da vino
WINE LIST   la lista dei vini
WITH   con
WITHOUT   senza
WRONG   sbagliato
YES   sì
YESTERDAY   ieri
YOU   Lei

Foods and Beverages

ALMOND   la mandorla
ANCHOVY   l'acciuga

APERITIF   l'aperitivo
APPETIZER   l'antipasto
APPLE   la mela
APPLE SAUCE   il purè di mele
APRICOT   l'albicocca
ARTICHOKE   il carciofo
ASPARAGUS   l'asparago
ASSORTED CHEESES   i formaggi assortiti
AVOCADOS   gli avocadi
BACON AND EGGS   le uova e pancetta
BACON   la pancetta
BANANA   la banana
BASKET OF FRUIT   il cestino di frutta
BEANS   i fagioli
BEEF   il manzo
BEEFSTEAK   la bistecca
BEER   la birra
BEER, BOTTLED   la birra in bottiglia
BEER, DARK   la birra scura
BEER, DRAFT   la birra alla spina
BEER, LIGHT   la birra chiara
BISCUIT   il biscotto
BRANDY   il brandy, il cognac
BREAD   il pane
BREAKFAST SAUSAGES   le salsicce
BROCCOLI   i broccoli
BURGUNDY   il borgogna
BUTTER   il burro
CABBAGE   il cavolo
CAKE   la torta
CANDY   la caramella
CARP   la carpa
CARROTS   le carote
CAULIFLOWER   il cavolfiore
CELERY   il sedano
CEREAL, COLD   i cereali
CEREAL, HOT   i cereali caldi

CHAMPAGNE   lo spumante, lo champagne
CHEESE   il cacio, il formaggio
CHERRIES   le ciliegie
CHICKEN FRICASSEE   il pollo alla cacciatora
CHICKEN   il pollo
CHICKEN, FRIED   il pollo fritto
CHICKEN, ROAST   il pollo arrosto
CHICKEN, SOUP   la minestra di pollo
CHIPS   le patatine fritte
CHOCOLATE BAR   la tavoletta di cioccolato
CHOCOLATE   la cioccolata
CHOP   la costoletta
CLAMS   le vongole
COCKTAIL   il cocktail
COD   il merluzzo
COFFEE   il caffè
COFFEE WITH CREAM   il caffè con panna
COFFEE WITH HOT MILK   il caffè con latte caldo
COFFEE WITH MILK   il caffè con latte
COFFEE, AMERICAN   il caffè americano
COFFEE, BLACK   il caffè nero
COFFEE, DECAFFEINATED   il caffè decaffeinato
COFFEE, ICED   il caffè freddo
COFFEE, INSTANT   il caffè istantaneo
COFFEE, ROLLS, BUTTER   il caffè, i panini, il burro
COGNAC   il cognac
COLD MILK   il latte freddo
COMPOTE, STEWED FRUIT   la composta di frutta
CONTINENTAL BREAKFAST   la colazione continentale
COOKED SAUSAGES   le salsicce cotte
COOKIES   i biscotti
CORN   il grano
CREAM   la panna
CUCUMBER   il cetriolo
CUP OF COFFEE   la tazza di caffè
CUSTARD   la crema
DESSERT   il dolce

DRINKS   le bibite
DRY   secco
DUCK   l'anitra
EEL   l'anguilla
EGGS, FRIED WITH BACON   le uova fritte con pancetta
EGGS, FRIED WITH HAM   le uova fritte con il prosciutto
EGGS, FRIED WITH POTATOES   le uova fritte con le
   patate
EGGS, FRIED WITH SAUSAGE   le uova fritte con la
   salsiccia
EGGS   le uova
EGGS WITH BACON   le uova e pancetta
EGGS, BOILED FIRM   le uova sode
EGGS, BOILED HARD   le uova molto sode
EGGS, BOILED   le uova sode
EGGS, BOILED SOFT   le uova alla coque
EGGS, FRIED   le uova al burro
EGGS, FRIED OVER   le uova al burro girate
EGGS, FRIED UP   le uova al burro girate
EGGS, POACHED FIRM   le uova in camicia ben cotte
EGGS, POACHED   le uova in camicia
EGGS, POACHED SOFT   le uova in camicia soffici
EGGS, SCRAMBLED   le uova strapazzate
EGGS, SCRAMBLED WITH BACON   le uova strapazzate
   con la pancetta
EGGS, SCRAMBLED WITH HAM   le uova strapazzate col
   prosciutto
EGGS, SCRAMBLED WITH POTATOES   le uova
   strapazzate con le patate
EGGS, SCRAMBLED WITH SAUSAGE   le uova
   strapazzate con le salsicce
EGGS, SHIRRED   le uova alla cocotte
ESPRESSO BLACK   il caffè espresso
ESPRESSO WEAK   il caffè espresso lungo
ESPRESSO WITH MILK   il caffè espresso macchiato
FISH   il pesce
FOOD   il cibo

FRENCH ROLL   il panino, la michetta
FRIED   fritto
FRIED POTATOES   le patate fritte
FROG'S LEGS   le cosce di rana
FRUIT DRINK   la bevanda alla frutta
FRUIT JUICE   il succo di frutta
FRUIT   la frutta
FRUIT SALAD   la macedonia
FULL-BODIED   pieno
GAME   la cacciagione
GARLIC   l'aglio
GIN AND TONIC   il gin e tonic
GIN   il gin
GLASS OF BEER   un bicchiere di birra
GLASS OF LIQUEUR   un bicchierino di liquore
GLASS OF MILK   un bicchiere di latte
GLASS OF WATER   un bicchiere d'acqua
GLASS OF WINE   un bicchiere di vino
GOOSE   l'oca
GOOSE LIVER PASTE   il patè di fegato d'oca
GRAPE   l'uva
GRAPEFRUIT   il pompelmo
GRAPEFRUIT JUICE   il succo di pompelmo
GRAVY   la salsa
GREEN BEANS   i fagiolini
GREEN PEPPER   i peperoni verdi
GREEN SALAD   l'insalata verde
GREEN VEGETABLES   la verdura
HADDOCK   il merluzzo
HALIBUT   il palombo
HAM   il prosciutto
HEN   la gallina
HERRING   l'aringa
HONEY   il miele
HOT CHOCOLATE   la cioccolata calda
HOT MILK   il latte caldo
HOT WATER   l'acqua calda

HOT, SPICY   piccante
ICE CREAM   il gelato
ICE CUBES   il ghiaccio
ICE   il ghiaccio
ICE WATER   l'acqua con ghiaccio
ITALIAN HAM   il prosciutto
JAM   la marmellata
JUICE   il succo
KETCHUP   la rubra, il ketchup
KIDNEYS   i rognoni
LAMB CHOPS   le cotolette d'agnello
LAMB   l'agnello
LEMON   il limone
LEMONADE   la limonata
LETTUCE   la lattuga
LIMA BEANS   i fagioli di spagna
LIQUEUR   il liquore
LIVER   il fegato
LOAF OF BREAD   la forma di pane
LOBSTER   l'aragosta
LOCAL RED WINE   il vino locale rosso
LOCAL WHITE WINE   il vino locale bianco
LOCAL WINE   il vino locale
MACARONI   i maccheroni
MACKEREL   gli sgombri
MARMALADE   la marmellata
MASHED POTATOES   il purè di patate
MAYONNAISE   la maionese
MEAT   la carne
MEATBALLS   le polpette
MILK   il latte
MINERAL WATER WITH OR WITHOUT GAS   l'acqua
   minerale
MIXED SALAD   l'insalata mista
MUSHROOMS   i funghi
MUSSELS   le cozze
MUSTARD   la senape

MUTTON   il castrato
NEAT, STRAIGHT   liscio
NOODLES   la pasta asciutta
NUT   la noce
OATMEAL   l'avena calda
OIL   l'olio
OLIVE   l'oliva
OLIVE OIL   l'olio d'oliva
OLIVES, BLACK   le olive nere
OLIVES, GREEN   le olive verdi
OMELET   la frittata
ON THE ROCKS   con ghiaccio
ONION   la cipolla
ORANGE JUICE   il succo d'arancia
ORANGE   l'arancia
OYSTERS   le ostriche
PANCAKES   le fritelle, i pancakes
PARMESAN CHEESE   il formaggio parmigiano
PARSLEY   il prezzemolo
PASTA SERVED FIRM BY UNDERCOOKING   al dente
PASTRY   la pasticceria
PEACH   la pesca
PEANUTS   le arachidi
PEAR   la pera
PEAS   i piselli
PEPPER   il pepe
PIE   la torta
PIGEON   il piccione
PINEAPPLE JUICE   il succo d'ananas
PINEAPPLE   l'ananas
PLUM   la prugna
PORK CHOPS   le cotolette di maiale
PORK   il maiale
PORT   il porto
POTATO SALAD   l'insalata di patate
POTATOES   le patate
POTATOES, BOILED   le patate bollite

POTATOES, FRIED   le patate fritte
POULTRY   il pollo, il pollame
PRAWNS   gli scampi
PRUNES   le prugne secche
RABBIT   il coniglio
RADISHES   i rapanelli
RASPBERRIES   i lamponi
RED CABBAGE   il cavolo rosso
RED WINE   il vino rosso
RICE   il riso
ROAST BEEF   il roast beef
ROAST CHICKEN   il pollo arrosto
ROAST PORK   l'arrosto di maiale
ROAST VEAL   l'arrosto di vitello
ROLL   il panino
ROSÉ WINE   il vino rosato
RUM   il rum
SACCHARIN   la saccarina
SALAD DRESSING   il condimento per l'insalata
SALAD   l'insalata
SALAMI   il salame
SALMON   il salmone
SALT   il sale
SANDWICH   il panino imbottito
SANDWICH ROLLS   i panini
SAUCE   la salsa
SAUERKRAUT   i crauti
SAUSAGE   la salsiccia
SCOTCH   lo scotch, il whiskey scozzese
SCRAMBLED EGGS   le uova strapazzate
SEAFOOD   i frutti di mare
SHARK   lo squalo
SHERRY   lo sherry
SHRIMP COCKTAIL   il cocktail di scampi
SHRIMP   i gamberi, gli scampi
SNAILS   le lumache
SODA   la soda, il selz

SODA WATER   l'acqua di selz
SOFT DRINKS   le bibite gassate
SOFT-BOILED EGG   l'uovo alla coque
SOLE   la sogliola
SOUP   il brodo
SPARKLING   spumante
SPICY SAUCE   la salsa piccante
SPICY SAUSAGE   la salsiccia piccante
SPINACH   gli spinaci
SQUID   i calamari
STEAK   la bistecca
STEAMED   cotto al vapore
STEWED   in umido
STRAWBERRIES   le fragole
SUGAR   lo zucchero
SWEETS   i dolci
TEA   il tè
TEA WITH CREAM   il tè macchiato, il tè con latte
TEA WITH LEMON   il tè al limone
TOAST   il pane tostato
TOMATO   il pomodoro
TOMATO JUICE   il succo di pomodoro
TONGUE   la lingua
TROUT   la trota
TRUFFLE   il tartufo
TUNA   il tonno
TURKEY   il tacchino
VANILLA   la vaniglia
VEAL   il vitello
VEGETABLE SOUP (THICK)   il minestrone
VEGETABLES   i legumi
VERMOUTH   il vermouth
VINEGAR   l'aceto
VODKA   la vodka
WATER   l'acqua
WATERMELON   l'anguria
WHIPPED CREAM   la panna montata

WHISKEY AND SODA   il whiskey e soda
WHISKEY   il whiskey
WINE   il vino
WINE, LOCAL RED   il vino locale rosso
WINE, LOCAL WHITE   il vino locale bianco
WINE, RED   il vino rosso
WINE, SPARKLING   il vino spumante
WINE, VERY DRY   il vino molto secco
WINE, VERY FULL-BODIED   il vino molto corposo
WINE, WHITE   il vino bianco
YOGHURT   lo yogurt

In the Restaurant: To Order or Make Requests

A TABLE FOR FOUR, PLEASE   Un tavolo per quattro persone, per favore
A TABLE FOR THREE, PLEASE   Un tavolo per tre persone, per favore
A TABLE FOR TWO, PLEASE   Un tavolo per due persone, per favore
A TABLE FOR..., PLEASE   Un tavolo per... persone, per favore
ANOTHER CHAIR   un'altra sedia
AT WHAT TIMES ARE MEALS SERVED?   A che ore servono i pasti?
BATHROOM   il bagno
BOTTLE OF GOOD LOCAL WINE   una bottiglia di buon vino locale
BRING ME THE MENU, PLEASE   Mi porti la lista, per favore
BRING ME THE WINE LIST, PLEASE   Mi porti la lista dei vini, per favore
BRING US COFFEE NOW, PLEASE   Ci porti il caffè adesso, per favore
CAN I HAVE...   Potrei avere...

CAN WE BE SERVED QUICKLY? Possiamo essere serviti in fretta?

CAN WE DINE NOW? Possiamo mangiare adesso?

CAN YOU HELP ME? Può aiutarmi?

CAN YOU RECOMMEND A GOOD RESTAURANT, NOT TOO EXPENSIVE? Può consigliare un buon ristorante non troppo caro?

CAN YOU RECOMMEND A GOOD RESTAURANT? Può consigliare un buon ristorante?

CAN YOU TELL ME WHAT THIS IS? Mi può dire che cos'è questo?

CARAFE OF LOCAL RED WINE, PLEASE Del vino rosso locale, per favore

CARAFE OF LOCAL WHITE WINE, PLEASE Del vino bianco locale, per favore

COOKED MORE, PLEASE Più cotto, per favore

COULD I HAVE A (AN)..., PLEASE Posso avere..., per favore

COULD WE HAVE A TABLE? Potremmo avere un tavolo?

COULD WE HAVE MORE..., PLEASE? Potremmo avere ancora..., per favore?

CUP la tazza

DINING ROOM la sala da pranzo

DO YOU ACCEPT AMERICAN MONEY? Accetta moneta americana?

DO YOU ACCEPT U.S. CURRENCY? Accettate valuta americana?

DO YOU ACCEPT TRAVELER'S CHECKS? Accettate i traveller's checques?

DO YOU ACCEPT DINERS CARD? Accetta la carta di credito Diners?

DO YOU ACCEPT MASTERCARD? Accetta la carta di credito MasterCard?

DO YOU ACCEPT THE AMERICAN EXPRESS CREDIT CARD? Accetta la carta di credito dell'American Express?

DO YOU ACCEPT VISA CARD?   Accetta la carta di credito Visa?

DO YOU HAVE A CHILDREN'S MENU?   Avete un menu per bambini?

DO YOU HAVE A DISH OF THE DAY?   C'è un piatto del giorno?

DO YOU HAVE A SET MENU?   Avete un menù a prezzo fisso?

DO YOU HAVE LOCAL DISHES?   Avete piatti locali?

DO YOU HAVE SANDWICHES?   Avete dei panini imbottiti?

DO YOU HAVE WINE BY THE GLASS?   Si può avere un bicchiere di vino?

DO YOU SPEAK ENGLISH?   Parla inglese?

DO YOU UNDERSTAND?   Capisce?

FORK   la forchetta

GLASS   il bicchiere

GLASS OF..., PLEASE   Un bicchiere di..., per favore

HAVE YOU A TABLE FOR... PEOPLE?   Ha un tavolo per... persone?

HAVE YOU ANY...?   Avete del (della, dello)...?

HAVE YOU COMPLETE DINNERS?   Avete menù completi?

HAVE YOU FIXED-PRICE DINNERS?   Avete menù a prezzo fisso?

HOT FIRST COURSES   i primi piatti caldi

HOT MAIN COURSES   i secondi piatti caldi

HOW LONG WILL IT TAKE?   Quanto tempo ci vorrà?

HOW LONG?   Per quanto tempo?

HOW MANY?   Quanti?

HOW MUCH IS OWED?   Quanto le devo?

HOW MUCH IS THAT?   Quanto costa?

HOW MUCH SHOULD THE TAXI CHARGE?   Quanto vuole il tassista? *or* Quanto costa il tassì?

I AM IN A HURRY   Ho fretta

I LIKE THE MEAT MEDIUM   Vorrei la carne abbastanza cotta

I LIKE THE MEAT RARE   Vorrei la carne al sangue

I LIKE THE MEAT WELL-DONE   Vorrei la carne ben cotta

I WANT A TABLE FOR... PEOPLE AT... O'CLOCK   Vorrei un tavolo per... persone alle...

I WANT SOMETHING SIMPLE, NOT TOO SPICY   Vorrei qualcosa semplice, non troppo piccante

I WANT...   Vorrei...

I WOULD LIKE A BOTTLE OF WINE   Vorrei una bottiglia di vino

I WOULD LIKE A GLASS OF MILK   Vorrei un bicchiere di latte

I WOULD LIKE A GLASS OF RED WINE   Vorrei un bicchiere di vino rosso

I WOULD LIKE A GLASS OF WHITE WINE   Vorrei un bicchiere di vino bianco

I'D LIKE A DESSERT, PLEASE   Vorrei del dolce, per favore

I'D LIKE AN APERITIF, PLEASE   Vorrei un aperitivo, per favore

I'D LIKE AN APPETIZER, PLEASE   Vorrei dell'antipasto, per favore

I'D LIKE SOME BEEF, PLEASE   Vorrei della carne di manzo, per favore

I'D LIKE SOME FISH, PLEASE   Vorrei del pesce, per favore

I'D LIKE SOME LAMB, PLEASE   Vorrei dell'agnello, per favore

I'D LIKE SOME PORK, PLEASE   Vorrei del maiale, per favore

I'D LIKE TO PAY   Vorrei pagare

I'D LIKE...   Vorrei...

I'LL TAKE THIS   Prenderò questo

IS THE TIP INCLUDED?   La mancia è compresa?

KOSHER   kosher

LADIES'   per signore

LARGE SPOON   il cucchiaio grande

LAVATORY   la toilette
LEAN   magro
LET'S CALL THE WAITER   Chiamiamo il cameriere
MAY I CHANGE THIS?   Posso cambiare questo?
MAY I HAVE OUR HATS AND COATS PLEASE?   Mi dia
   i cappelli e le giacche, per favore
MAY I HAVE THE MENU?   La lista, per favore
MAY I HAVE THE WINE LIST?   La lista dei vini, per favore
MAY I HAVE THIS?   Vorrei questo
MAY I PLEASE HAVE THE MENU?   Per favore, mi può
   dare il menù
MEDIUM   non troppo cotto
MEN'S   per signori
MENU   la lista delle vivande
MENU, PLEASE   La lista, per favore
MORE BEER, PLEASE   Ancora della birra, per favore
MORE BREAD, PLEASE   Ancora del pane, per favore
MORE COFFEE, PLEASE   Ancora del caffè, per favore
MORE   più
MORE WATER, PLEASE   Ancora dell'acqua, per favore
NO SAUCE, PLEASE   Senza la salsa, per favore
NOTHING MORE, THANKS   Nient'altro, grazie
PASTRY CART   il carrello della pasticceria
PAY, TO   pagare
PEPPER MILL   il macinapepe
PLATE   il piatto
PLEASE BRING ME   per piacere, mi porti
PLEASE CALL THE HEADWAITER   Per favore (piacere),
   chiami il capocameriere
PLEASE CHANGE THIS BILL   Mi cambia questi soldi,
   per favore
PLEASE HURRY   Per favore, faccia presto
PLEASE SERVE US QUICKLY   Per favore, ci serva in
   fretta
PLEASE TAKE IT AWAY   Lo porti via, per favore
PLEASE TELL ME THE WAY TO...   Prego, qual'è la via
   per andare a...

PREPARED AT THE TABLE   preparato al tavolo
QUICKLY   subito
RARE   poco cotto
SLICE OF   una fetta di
SMALL BOTTLE OF   una mezza bottiglia di
SOMETHING LIGHT, PLEASE   Qualcosa di leggero, per favore
SOUP SPOON   il cucchiaio da minestra
SPOON   il cucchiaio
SUGAR BOWL   la zuccheriera
TABLE BY THE WINDOW   Un tavolo vicino alla finestra
TABLE FOR TWO, PLEASE   Un tavolo per due, per favore
TABLE OUTSIDE   un tavolo all'aperto
TABLESPOON   il cucchiaio da tavola
TAKE IT AWAY, PLEASE   Lo porti via, per favore
TEASPOON   il cucchiaino
THE MENU, PLEASE   La lista, per favore
TOILET FOR LADIES   la toilette per signore
TOILET FOR MEN   la toilette per signori
TOILET   il gabinetto
TOOTHPICK   uno stuzzicadenti
VERY WELL-DONE   molto ben cotto
WATER   l'acqua
WE WOULD LIKE A BOTTLE OF DRY WINE   Vorremmo una bottiglia di vino secco
WE WOULD LIKE A BOTTLE OF RED WINE   Vorremmo una bottiglia di vino rosso
WE WOULD LIKE A BOTTLE OF SWEET WINE   Vorremmo una bottiglia di vino dolce
WE WOULD LIKE A BOTTLE OF WHITE WINE   Vorremmo una bottiglia di vino bianco
WE WOULD LIKE A GLASS OF DRY WINE   Vorremmo un bicchiere di vino secco
WE WOULD LIKE A GLASS OF RED WINE   Vorremmo un bicchiere di vino rosso
WE WOULD LIKE A GLASS OF SWEET WINE   Vorremmo un bicchiere di vino dolce

WE WOULD LIKE A GLASS OF WHITE WINE
  Vorremmo un bicchiere di vino bianco
WE'LL COME AT... O'CLOCK   Verremo alle...
WELL-COOKED   ben cotto
WELL-DONE   ben cotto
WHAT ARE THE LOCAL DISHES?   Qual'è la specialità
  locale?
WHAT CREDIT CARDS DO YOU HONOR?   Quali carte
  di credito accetta?
WHAT DO YOU RECOMMEND?   Cosa consiglia?
WHAT IS THAT?   Che cos'è?
WHAT IS THE SPECIALTY OF THE HOUSE?   Qual è la
  specialità della casa?
WHAT IS THE TIME?   Quanto ci vuole?
WHAT SALADS DO YOU HAVE?   Che insalate avete?
WHAT SEAFOOD DO YOU HAVE?   Che tipo di pesce
  avete?
WHAT SHALL WE ORDER TO BE SERVED QUICKLY?
  Che cosa può essere servito subito?
WHAT WINE DO YOU RECOMMEND?   Che vino ci
  consiglia?
WHAT'S THIS?   Cos'è questo?
WHERE CAN I EXCHANGE CURRENCY?   Dove posso
  cambiare della valuta?
WHERE IS THE TELEPHONE?   Dov'è il telefono?
WHERE IS THE TOILET?   Dov'è il gabinetto?
WILL YOU ACCEPT AMERICAN MONEY?   Accettate
  denaro americano?
WINE GLASS   il bicchiere da vino
WINE LIST, PLEASE   La lista dei vini, per favore
WINE, LOCAL RED   il vino locale rosso
WINE, LOCAL WHITE   il vino locale bianco
WINE, VERY FULL-BODIED   il vino molto corposo
WITH POTATOES, PLEASE   con delle patate, per favore
WITH SODA WATER, PLEASE   con selz, per favore
WITHOUT ICE   senza ghiaccio

Problems

AIR IS BLOWING ON ME   C'è della corrente d'aria
BAD   male, cattivo
BITTER   amaro
BITTER, THIS IS TOO   Questo è troppo amaro
COOKED MORE, PLEASE   Più cotto, per favore
DIRTY   sporco
FOOD IS COLD   Il cibo è freddo
HOTTER   più caldo
I AM COLD   Ho freddo
I AM HOT   Ho caldo
I AM ILL   Sono ammalato
I AM IN A HURRY   Ho fretta
I AM LOST   Ho perso la strada
I AM WARM   Ho caldo
I ASKED FOR...   Avevo chiesto...
I DID NOT ORDER THIS   Non ho ordinato questo
I DO NOT LIKE THAT   Non mi piace quello
I DON'T UNDERSTAND   Non capisco
I HAVE A TERRIBLE TOOTHACHE   Ho un fortissimo
    mal di denti
I HAVE LOST MY COAT   Ho perduto il cappotto
I HAVE LOST MY MONEY   Ho perduto il denaro
I HAVE LOST MY PASSPORT   Ho perduto il passaporto
I SPEAK ONLY ENGLISH   Parlo solo inglese
I THINK THERE IS A MISTAKE HERE   Credo che ci sia
    uno sbaglio qui
I'M HUNGRY   Ho fame
I'M THIRSTY   Ho sete
IS THERE ANYONE HERE WHO KNOWS FIRST AID?
    C'è qualcuno qui che sappia prestare pronto soccorso?
IT DOES NOT TASTE RIGHT   Non ha un buon sapore
IT IS NOT GOOD   Non è buono
IT ISN'T HOT ENOUGH   Non è abbastanza caldo
MAY I CHANGE THIS?   Posso cambiare questo?
OVERDONE, THE MEAT IS   La carne è troppo cotta

PLEASE CALL THE HEADWAITER   Per favore (piacere), chiami il capocameriere

PLEASE TAKE IT AWAY   Lo porti via, per favore

RAW   crudo

SOUR   agro

STOP   la fermata

STRONG   forte

SWEET, THIS IS TOO   Questo è troppo dolce

TASTELESS   insipido

THAT IS BAD   È cattivo

THAT'S NOT WHAT I ORDERED   Non è ciò che avevo ordinato

THE BILL IS INCORRECT   Il conto non è giusto

THE FISH IS BAD   Il pesce è cattivo

THE MEAT IS BAD   La carne è cattiva

THE MEAT IS OVERDONE   La carne è troppo cotta

THE MEAT IS TOO TOUGH   La carne è troppo dura

THE MEAT IS UNDERDONE   La carne non è cotta abbastanza

THE WINE IS CORKED   Il vino ha il turacciolo

THERE'S A MISTAKE IN THIS BILL   C'è un errore nel conto

THIS IS COLD   Questo è freddo

THIS IS NOT CLEAN   Questo non è pulito

THIS IS NOT FRESH   Questo non è fresco

THIS IS OVERCOOKED   Questo è troppo cotto

THIS IS TOO SOUR   Questo è troppo acido

THIS IS TOO SWEET   Questo è troppo dolce

THIS IS TOO TOUGH   Questo è troppo duro

THIS IS UNDERCOOKED   Questo non è abbastanza cotto

TOO RARE, THE MEAT IS   La carne è troppo al sangue

TOO TOUGH, THE MEAT IS   La carne è troppo dura

TOUGH   duro

UNDERDONE, THE MEAT IS   La carne è poco cotta

WHAT'S TAKING YOU SO LONG?   Perchè avete impiegato tanto tempo?

WHAT'S THIS AMOUNT FOR?   Perchè (Cos'è) questo
    importo?
WRONG   sbagliato

To Pay

BILL   il conto
CHANGE   il cambio
CHARGE FOR BREAD & TABLE   il pane e il coperto
CHECK   il conto
DO YOU ACCEPT AMERICAN MONEY?   Accetta
    moneta americana?
DO YOU ACCEPT DINERS CARD?   Accetta la carta di
    credito Diners?
DO YOU ACCEPT MASTERCARD?   Accetta la carta di
    credito MasterCard?
DO YOU ACCEPT VISA CARD?   Accetta la carta di
    credito Visa?
DOES NOT INCLUDE TIP   Il servizio non è compreso
EVERYTHING INCLUDED   tutto compreso, tutto incluso
FIXED PRICE   il prezzo fisso
HOW MUCH IS OWED?   Quanto le devo?
HOW MUCH?   Quanto?
I THINK THERE IS A MISTAKE HERE   Credo che ci sia
    uno sbaglio qui
I'D LIKE TO PAY   Vorrei pagare
INCLUDES TIP   Il servizio è compreso
IS EVERYTHING INCLUDED?   È tutto compreso?
IS SERVICE INCLUDED?   È compreso il servizio?
IS THE TIP INCLUDED?   La mancia è compresa?
KEEP THE CHANGE   Tenga il resto
PAY, TO   pagare
PLEASE CHANGE THIS BILL   Mi cambia questi soldi
SERVICE INCLUDED   servizio compreso
SERVICE NOT INCLUDED   servizio non compreso
THANK YOU, THIS IS FOR YOU   Grazie, questo è per
    Lei

THE BILL FOR THE WHOLE PARTY   il conto completo
THE BILL IS INCORRECT   Il conto non è giusto
THE CHECK, PLEASE   Il conto, per piacere
THERE'S A MISTAKE IN THIS BILL   C'è un errore nel
    conto
TIP IS FOR THE CAPTAIN   La mancia è per il
    capocameriere
TIP IS FOR THE WARDROBE   La mancia è per la
    guardarobiera
TIP IS FOR THE WINE WAITER   La mancia è per il
    cameriere addetto ai vini
TIP   la mancia
WE'D LIKE TO PAY SEPARATELY   Vorremmo pagare
    separatamente
WHAT CREDIT CARDS DO YOU HONOR?   Quali carte
    di credito accetta?
WHAT'S THIS AMOUNT FOR?   Perchè (Cos'è) questo
    importo?
WHERE CAN I EXCHANGE CURRENCY?   Dove posso
    cambiare della valuta?
WHO DO I PAY?   Chi pago?
WILL YOU ACCEPT AMERICAN MONEY?   Accettate
    denaro americano?

Doctor/Dentist/Emergency

CALL A DOCTOR   Chiami il medico
CALL A POLICEOFFICER   Chiami un poliziotto
CALL AN AMBULANCE   Chiamate un'ambulanza
CAN YOU RECOMMEND A GOOD DENTIST?   Può
    consigliare un buon dentista?
DENTIST   il dentista
DENTIST, JUST FIX IT TEMPORARILY   Dentista, faccia
    una medicazione provvisoria
DOCTOR WHO SPEAKS ENGLISH, A   un dottore che
    parla inglese
DOCTOR, IT HURTS HERE   Dottore, fa male qui

DOES ANYONE SPEAK ENGLISH? Qualcuno parla
inglese?
EMERGENCY l'emergenza
FIRE il fuoco
HEART ATTACK l'attacco cardiaco
HELP l'aiuto
HOSPITAL l'ospedale
I AM HOT Ho caldo
I AM ILL Sono ammalato
I HAVE A TERRIBLE TOOTHACHE Ho un fortissimo
mal di denti
IS THERE A DOCTOR HERE? C'è un dottore qui?
IS THERE ANYONE HERE WHO KNOWS FIRST AID?
C'è qualcuno qui che sappia prestare pronto soccorso?
PHARMACY la farmacia
SICKNESS la malattia
STOP la fermata
THERE HAS BEEN AN ACCIDENT C'è stato un incidente
THIS IS AN EMERGENCY È un caso urgente
URGENT urgente

Telephone

CALL A TAXI Chiamate un tassì
CAN I DIAL THIS NUMBER? Posso fare questo numero?
DO I NEED TELEPHONE TOKENS? Mi occorrono dei
gettoni?
HOW MUCH IS A TELEPHONE CALL TO...? Quanto
costa una telefonata a...?
I HAVE BEEN DISCONNECTED È caduta la linea
I WANT THE TELEPHONE NUMBER... Desidero il
numero di telefono...
I WANT TO MAKE A COLLECT CALL TO NUMBER...
Vorrei fare una telefonata a carico del destinatario al
numero...
I WANT TO MAKE A LOCAL CALL TO NUMBER...
Vorrei fare una telefonata urbana al numero...

I WANT TO MAKE A LONG-DISTANCE CALL   Vorrei
fare una telefonata interurbana

I WOULD LIKE TO TELEPHONE...   Vorrei fare una
telefonata...

MAY I HAVE SOME TELEPHONE TOKENS   Mi dia
qualche gettone

MAY I SPEAK TO...   Potrei parlare con...

MY NUMBER IS...   Il mio numero è...

NUMBER IS OCCUPIED   Il numero è occupato

OPERATOR   il centralino

PLEASE ASK HIM (HER) TO CALL ME AT...   Per favore,
gli (Le) dica di chiamarmi a...

PLEASE RECONNECT ME   Mi rimetta in linea, per
favore

PLEASE SPEAK MORE SLOWLY   Per favore, parli più
lentamente

PLEASE TELEPHONE MY HOTEL   Telefoni al mio
albergo

PLEASE TELL HIM (HER)... CALLED   Gli (Le) dica che...
ha chiamato

REPEAT, PLEASE   Ripeta, per favore

SPEAKING IS...   Parla...

TELEPHONE   il telefono

THIS PHONE IS NOT WORKING   Questo telefono non
funziona

WHAT COIN DO I PUT IN?   Quale moneta devo inserire?

WHAT IS THE TELEPHONE NUMBER?   Qual è il
numero di telefono?

WHEN CAN THE DOCTOR COME?   Quando può venire
il dottore?

WHERE IS THE TELEPHONE BOOK?   Dov'è la guida
telefonica?

WHERE IS THE TELEPHONE?   Dov'è il telefono?

3

How to Understand It: Italian to English

Appetizers

A PIACERE   to your own choosing or pleasure

A SCELTA   of your choosing

ABBACCHIO BRODETTATO   pieces of lamb cooked in a sauce of egg yolks flavored with lemon peel

ACCIUGHE   anchovies

ACCIUGHE AL POMODORO   anchovies with tomato and breadcrumbs

ACCIUGHE E FUNGHI   anchovies and mushrooms

ACCIUGHE RIPIENE   deep-fried anchovies stuffed with cheese and bread crumbs

ACCIUGHE TARTUFATE   anchovies prepared with garlic and truffles

AFFETTATI MISTI   mixture of sliced cold meats, ham, sausages

AFFETTATO   sliced cold meat

ALICI   salt cured anchovies

ALICI AL LIMONE   fresh anchovies baked with olive oil and lemon juice

ANGUILLA   eel

ANTIPASTI   appetizers, first course (see ANTIPASTO)

ANTIPASTI ASSORTITI   assorted appetizers of vegetables, cold cuts, olives

ANTIPASTI DI MOLLUSCHI   plate of assorted shellfish

ANTIPASTO   hors d'oeuvre, appetizer

ANTIPASTO A SCELTA   appetizer to one's own choosing
ANTIPASTO AI FUNGHI   marinated mushrooms
ANTIPASTO ALLA GENOVESE   raw young broad beans, salami and cheese
ANTIPASTO DI BURANELLA   assorted seafood appetizer
ANTIPASTO DI MARE   seafood appetizer
ANTIPASTO DI PESCE   appetizer of fish
ANTIPASTO MAGRO   assorted meatless appetizers
ANTIPASTO MISTO   assorted appetizers of cured meats and marinated vegetables
ANTIPASTO MISTO NAVE   assorted seafood appetizer
ARAGOSTA   spiny lobster
ARINGA   herring
ARINGA ALLA CALABRESE   fresh herring braised in garlic oil, mashed and spread on toast
ARINGA, CETRIOLI E BARBABIETOLE   herring in thick cream, cucumber, beets
ARROSTI MISTI FREDDI   cold sliced roast meat
ASTACO   lobster (also ASTICE)
BABBALUCI   snails in olive oil with tomatoes and onions
BACCELLI   raw, broad beans
BAGNA CAUDA   hot sauce for dipping raw vegetables with anchovies, wine, garlic
BIANCHETTI   just hatched anchovies or sardines boiled, served cold
BIANCHETTI FRITTI   fried small sardines
BONDIOLA DI PARMA   pork sausage from Parma
BOTARGUE   smoked or dried tuna or mullet roe, served with oil and lemon
BOTTARGA   hard roe of tuna fish, eaten with olive oil and lemon or lightly baked
BRESAOLA AL LIMONE   salted, dried beef with lemon juice
BURANELLA   mixed seafood antipasto
BUTTARIGA   tuna *or* mullet roe
CALAMARI   squid

CALAMERETTI FRITTI   baby squid, lightly floured

CALZONCINO MEZZADRO   turnover filled with scrambled eggs, sausage, onions, potatoes, Parmesan cheese

CAODA   hot herb oil and anchovy dip for raw vegetables

CAPONATA   chopped eggplant, cooked in open pan with sauce of tomatoes, onion and herbs

CAPONATA ALLA MARINARA   hard biscuits covered with oil, garlic, anchovies, black olives, onions, marinated eggplant, pimentos, herbs

CAPPELLE DI FUNGHI RIPIENE   baked stuffed mushroom caps

CAPPERI   capers

CARCIOFI   artichokes

CARCIOFI AI FUNGHI   artichokes stuffed with mushrooms, bread crumbs, onion and herbs

CARCIOFI AL FORNO   artichokes baked in a covered pan with olive oil, garlic and parsley

CARCIOFI AL VINO BIANCO   artichokes stewed in oil, white wine and herbs

CARCIOFI ALLA CONTADINA   artichokes stuffed with bread crumbs, garlic, anchovies, capers, stewed in oil

CARCIOFI ALLA FIORENTINA   artichoke hearts with a cheese sauce, mushrooms and cauliflower

CARCIOFI ALLA VENEZIANA   artichokes stewed in oil and white wine

CARCIOFI ARROSTITI   roasted artichokes with garlic, olive oil and parsley

CARCIOFI BOLLITI   hot *or* cold boiled artichokes served with a dressing

CARCIOFI CON MAIONESE   artichoke hearts with mayonnaise

CARCIOFI DORATI   artichokes dipped in egg and flour and fried

CARCIOFI RIPIENI   cheese-stuffed artichokes

CARCIOFO RIPIENO   cold artichoke stuffed with marinated artichoke hearts, tomato, bread, lemon vinaigrette

CARDOONS   thistle-like plant, leaves and stalks eaten as
   celery (see CARDI)
CARPACCIO   thinly-sliced raw beef fillet, usually served
   with a piquant sauce
CARRELLO VARIO   assorted antipasti from a rolling cart
CAVIALE   caviar
CAVOLFIORE   cauliflower
CECI   chick-peas
CESTINI   small cases of puff or flaky pastry with tasty
   fillings
CETRIOLI   cucumbers
CETRIOLI ALL'ACETO   pickled cucumbers
CETRIOLINI   small pickles
CHIOCCIOLE   snails
CHIZZE   squares of pastry filled with anchovy or cheese
CIPOLLINA   pearl onion
CIPOLLINE D'IVREA   pearl onions sautéed in herb wine
CIPOLLINE NOVELLE   green onions (scallions)
COCKTAIL DI PESCE   fish cocktail
COPPA   kind of raw ham, usually smoked, sliced and
   served cold
COPPA DI FRUTTA   cup of fruit cocktail
COPPA DI GAMBERETTI   shrimp cocktail
COZZE   mussels
COZZE ALLA MARINARA   mussel stew with garlic,
   pepper or ginger and gravy, in which there is some of
   the sea water taken up with the mussels themselves
COZZE CON RISO   mussels pan fried with tomatoes, rice,
   garlic, oil
COZZE E VONGOLE   baby clams and mussels
COZZE FRITTE   mussels breaded and deep fried
COZZE IMPEPATE   mussels highly flavored with pepper
CROCCHETTA DI RISO   rice croquette with cheese
   center, deep fried
CROSTACEO   shellfish
CROSTINI   small pieces of toast, croutons

CROSTINI ALLA NAPOLETANA   small toast with anchovies and melted cheese

CROSTINI ALLA PROVATURA   slices of bread dipped in egg and put in oven with a slice of cheese melted on top

CROSTINI CON FEGATINI DI POLLO E PROSCIUTTO toasts with chicken liver and ham

CROSTINI CON TARTUFI BIANCHI   rarebit with white truffle

CROSTINI DI MOZZARELLA   cheese toast

CROSTINI MARCHESE   toast with chicken liver

CULATELLO   type of raw ham cured in white wine

DATTERI DI MARE   mussels *or* small clams

DATTERI MARINATI   little shellfish in sauce of olive oil, vinegar, sage and garlic

DORATINI DI RICOTTA   cheese fritters served without sugar at beginning of meal, with sugar at end of meal

FAGIOLI   beans

FAGIOLI AL TONNO   French beans with tuna fish

FAGIOLINI   green string beans

FEGATELLI DI POLLO AL MARSALA   chicken livers with Marsala wine

FEGATO DI OCA   goose liver

FEGATO DI VOLATILI   various fowl livers

FICHI CON PROSCIUTTO   figs with prosciutto ham

FINOCCHIO   fennel

FINOCCHIO IN PINZIMONIO   raw fennel dipped in herb olive oil

FINOCCHIONA ALLA TOSCANA   pork salami flavored with fennel

FOIE GRAS DI POLLO   chicken liver pâté

FRAGOLINE DI MARE   tiny squids, "little sea strawberries"

FRITTELLE ALLA VALTELLINA   cheese fritters deep fried

FRITTELLE DI MITILI   mussel fritters in batter

FRITTELLE DI RICOTTA   deep-fried ricotta cheese balls

FRITTO DI FIORI DI ZUCCA   fried squash flowers

FRUTTI DI MARE   small shellfish

FUNGHETTI ALLA GIUDIA   mushrooms in oil with
garlic and parsley
FUNGHI   mushrooms
FUNGHI AL FUNGHETTO   mushrooms with garlic and herbs
FUNGHI ALLA GRIGLIA   grilled mushrooms
FUNGHI ARROSTO   grilled mushrooms seasoned with
garlic, olive oil, parsley
FUNGHI FRITTI   mushrooms batter dipped and deep
fried
FUNGHI IMBOTTITI   stuffed mushroom caps
FUNGHI PORCINI   wild mushrooms
FUNGHI PORCINI AL TEGAME   wild mushrooms
sautéed in garlic and mint
GALANTINA DI CAPPONE   fine chopped capon loaf in
meat gelatine
GALANTINA DI POLLO   fine chopped chicken loaf in
meat gelatine
GALANTINA DI PROSCIUTTO   fine chopped ham loaf
in meat gelatine
GALANTINA IN GELATINA   fine chopped meat loaf in
meat gelatine
GAMBERETTI   very small shrimp
GAMBERI   shrimp (also SCAMPI)
GIANCHETTI   tiny white boneless fish for antipasti
GRANCHIO   crab (see GRANCEOLA)
INSALATA DI ARINGHE   herring salad
INSALATA DI CARNI   chopped up meat salad with cold
cooked vegetables and hard-boiled eggs
INSALATA DI CAVOLFIORE   cauliflower salad
INSALATA DI CECI   chick-pea salad
INSALATA DI FRUTTI DI MARE   seafood salad, dressing
of oil, lemon juice, mustard, garlic
INSALATA DI GAMBERETTI   shrimp salad in
mayonnaise sauce
INSALATA DI LENTICCHIE   lentil salad
INSALATA DI PESCE   seafood salad with oil and lemon
sauce

INVOLTINI DI ASPARAGI E PROSCIUTTO   asparagus and cheese wrapped in ham slices

LINGUA AL PROSCIUTTO E MADERA   boiled tongue slices with ham served in wine sauce

LINGUA ALL'ESCARLATE   boiled tongue sliced, served cold

LINGUA IN SALSA VERDE   boiled tongue served cold in sauce of capers, anchovy, oil

LINGUA PICCANTE   spiced *or* pickled tongue

LINGUA SALMISTRATA   pickled beef tongue served cold

LUMACHE   boiled snails cooked in sauce of tomatoes and ginger

LUMACHE ALLA BORGOGNONA   snails stuffed with garlic and parsley butter

LUMACHE ALLA BOURGUIGNONNE   snails cooked in garlic butter

LUMACHE ALLA FRANCESE   snails filled with onion, carrot, celery, parsley, butter, garlic, bread crumbs and leeks, served in their shells

LUMACHE ALLA MILANESE   snails sautéed in garlic, oil, butter, anchovies, onions

LUMACHE ALLA PARIGINA   snails cooked in garlic butter

LUMACHE ALLA ROMANA   snails cooked in tomato, anchovy and garlic

LUMACHE ALLA VALDOSTANA   snails braised in oil, garlic, mushrooms, tomato and herbs

MACCHERONI ALLA CHITARRA   macaroni spread over an object resembling a "guitar" and cut into square strips

MAGRO   lean meat *or* vegetarian antipasti

MAIONESE   mayonnaise

MARINATO   marinated

MELANZANE AI FERRI   eggplant slices, grilled

MELANZANE AI FUNGETIELLI   slices of eggplant sautéed with tomatoes, oil, olives, capers, oregano

MELANZANE AL FUNGHETTO   eggplant prepared like mushrooms, chopped small, seasoned with garlic, oil, parsley and pepper

MELANZANE ALL'AGRODOLCE   eggplant in a sweet-sour sauce

MELANZANE ALL'OLIO   eggplant marinated in wine vinegar, garlic, pepper

MELANZANE ALLA FIORENTINA   eggplant slices cooked in layers with cheese and tomatoes

MELANZANE ALLA LIGURE   eggplant sautéed with tomatoes and eggs

MELANZANE ALLA MARINARA   marinated eggplant with garlic and peppers

MELANZANE ALLA NAPOLETANA   eggplant slices layered with cheese, then baked

MELANZANE ALLA PARMIGIANA   eggplant cut into thin slices, dipped in oil, spices, buffalo cheese, tomato sauce, powdered with Parmesan cheese, browned slowly in oven

MELANZANE E PEPERONI FRITTI   deep-fried eggplant and peppers

MELANZANE FARCITE   eggplant stuffed with tomato, anchovies, garlic, oil, parsley, baked in oven

MELANZANE GRATINATE   eggplant fried, pulp mixed with grated cheese, replaced and oven baked

MELANZANE IMBOTTITE   eggplant stuffed with rice, cheese, parsley

MELANZANE RIPIENE ALLA CALABRESE   eggplant stuffed with mince, onion, chopped basil, rice or bread crumbs, grated cheese, tomato sauce, baked in oven

MELANZANE RIPIENE ALLA ROMAGNA   fried eggplant alternating with slices of cheese, then oven browned

MELANZANE RIPIENE ALLA SICILIANA   eggplant with chopped meat and tomato sauce, beaten egg and grated cheese

MELONE COL PROSCIUTTO   melon with prosciutto ham

MISTO   mixed

MISTO NAVE   mixed seafood antipasto

MITILI   mussel

MONZETTE   snails (see LUMACHE)

MORTADELLA   pork sausage made of pork fat, pepper-corns and pistachio nuts

MOSCARDINI   small squid

MOSCARDINO   small squid

MOZZARELLA ALLA ROMANA   cheese slices breaded and pan fried

MOZZARELLA COI CROSTINI   bread and cheese pieces baked and served with butter and anchovies

MOZZARELLA CON POMODORI E ACCIUGHE   mozzarella cheese with tomatoes and anchovies

MOZZARELLA CON RICOTTA E PROSCIUTTO   mozzarella with ricotta and ham

MOZZARELLA CON UOVA E ACCIUGHE   mozzarella with egg, cheese and anchovies

MUSCOLI   mussel type shellfish

OLIVE AGRODOLCI   olives in vinegar and sugar

OLIVE AL FORNO   olives wrapped in bacon and baked

OLIVE ALL'AGLIO   garlic black olives

OLIVE CONDITE CON CAPPERI   olives with capers

OLIVE NERE   black olives

OLIVE RIPIENE   olives stuffed with meat, cheese or pimento

OLIVE VERDI   green olives

OSTRICHE   oysters

OSTRICHE ALLA TARANTINA   baked fresh oysters

PANCETTA   bacon, salted and spiced then rolled, eaten raw

PASSATEMPI   small portions of seafood, pizza, vege-tables, from pushcarts

PATÉ   finely ground meat *or* liver paste served cold

PATÉ D'OCA   fine ground goose liver loaf sliced and served cold

PATÉ DI FEGATO   fine liver paste usually served cold

PATÉ DI POLLO TARTUFATO   fine chicken liver with truffles

PEOCI   mussels

PEPERONATA   sautéed sweet peppers, onions and tomatoes

PEPERONCINI   small pickled green peppers

PEPERONI   green *or* red sweet peppers

PEPERONI AL FORNO   sweet peppers baked in the oven with olive oil

PEPERONI ARROSTITI   roasted sweet peppers

PEPERONI IMBOTTITI PICCANTI   stuffed sweet peppers

PESCE IN CARPIONE   fried fish marinated with onions in vinegar

PETITS PATÉS   little filled pastry cases

POLPO   octopus *or* small squid

POLPO AL PURGATORIO   octopus cooked in oil, tomato, parsley, garlic and pepper

POMODORO   tomato

POMODORO CON ACCIUGHE E MANDORLE   tomato with anchovies and almonds

POMPELMO   grapefruit

PROSCIUTTO   salted air-cured ham

PROSCIUTTO AFFUMICATO   cured, smoked ham

PROSCIUTTO COI FICHI   ham with ripe figs

PROSCIUTTO COI FUNGHI   ham with cheese and mushrooms

PROSCIUTTO COTTO   cured smoked ham which is cooked

PROSCIUTTO CRUDO   salt cured ham which is air-dried

PROSCIUTTO DI CINGHIALE   smoked wild boar

PROSCIUTTO DI LANGHIRANO   ham from the province of Parma

PROSCIUTTO DI MONTAGNA   ham from a mountain district

PROSCIUTTO DI PARMA   cured ham from Parma

PROSCIUTTO E MELONE   ham with melon

PROVATURA ALLO SPIEDO   diced bread and provatura cheese toasted on a spit

RADICI   radishes

RAFANO   horseradish

RANE   frog *or* frog's legs

RANE DORATE   skinned frogs' legs dipped in egg and fried in olive oil

RAPANELLI   radishes

RAVANELLI   radishes

RICCI DI MARE   sea urchins, served raw with lemon
RIFREDDO MISTO   assorted cold roast meat
RIPIENE   stuffed
SALAME   salami
SALAME ALL'UNGHERESE   Hungarian salami of pork and beef
SALAME ALLA CACCIATORA   hard, dried salami
SALAME ALLA FINOCCHIONA   salami from Tuscany, flavored with fennel seed
SALAME ALLA GENOVESE   salami with a mixture of pork, veal and pork fat
SALAME DI FABRIANO   salami with a mixture of pork and veal, from Marches
SALAME DI FELINO   pure pork salami from village of Felino near Parma
SALMONE   salmon fish
SALMONE AFFUMICATO   smoked salmon
SALMONE SCOZZESE   Scotch salmon
SALSICCE   sausages eaten newly made and fried, *or* dry and seasoned
SALUMI   sausage served sliced cold
SALUMI NOSTRANI   local salami
SARDE   sardines
SARDE AL BECCAFICCU   stuffed, baked sardines
SARDE AL FINOCCHIO   fresh sardines baked in tomato wine sauce
SARDE AL VINO BIANCO   sardines baked with wine, anchovies
SARDE ALL'OLIO E ORIGANO   sardines baked in olive oil and oregano
SARDE ALLA BRACE   grilled sardines
SARDE IN CARPIONE   fried, marinated sardines
SARDE IN TORTIERA   baked sardines with garlic, oil, lemon
SARDE RIPIENE   stuffed sardines
SARDELLE   sardines
SARDELLINE   young sardines
SARDINA   small sardine (also see SARDE)

SCAMPI   shrimp *or* prawns (also see GAMBERI)

SCAMPI ALLA VENEZIANA   shrimp boiled and served cold with lemon juice

SCAMPI DORATI   breaded and deep-fried shrimp

SEDANO   celery

SEPPIA IN UMIDO   stewed squid

SFORMATO FREDDO DI TONNO E PATATE   cold tuna and potato mold

SOTTACETO   pickled

SPIEDINI DI MOZZARELLA   bread and cheese pieces baked and served with butter and anchovies

STRUFFOLI   pastries of sweet dough with a thin slice of onion, fried in olive oil

STUZZICA APPETITO   antipasti of vegetables pickled in oil and vinegar

SUCCO DI POMODORO   tomato juice

TARTUFI   truffles

TARTUFI ALLA PIEMONTESE   truffles baked with Parmesan cheese

TARTUFI BIANCHI   white truffles

TARTUFI DI MARE   cockles *or* small clams with truffles

TARTUFI FRESCHI   fresh white truffles with butter

TARTUFI NERI   black truffles

TIMBALLO DI LEGUMI   thin layers of zucchini, ricotta, tomato, rice, vegetable puree

TONNO   tuna

TONNO DI BOTTARGA   tuna roe, grilled *or* boiled and served with oil and lemon

TONNO SOTT'OLIO   tuna fish in oil

TOPINAMBUR   Jerusalem artichoke

TOPINAMBUR AL POMODORO   Jerusalem artichoke smothered with tomato and onion

TROTA AFFUMICATA   smoked trout

UOVA ALLA RUSSA   stuffed, hard eggs with mayonnaise sauce

UOVA FARCITE AL LIMONE   hard-boiled, lemon-stuffed eggs

UOVA FARCITE AL PROSCIUTTO   hard-boiled, ham-
stuffed eggs
UOVA RIPIENE   stuffed hard-boiled eggs
VENTRESCA DI TONNO   belly of tuna fish often canned
with oil
VERDURE MARINATE   pickled green vegetables
VITELLO ARROSTO   roast veal, usually leg
VITELLO ARROSTO AL SOAVE   roast veal in white wine
VITELLO TONNATO   thin veal slices served cold, after
sautéed with tuna, anchovies, olive oil, wine
VONGOLA   small clam
ZUCCHINE   Italian squash
ZUCCHINE FRITTE   squash batter dipped and deep fried
ZUCCHINE IMBOTTITE DI CARNE   squash stuffed with
meat

Beverages

ACQUA   water
ACQUA CON GAS   water with gas (carbonated)
ACQUA CON GHIACCIO   ice water
ACQUA FREDDA   ice-cold water
ACQUA GASSATA   soda water
ACQUA MINERALE   mineral water with or without gas
ACQUA NATURALE   well *or* tap water
ALTRE BEVANDE   other kinds of beverages
ARANCIATA   orangeade
BEVANDE   beverages
BIBITE   beverages *or* drinks
BICCHIERE D'ACQUA   glass of water
BICCHIERE DI LATTE   glass of milk
CAFFÉ   coffee
CAFFÉ CORRETTO   espresso made with liquor or brandy
CAFFÉ E LATTE   coffee with half milk
CAFFÉ ESPRESSO   strong aromatic coffee
CAFFÉ FREDDO   iced coffee

CAFFÉ MACCHIATO   espresso made with a few drops of
  warm milk
CAFFÉ NERO   black coffee
CAFFÉ RISTRETTO   small concentrated cup of coffee
CAPPUCCINO   black coffee with steamed milk on top
CREMA   cream
FRAPPÉ   milk shake
GHIACCIATO   iced, chilled
GHIACCIO   ice cubes
GRANITA   water ice crystals made with flavorings
GRANITA DI CAFFÉ   cold coffee poured over crushed ice
GRANITA DI CAFFÉ CON PANNA   coffee ice crystals
  served with whipped cream
GRANITA DI FRAGOLE E LAMPONI   strawberry *or*
  raspberry ice crystals
LATTE   milk
LATTE AL CACAO   chocolate milk drink
LIMONATA   lemonade
PANNA   cream
SCIROPPO   fruit syrup diluted with water
SIDRO   cider
SPREMUTA   fresh fruit drink
SPREMUTA D'ARANCIA   orange-flavored drink
SUCCO   juice
SUCCO DI FRUTTA   thick fruit juice
SUCCO DI POMODORO   tomato juice
SUGO DI ARANCIA   orange juice
TÉ   tea
TÉ AL LATTE   tea with milk
TÉ AL LIMONE   tea with lemon

Bread

BAICOLI   dry biscuits made of flour, sugar, salt and
  butter, flavored with orange
BRUSCHETTA   thick slice of bread, grilled with garlic and
  olive oil

CARASAU   paper thin shepherds' bread from Sardinia

CARTA DI MUSICA   white bread of thin, unleavened layers, "music paper" put one on top of another

CIAMBELLA   ring-shaped bun

CORNETTI   crescent rolls

CRESCENTE   savory bread, baked with ham or bacon bits

CRESCENTINE   eggless pie dough snack, eaten by itself or with salami or ham

CROSTINI   small pieces of toast, croutons

CROSTINI ALLA NAPOLETANA   small toast with anchovies and melted cheese

CROSTINI ALLA PROVATURA   slices of bread dipped in egg and put in oven with a slice of cheese melted on top

CROSTINI DI MOZZARELLA   cheese toast

CUSCINETTI PANDORATI   egg-fried bread stuffed with ham, anchovy, cheese, deep fried

FITASCETTA   baked onion bread ring

FOCACCIA   flat bread with olive oil, onions or cheese

FOCACCIA ALLA SALVIA   bread baked with sage

FOCACCIA COI CICCIOLI   flat bacon bread

FRITTELLE DI SEGALA   little rolls of dark rye flour and egg, spiced and fried in olive oil

GRISSINI   dry bread sticks

MARITOZZO   soft roll

MARITOZZO FORNAIO ALLA ROMANA   buns baked with raisins, pine nuts, orange peel

MIASCIA TREMAZZO   bread and grape cake

MICHETTE   sweet cakes, bread rolls

PAGNOTTA   loaf of bread

PAGNOTTINE BRUSCHE   bread baked with fine diced salami and cheese

PAN DEI SANTI   bread with lemon, raisins, almonds (Saints' Bread)

PAN DI RAMERINO   baked buns with raisins and rosemary

PAN TOSTATO   toasted Italian bread

PANDOLCE ALLA GENOVESE   baked sweet bread

PANDORATO   bread dipped in whipped egg and fried (French Toast)
PANDORO   golden bread
PANE   bread
PANE CASARECCIO   homemade bread
PANE DI SEGALE   rye flour bread
PANE GIALLO DI GRANO DURO   hard wheat bread
PANE INTEGRALE   whole wheat bread
PANE SCURO   dark bread
PANGRATTATO   bread crumbs
PANINI   various bread and rolls
PANINO   like a French hard roll
PANINO IMBOTTITO   sandwich made with hard roll
PANZENELLA   special bread dish made with olive oil, tomato, onion and French dressing
PIADINA ALLA ROMAGNOLA   griddle-baked, thin flat bread
QUARESIMALI   dry biscuits of flour, egg and toasted almond
SPIEDINI DI MOZZARELLA   bread and cheese pieces baked and served with butter and anchovies
TARTINA   open-faced sandwich
TORTA SUL TESTO   bread made on heated slab
TOSTATO   toasted
TOSTO FRANCESE   French toast, mascarpone cheese, maple syrup
TRAMEZZINO   small sandwich

Cakes and Pastries

AMARELLI MODENA   dry biscuits of egg white, sweet and bitter almonds
AMARETTI   macaroons
ANICINI   aniseed cookies
BIGNÉ   baked *or* fried pastry filled with custard
BISCOTTINI AL MIELE   baked honey cookies
BISCOTTO   rusk, biscuits *or* cookies

BOCCONOTTA   chocolate cookies baked with fruit, coffee and liqueur

BOCCONOTTI   pastry filled with custard

BOMBOLONI   fried cookies filled with cream

BRIGIDINI   anise seed wafers

BUSSOLA   baked doughnut-shaped cake made with lemon peel

CALCIONETTI   cookies with chestnut filling

CANNARICULI   deep-fried honey cookies

CANNOLI   round pastry cases filled with cottage cheese, candied fruit or chocolate

CANNOLI ALLA CREMA DI CAFFÉ   fried pastry roll filled with coffee-flavored ricotta cheese

CANNOLI ALLA SICILIANA   pastry shell filled with ricotta cream

CARTEDDATE   honey-coated, fried *or* baked pastries made with wine

CASSATA ALLA SICILIANA   refrigerator cake with ricotta cheese, candied fruit, chocolate, almonds, Marsala wine

CASSATELLA   chocolate icebox cake

CASSATINE   tarts (also see TORTA)

CASSATINE DI RICOTTA   baked ricotta cheese filled tarts

CASTAGNACCIO   chestnut flour tart with nuts, raisins, candied fruits

CASTAGNACCIO ALLA TOSCANA   chestnut cake

CENCI   fried cookies

CIALZON DI FRUTTA   turnover filled with assorted fruits, sprinkled with crystallized sugar and cinnamon

CIAMBELLA ALLA BOLOGNESE   fruit and nut cake made with wine

CIAMBELLA DI PASQUA   sweet Easter bread

CIARAMICOLA   cake with liqueur, lemon rind, covered with meringue

CICERCHIATA   deep-fried honey cake balls

COPATA   small wafer of honey and nuts

CRISPELLE   pastry deep fried then honey coated

CROSTATA   pie *or* tart
CROSTATA DI CREMA   custard tart
CROSTATA DI VISCIOLE   sour cherry tart
CROSTOLI   fried ribbon cookies
DOLCI   pastries, cakes, sweets, desserts
DOLCI DI MELE   apple cake
DOLCI DI TORINO   rich chocolate dessert
FAVE DEI MORTI   All Soul's Day cookies with almonds
    and pine nuts
FAVE DOLCI   "bean" size and shape almond cinnamon cookies
FAVETTE   rum cookies
FOCACCIA DOLCE   sweet ring-shaped cake
FREGOLATA   almond cookies
FRUSTENGA   cornmeal fruit cake with figs
FRUTTA MARTURANA   almond paste baked in fruit
    shapes and colored
GERMINUS   baked almond macaroons
GIALLETTI   fruited cornmeal cookies
MIASCIA TREMEZZO   bread and grape cake
MICHETTE   sweet cakes, bread rolls
MOSTACCIOLI   hard sweets made of flour and honey
MUSTACCIOLI DI ERICE   baked almond cookies
MUSTACCIOLI DI NATALE   Christmas spice cookies
NEPITELLE   sweet Christmas pies
NESPOLA   a tart wild fruit
OSS DA MORD   anise-flavored buns
PAN DEMEI   anise-flavored buns
PAN DI GENOVA   almond cake
PAN DI RAMERINO   baked buns with raisins and rosemary
PAN DI SPAGNA   spongecake
PAN PEPATO   spicy nut bread cookies
PANDOLCE   heavy cake with dried fruit and pine kernels
PANDORO DI VERONA   very light fluffy cake usually
    star shaped
PANE ALLA TIROLESE   confection of flour, eggs, butter,
    almonds, cinnamon and lemon peel
PANETTONE   tall light cake with raisins and crystallized fruit

PANETTONE CERTOSINO   Christmas fruit bread

PANFORTE   a hard cake of nuts, cocoa, spices, candied orange and lemon peel, melon and honey

PANFORTE DI SIENA   dry, nougat-like sweet made of almonds, candied fruits, spices, flour, butter and eggs

PARROZZO   baked almond and chocolate cake

PASTA FROLLA   sweet pastry dough

PASTICCERIA   cake and pastry shop

PASTICCINO   tart, cake, small pastry

PASTIERA   short pastry containing filling of cottage cheese and candied fruit

PASTINE RUSTICHE   pie filled with ricotta cheese, eggs, citron, raisins, pine nuts, chocolate

PESTRINGOLO   baked fruit cake with figs

PINOCCHIATE   pine kernel and almond cake

PRESNITZ   Easter fruitcake

PROFITEROLE AL CIOCCOLATO   cream puff pastry with chocolate frosting

RICCIARELLI DI SIENA   marzipan cookies from Siena

ROCCIATA DI ASSISI   fruit roll with raisins, walnuts, dry figs, almonds, citrus

SAINT HONORÉ   custard-filled pastry with cream puffs

SAVARIN   liquor-soaked cake ring filled with fruit and topped with whipped cream

SCIUSCELLO   ricotta cheesecake with fruit, almonds, brandy, chocolate, lemon peel

SEMIFREDDO   ice cream cake

SFOGLIATELLE   cakes made of thin flakes of pastry wrapped around a filling of spiced cottage cheese and candied fruit

SFOGLIATELLE FROLLE   baked pastry filled with ricotta cheese, fruits, cinnamon

SILVANO   chocolate meringue *or* tart

STACCIATA UNTA   cake with sugar icing

STRANGOLA PRETI   baked nut cake

STRUFFOLI ALLA NAPOLETANA   fried pastry with honey, various fruits, ricotta cheese

STRUFFOLI DI NATALE   fried honey cookies

TORTA   pie, tart *or* cake

TORTA AL GIANDUIA   chocolate cake with jam, brandy, hazelnuts, honey, etc.

TORTA CASERECCIA DI POLENTA   cornmeal shortcake with dried fruit and pine nuts

TORTA DI FRUTTA SECCA   baked fruit cake with nuts, figs, chocolate, eggs, candied fruit peel

TORTA DI MANDORLE   almond cake

TORTA DI MELE   apple pie *or* torte

TORTA DI MERINGA   fruit pie with whipped cream

TORTA DI NOCCIUOLE   hazelnut cake

TORTA DI NOCI   walnut cake

TORTA DI PERE ALLA PAESANA   plain cake with fresh pears

TORTA DI PRUGNE   baked spongecake with wine, prunes, sugar, eggs

TORTA DI RICOTTA   ricotta cheesecake

TORTA DI RISO   rice cake

TORTA MILLE FOGLIE   thin cake layers separated with custard

TORTA PARADISO   spongecake

TORTA ZUCCOTTO   liquor-soaked cake ring filled with fruit, ice cream, chocolate, whipped cream

TORTANO   baked savory cake made with pork renderings

TORTIGLIONE   almond cake

TORTINA DI MARMELLATA   jam-filled tart

TORTINI AL CASTAGNACCIO   chestnut flour cake

TORTINO DI MOZZARELLA   cheese tart

TORTIONATA ALLA LODIGIANA   almond cake

TURIDDU   biscuits made of flour, egg and almonds, powdered with sugar icing

ZALETI   cake with white raisins, eggs, cornmeal, rum, sugar, pine nuts, lemon rind

ZEPPOLA   deep-fried fritter *or* doughnut

ZEPPOLE DI SAN GIUSEPPE   dessert fritters with cinnamon and sugar

ZUCCOTTO   creamy icebox cake made with fruit and liquor

ZUPPA ALL'EMILIANA   spongecake, custard, chocolate
and cherry preserve

ZUPPA INGLESE   cake steeped in custard sauce and rum
and cordials

Cheese and Butters

ABBESPATA   soft, mild ricotta cheese

AL GRATIN   covered with grated cheese and bread
crumbs and oven baked

ASIAGO   cheese made of skimmed milk

BEL PAESE   mild soft cheese

BUDINO DI RICOTTA   ricotta cheese pudding

BURRO   butter

BURRO E ACCIUGHE   butter and anchovies

BURRO E SALVIA   butter and sage

BURRO MAGGIORDOMO   butter with lemon juice and
parsley

BURRO, LATTE E PARMIGIANO   with butter, milk and cheese

BURRO, PANNA E UOVA   with butter, cream and eggs

CACIO   cheese

CACIOCAVALLO   firm, slightly sweet cheese from cow's
or sheep's milk

CACIOCAVALLO AL FUMO   sweet cheese melted by
steaming

CACIOCAVALLO DI PESCOCOSTANZO   highly-spiced
strong buffalo cheese

CACIOTTE   small ewe milk cheese stuffed with butter

CAPRINO   soft goat's cheese

CAPRINO ROMANO   hard goat's milk cheese

CARNIA   hard provolone type cheese

CREMA DI MASCARPONE   soft cream cheese with rum
and sugar added

CREMINO   soft cheese *or* type of ice cream bar

CROSTINI CON TARTUFI BIANCHI   rarebit with white
truffle

FIADONE   baked cheese pie

FONDUA ALLA PIEMONTESE   melted Fontina cheese with white truffles

FONDUTA - FONDUA   fondue melted with Fontina cheese, white truffle

FONTINA   soft, creamy cheese used in cooking

FORMAGGI ASSORTITI   assorted cheeses

FORMAGGIO   cheese

FORMAGGIO ALL'ARGENTIERA   sweet cheese melted by pan frying

FRITTELLE DI RICOTTA   deep-fried ricotta cheese balls

GARGONZOLA   creamy mild cheese

GNOCCHI ALLA BAVA   potato dumplings with cheese

GNOCCHI ALLA PIEMONTESE   dumplings with Parmesan cheese, Emmenthal cheese and white truffle

GORGONZOLA   blue veined salad cheese, tangy flavored

GRANA   hard, tasty cheese

GRANA LODIGIANO   goat milk strong-flavored cheese

GRATINATA   sprinkled with bread crumbs and cheese and oven-browned

GRATTUGIATO   grated

GROVIERA SVIZZERA   Swiss cheese

GRUVIERA   mild cheese with holes, like Swiss Gruyère

INCANESTRATO   hard, salty cheese, usually grated

LODIGIANO   kind of Parmesan cheese

MASCARPONE   delicate cream cheese

MOZZARELLA   cheese made from whey

MOZZARELLA ALLA MILANESE   cheese slices battered with bread crumbs, deep fried

MOZZARELLA ALLA ROMANA   cheese slices breaded and pan fried

MOZZARELLA COI CROSTINI   bread and cheese pieces baked and served with butter and anchovies

MOZZARELLA CON POMODORI E ACCIUGHE   mozzarella cheese with tomatoes and anchovies

MOZZARELLA CON RICOTTA E PROSCIUTTO   mozzarella with ricotta and ham

MOZZARELLA CON UOVA E ACCIUGHE   mozzarella
with egg, cheese and anchovies
MOZZARELLA DI BUFALA   pear-shaped mild buffalo
milk cheese
MOZZARELLA FRITTA   fried mozzarella cheese
MOZZARELLA IN CARROZZA   like Welsh rarebit, made
of buffalo cheese
OVALINA   small mozzarella cheese from buffalo's milk
PAGLIARINO   medium-soft cheese
PARMIGIANO   Parmesan cheese
PARMIGIANO REGGIANO   hard, strong-flavored cheese,
generally grated
PECORINO   hard, strong-flavored cheese
PIACENTINO   hard, peppery cheese, usually grated
PICONI   baked turnovers filled with ricotta cheese
PIZZA DOLCE   ricotta pie
POLENTA ALLA LODIGIANA   cooked cornmeal slices
with Gruyère cheese, battered, pan fried
POMODORO CON MOZZARELLA   tomatoes and mozzarella
PROVATURA   soft, mild cheese made from buffalo's milk
PROVATURA ALLO SPIEDO   diced bread and provatura
cheese toasted on a spit
PROVOLE DI BUFALA   hard cheese of buffalo milk
PROVOLONE   white, medium-hard cheese
RAGUSANO   hard sweet cheese
RAVIGGIOLO   sharp cheese from sheep or goat milk
RICOTTA   cottage cheese made from whey
RICOTTA CON SALSICCE   cottage cheese with sausage
RICOTTA CON SPINACI E CERVELLA   cottage cheese
with spinach and brains
RICOTTA FRITTA   ricotta cheese fritters
ROBIOLA   soft, sweet sheep milk cheese
ROQUEFORT   strong-flavored cheese used mainly in
salads and dressings
SARDO   strong-flavored sheep cheese
SCAMORZA   aged mozzarella cheese
SCAMORZE RIVISONDOLI   soft cream cheese

SCAMORZINE   cheese from sheep's milk, sometimes
   roasted
SFORMATO   baked mold
SFORMATO ALLA BESCIAMELLA   baked mold of egg
   whites, milk, cheese, meat sauce
SOUFFLÉ DI SPINACI E RICOTTA   spinach and cheese
   soufflé
SPIEDINI DI MOZZARELLA   bread and cheese pieces
   baked and served with butter and anchovies
STRACCHINO   creamy white soft cheese
TALEGGIO   medium-hard mild cheese
TORTA DI POLENTA E FONTINA   cornmeal and cheese
   pudding
TORTINO   tart filled with cheese and vegetables
TORTINO DI MOZZARELLA   cheese tart
TORTINO DI PATATE   potato and cheese tart
VALDOSTANA   ham and fontina cheese

Desserts, Fruits, Nuts

ALBICOCCA   apricot
AMARETTI   macaroons
ANANAS   pineapple
ANANAS AL LIQUORE   pineapple served with a liqueur
ANGURIA   watermelon
ANICINI   aniseed cookies
ARACHIDE   peanut
ARANCIA   orange
ARANCIA AFFETTATA   slices of orange poached in liqueur
ARANCIA AL MARSALA   sliced oranges in Marsala wine
ARANCIATA DI NUORO   orange rind candy
ATTORTA   flaky pastry filled with fruit and almonds
AVELLANA   hazelnut
BACCHE DI SOTTOBOSCO   seasonal berries
BANANE   bananas
BERGAMOT   small sweet, aromatic rind orange
BICCIOLANI DI VERCELLI   spiced sweet cookies

BIGNÉ   baked *or* fried pastry filled with custard

BISCOTTINI AL MIELE   baked honey cookies

BISCOTTO   rusk, biscuits *or* cookies

BISCOTTO DI SAVONA   light potato flour cake with orange and lemon peel

BISCUIT TORTONI   dessert of whipped egg whites, whipped cream, macaroon crumbs and bits of almond

BOCCONOTTA   chocolate cookies baked with fruit, coffee and liqueur

BOCCONOTTI   pastry filled with custard

BOMBOLETTE DI RICOTTA   ricotta fritters

BOMBOLONI   fried cookies filled with cream

BONGO BONGA   profiteroles

BRIGIDINI   anise seed wafers

BUDINO   custard, pudding

BUDINO DI MANDORLE   almond pudding

BUDINO DI PANE   bread pudding

BUDINO DI PANETTONE   rum and wine soaked bread pudding

BUDINO DI RICOTTA   ricotta cheese pudding

BUDINO FREDDO AL GIANDUIA   chocolate custard, hazelnuts

BUSECCHINA   chestnuts stewed in wine and cream

BUSSOLA   baked doughnut shaped cake made with lemon peel

CACHI   persimmon

CAFFÉ AFFOGATO   white chocolate ice cream, espresso, whipped cream

CALCIONETTI   cookies with chestnut filling

CANDITO   candied

CANNARICULI   deep-fried honey cookies

CANNOLI   round pastry cases filled with cottage cheese, candied fruit or chocolate

CANNOLI ALLA CREMA DI CAFFÉ   fried pastry roll filled with coffee-flavored ricotta cheese

CANNOLI ALLA SICILIANA   pastry shell filled with ricotta cream

CARAMELLATO   caramelized sugar coating

CARTEDDATE   honey-coated fried or baked pastries made with wine

CASEATA GELATA   dessert with custard ice cream and whipped cream

CASSATA   ice cream cake with chocolate, custard and almonds

CASSATA ALLA SICILIANA (DOLCE)   mould of ricotta cheese, candied fruit, chocolate, flavored with vanilla and maraschino cherries supported with sponge cakes

CASSATA ALLA SICILIANA (GELATA)   ice cream made in several different colored layers with candied fruit and almonds

CASSATA ALLA SICILIANA   refrigerator cake with ricotta cheese, candied fruit, chocolate, almonds, Marsala wine

CASSATELLA   chocolate icebox cake

CASSATINE   tarts (also see TORTA)

CASSATINE DI RICOTTA   baked ricotta cheese filled tarts

CASTAGNACCIO   chestnut flour tart with nuts, raisins, candied fruits

CASTAGNACCIO ALLA TOSCANA   chestnut cake

CASTAGNE   chestnuts

CASTAGNE AL MARSALA   chestnuts with Marsala wine

CASTAGNE ALLA ROMAGNOLA IN VINO ROSSO   chestnuts boiled in red wine

CASTAGNE STUFATE   chestnuts stewed in wine

CASTAGNOLE FRITTE   sweet lemon fritters

CENCI   fried cookies

CESTINO DI FRUTTA   large basket of fruit

CIALDE   wafers *or* cookies

CIALZON DI FRUTTA   turnover filled with assorted fruits, sprinkled with crystallized sugar and cinnamon

CIAMBELLA ALLA BOLOGNESE   fruit and nut cake made with wine

CIAMBELLA DI PASQUA   sweet Easter bread

CIARAMICOLA   cake with liqueur, lemon rind, covered with meringue

CICERCHIATA   deep-fried honey cake balls
CILIEGE AL BAROLO   cherries, sautéed in wine, sugar
   and cream
CILIEGIA   cherry
CIOCCOLATA   chocolate
COCOMERO   watermelon
COMPOSTA   stewed fruit
COMPOSTA DI FRUTTA   fruit compote
COPATA   small wafer of honey and nuts
COPPA DI FRUTTA   cup of fruit cocktail
CREMA   cream soup *or* custard
CREMA CARAMELLA   custard topped with caramel sauce
CREMA DI MASCARPONE   soft cream cheese with rum
   and sugar added
CREMA FREDDA DI UVA NERA   chilled grape pudding
CREMA FRITTA   fried cream
CREMA PASTICCERA   custard cream sauce
CREMINO   soft cheese *or* type of ice cream bar
CRISPELLE   pastry deep fried then honey coated
CROCCANTE DI MANDORLE   almond brittle
CROSTATA   pie *or* tart
CROSTATA DI CREMA   custard tart
CROSTATA DI VISCIOLE   sour cherry tart
CROSTOLI   fried ribbon cookies
CUSCINETTI   pasta dumplings stuffed with jam
DATTERO   date
DOLCE   sweet, soft, mild
DOLCE DI CASTAGNE   chestnut chocolate soufflé
DOLCE DI CASTAGNE E RISO   sweet chestnut and rice
   pudding
DOLCI   pastries, cakes, sweets, desserts
DOLCI DI MELE   apple cake
DOLCI DI TORINO   rich chocolate dessert
DORATINI DI RICOTTA   cheese fritters served without
   sugar at beginning of meal, with sugar at end of meal
FAVE DEI MORTI   All Soul's Day cookies with almonds
   and pine nuts

FAVE DOLCI   "bean" size and shape, almond cinnamon cookies

FAVETTE   rum cookies

FIAMMA   flamed, usually with brandy

FICHI   figs

FICHI AL CIOCCOLATO   chocolate-covered, nut-stuffed figs

FICHI ALLO SCIROPPO   cooked, rum-soaked fresh figs

FICO   fig (see FICHI)

FLUMMERI AL CIOCCOLATO   whipped chocolate pudding

FOCACCIA DOLCE   sweet ring-shaped cake

FRAGOLE   strawberries

FRAGOLE AL VINO   strawberries with wine

FRAGOLINE   wild strawberries

FRAGOLINE DI BOSCO   wild small strawberries

FRAGOLONE   very large strawberries

FREGOLATA   almond cookies

FRITOLE   spiced rum fritters

FRITTELLE DI FRUTTA   fried fruit fritters

FRITTELLE DI RICOTTA DOLCE   pan-fried ricotta cheese sweet fritters

FRITTURA DI RICOTTA   fried fritters of ricotta cheese with almond macaroon flour

FRUSTENGA   cornmeal fruit cake with figs

FRUTTA   fruit

FRUTTA CANDITA   crystallized oranges, tangerines, figs, or other fruits

FRUTTA COTTA   stewed fruit

FRUTTA FRESCA   fresh fruit

FRUTTA MARTURANA   almond paste baked in fruit shapes and colored

FRUTTA SCIROPPATA   fruit in syrup, usually canned

GELATI MISTI   assortment of Italian ice creams and sorbets

GELATINI DI CREMA   biscuit tortoni

GELATO   ice cream, iced dessert often with fresh fruit

GELATO AL COCOMERO   watermelon ice

GELATO AL TARTUFO   ice cream with chocolate sauce

GELATO ALL'UVA NERA   black grape ice cream

GELATO ALLA BANANA COL RUM   banana ice cream with rum

GELATO ALLA CREMA   custard cream ice cream

GELATO ALLA FRAGOLA   strawberry ice cream

GELATO ALLA NOCCIOLA   hazelnut ice cream

GELATO ALLA PRUGNA   prune ice cream

GERMINUS   baked almond macaroons

GIALLETTI   fruited cornmeal cookies

GINEPRO   juniper berry

GRANATINA   fruit syrup on crushed ice

GRANITA   water ice crystals made with flavorings

GRANITA DI CAFFÉ CON PANNA   coffee ice crystals served with whipped cream

GRANITA DI FRAGOLE E LAMPONI   strawberry *or* raspberry ice crystals

GRANITE   general term to describe iced sweets

LACIADITT   deep-fried apple fritters

LAMPONE   raspberry

LATTE ALLA PORTOGHESE   baked custard with liquid caramel

LIMONE   lemon

MACEDONIA D'UVA BIANCA E NERA   bowl of white and black grapes

MACEDONIA DI FRUTTA   fruit salad

MANDARINO   mandarin orange *or* tangerine

MANDARINO FARCITO   frozen tangerine dessert with rum

MANDORLA   almond

MANDORLATO   made with almonds

MANGO E FRAGOLE AL VINO BIANCO   mangoes and strawberries steeped in white wine

MANTECATO   very fluffy air-filled ice cream

MARMELLATA   jam

MARMELLATA DI ARANCE   orange marmalade

MARRONE   chestnut

MELAGRANA   pomegranate

MELE   apple

MELE COTOGNE   sour quince apple

MELE RENETTE AL FORNO CON AMARETTI   baked
  apples with macaroons
MELONE   melon
MERINGA   meringue
MERINGA AL CHANTILLY   meringue shells filled with
  whipped cream
MERINGA AL GELATO   meringue shells filled with ice cream
MIASCIA TRAMEZZO   bread and grape cake
MICHETTE   sweet cakes, bread rolls
MIELE   honey
MILLEFOGLIE   custard slice
MIRABELLA   yellow plum
MIRTILLO   blueberry *or* huckleberry
MONTE BIANCO   chestnuts cooked and grated covered
  with chilled whipped cream
MORA   blackberry *or* mulberry
MOSTACCIOLI   hard sweets made of flour and honey
MUSTACCIOLI DI ERICE   baked almond cookies
MUSTACCIOLI DI NATALE   Christmas spice cookies
NEPITELLE   sweet Christmas pies
NESPOLA   a tart wild fruit
NOCCIOLA   hazelnut *or* filbert
NOCE   walnut
NOCE DI COCCO   coconut
OMELETTE ALLA FIAMMA   a fluffy, sweet omelette
  with jam, flambeed with brandy at the table
OSS DA MORD   anise-flavored buns
PAN DEMEI   anise-flavored buns
PAN DI GENOVA   almond cake
PAN DI SPAGNA   spongecake
PAN PEPATO   spicy nut bread cookies
PANDOLCE   heavy cake with dried fruit and pine kernels
PANDORO DI VERONA   very light fluffy cake usually
  star shaped
PANETTONE   tall light cake with raisins and crystallized
  fruit
PANETTONE CERTOSINO   Christmas fruit bread

PANFORTE   a hard cake of nuts, cocoa, spices, candied orange and lemon peel, melon and honey

PANFORTE DI SIENA   dry, nougat-like sweet made of almonds, candied fruits, spices, flour, butter and eggs

PANNA MONTATA   whipped cream

PANNA MONTATA CON I CIALDONI   whipped cream served with wafers

PARROZZO   baked almond and chocolate cake

PASSATO DI MARRONI   puree of chestnuts

PASTA FROLLA   sweet pastry dough

PASTA GENOVESE CLASSICA   baked dessert from eggs, sugar, flour

PASTICCERIA   cake and pastry shop

PASTICCINO   tart, cake, small pastry

PASTIERA   short pastry containing filling of cottage cheese and candied fruit

PASTINE RUSTICHE   pie filled with ricotta cheese, eggs, citron, raisins, pine nuts, chocolate

PERE   pears

PERE AL FORNO   baked pears

PERE CARAMELLATE   pears dipped in boiling sugar

PERE COTTE ALLA CREMA E CIOCCOLATO   cooked pears with custard cream sauce and chocolate

PERE COTTE BIANCHE/ROSSE   pears baked in white *or* red wine

PERE HELÉNE   pears poached in vanilla syrup served with ice cream and chocolate sauce

PESCA   peach (also PESCHE)

PESCA AL BAROLO   peach baked in wine

PESCA ALLA PIEMONTESE   peach stuffed with macaroons and baked

PESCA MELBA   peach poached in syrup, vanilla ice cream, raspberry sauce

PESCANOCE   nectarine

PESCHE   peaches (see PESCA)

PESCHE RIPIENE   stuffed baked peaches

PESTRINGOLO   baked fruit cake with figs

PICONI   baked turnovers filled with ricotta cheese
PIGNOLI   pine kernels
PINOCCHIATE   pine kernel and almond cake
PINOCCHIO   pine nuts
PISTACCHI   pistachio nuts
PIZZA DOLCE   ricotta pie
POMPELMO   grapefruit
PONCE GELATO ALLA ROMANA   frozen fruit juices
   with rum and wine
POPONE   melon
PRESNITZ   Easter fruitcake
PRIMIZIE   first fruits *or* vegetables of season
PROFITEROLE   cream puff pastry with hot chocolate sauce
PROFITEROLE AL CIOCCOLATO   cream puff pastry
   with chocolate frosting
PRUGNE   plums
PRUGNE FARCITE   prunes stuffed with walnuts and chocolate
PRUGNE SECCHE   prunes
RAVIOLI DI SAN GIUSEPPE   baked pasta stuffed with jam
RAVIOLI DOLCI   sweet pasta made with jam and brandy
RIBES   currants
RIBES NERO   black currants
RIBES ROSSO   red currants
RICCIARELLI DI SIENA   marzipan cookies from Siena
ROCCIATA DI ASSISI   fruit roll with raisins, walnuts, dry
   figs, almonds, citrus
SAINT HONORÉ   custard-filled pastry with cream puffs
SAVARIN   liquor-soaked cake ring filled with fruit and
   topped with whipped cream
SAVOIARDI   ladyfingers, cookies
SCIUSCELLO   ricotta cheesecake with fruit, almonds,
   brandy, chocolate, lemon peel
SEMIFREDDO   ice cream cake
SEMIFREDDO ALLA CREMA   ice cream with almonds
SEMIFREDDO ALLO ZABAGLIONE   half frozen dessert
   of cream, eggs, sugar, wine

SFOGLIATELLE   cakes made of thin flakes of pastry
  wrapped around a filling of spiced cottage cheese and
  candied fruit

SFOGLIATELLE FROLLE   baked pastry filled with ricotta
  cheese, fruits, cinnamon

SILVANO   chocolate meringue *or* tart

SORBETTO   sherbet, flavored water ice

SPUMA GELATA ALLA CREMA   iced fruit vanilla mousse

SPUMONE   ice cream with nuts and strawberries or raspberries

SPUMONI   multi-flavored ice cream dessert, usually with
  fruit pieces

SPUMONI AL CROCCANTE   candied, chopped, toasted
  almond in and on ice cream dessert

STACCIATA UNTA   cake with sugar icing

STRANGOLA PRETI   baked nut cake

STRUFFOLI ALLA NAPOLETANA   fried pastry with
  honey, various fruits, ricotta cheese

STRUFFOLI DI NATALE   fried honey cookies

SUSINA   plum

TARTUFI DI CIOCCOLATA   coffee-flavored chocolate
  balls served cold

TORRONE   nougat

TORRONE AL CIOCCOLATO   chocolate nougat

TORRONE DI CREMONA   hard nougat made of egg white,
  honey, sugar, spices, toasted almonds and candied peel

TORRONE GELATO   iced nougat pudding

TORTA   pie, tart *or* cake

TORTA AL GIANDUIA   chocolate cake with jam, brandy,
  hazelnuts, honey, etc.

TORTA CASERECCIA DI POLENTA   cornmeal shortcake
  with dried fruit and pine nuts

TORTA DI FRUTTA   fruit flan

TORTA DI FRUTTA CON LA PANNA   fruit flan with cream

TORTA DI FRUTTA SECCA   baked fruit cake with nuts,
  figs, chocolate, eggs, candied fruit peel

TORTA DI MANDORLE   almond cake

TORTA DI MELE   apple pie *or* torte
TORTA DI MERINGA   fruit pie with whipped cream
TORTA DI NOCCIUOLE   hazelnut cake
TORTA DI NOCI   walnut cake
TORTA DI PERE ALLA PAESANA   plain cake with fresh
   pears
TORTA DI PRUGNE   baked spongecake with wine,
   prunes, sugar, eggs
TORTA DI RICOTTA   ricotta cheesecake
TORTA DI RISO   rice cake
TORTA DI VERMICELLI   sweet noodle dessert with
   honey, raisins, powdered sugar, eggs, cinnamon
TORTA GELATA   ice cream cake
TORTA MILLE FOGLIE   thin cake layers separated with
   custard
TORTA PARADISO   spongecake
TORTA ZUCCOTTO   liquor-soaked cake ring filled with
   fruit, ice cream, chocolate, whipped cream
TORTIGLIONE   almond cake
TORTINA DI MARMELLATA   jam-filled tart
TORTINI AL CASTAGNACCIO   chestnut flour cake
TORTINO DI MOZZARELLA   cheese tart
TORTIONATA ALLA LODIGIANA   almond cake
TRANCIA DI TORTA FARCITA   slice of fruit tart
UOVA ALLA MONACELLA   hard-boiled eggs stuffed
   and coated with chocolate
UVA   grapes
UVA CON PASSA E PROVOLA   grapes with raisins and
   cheese
UVA PASSA   raisins
UVA SPINA   gooseberries
VISCIOLI   wild cherries
ZABAGLIONE   dessert of egg yolks, sugar and Marsala
   wine, served warm
ZALETI   cake with white raisins, eggs, cornmeal, rum,
   sugar, pine nuts, lemon rind
ZEPPOLA   deep-fried fritter *or* doughnut

ZEPPOLE DI SAN GIUSEPPE   dessert fritters with cinnamon and sugar

ZUCCOTTO   creamy icebox cake made with fruit and liquor

ZUPPA AI DUE COLORI   vanilla and chocolate pudding on spongecake

ZUPPA ALL'EMILIANA   spongecake, custard, chocolate and cherry preserve

ZUPPA INGLESE   cake steeped in custard sauce, rum and cordials

Dumplings, Polenta

AVENA CALDA   warm oatmeal

BACCALÀ ALLA MILANESE   pan-fried dried cod fritters

CANEDERLI   large dumpling of bread with bacon in soup

CONSUM   dough dumplings filled with sautéed greens

CROCCHETTA   potato *or* rice croquette

CROCCHETTA DI PATATE   potato croquette with salami and cheese

CROCCHETTA DI POLLO   fried chicken croquette

CROCCHETTA DI RISO   rice croquette with cheese center, deep fried

CROCCHETTE DI PATATE   potato croquettes

CROCCHETTE DI PATATE ALLA ROMAGNOLA   potato and ham croquettes

CROCHETTE DI RISO   rice croquettes

FOCACCETTE FRITTE   cheese-filled pasta fritters

GNOCCHI   potato dumplings boiled and served with meat sauce and grated cheese

GNOCCHI AL PESTO   dumplings of dough boiled and served with pesto

GNOCCHI ALLA BAVA   potato dumplings with cheese

GNOCCHI ALLA FONTINA   dumplings of semolina, boiled in spiced milk with melted Fontina cheese, rolled in bread crumbs and fried

GNOCCHI ALLA PARMIGIANA   potato dumplings with Parmesan cheese

GNOCCHI ALLA PIEMONTESE   dumplings with Parmesan cheese, Emmenthal cheese and white truffle

GNOCCHI ALLA ROMANA   potato dumplings with Parmesan cheese

GNOCCHI DI LATTE   milk dumplings

GNOCCHI DI MAIS   dumplings of corn flour, served with tomato sauce and Parmesan cheese

GNOCCHI DI PATATE   potato dumplings

GNOCCHI DI POLENTA   baked pie of cornmeal, mushrooms, meat

GNOCCHI VERDI   spinach and cheese-filled potato dumplings

GRANOTURCO   corn meal (polenta)

MALLOREDDUS   dumplings of corn flour and saffron, served with spiced sauce and sprinkled with grated goat cheese

MIGLIACCIO ALLA NAPOLETANA   baked casserole of cornmeal, sausage, cheeses

POLENTA   baked, thick, cornmeal porridge

POLENTA ALLA LODIGIANA   cooked cornmeal slices with Gruyère cheese, battered, pan fried

POLENTA ALLA SARDA   cornmeal mixed with parsley, basil, tomatoes, sausages, pecorino cheese

POLENTA CON SALCICCE   cornmeal porridge and sausages

POLENTA CON STUFATINO   cornmeal baked with sausage, cheese, chili

POLENTA E UCCELLETTI   spit-roasted birds served on cornmeal

POLENTA E UCCELLI   small birds spit roasted with dumplings

POLENTA OROPA   cornmeal porridge with cheeses

POLENTA PASTICCIATA   dumpling with meat sauce, mushrooms, butter and cheese

POLENTA PASTICCIATA AI FUNGHI   baked cornmeal porridge with mushrooms

POLENTA STUFATA   cornmeal baked with sausage, cheese, tomato, chili

POLENTA TARAGNA   cooked cornmeal with cheese

POLPETTE DI GNOCCHI   dumplings stuffed with chopped meat or vegetables

POLPETTINE DI POLENTA   cornmeal croquettes

RIPIENI FRITTI   fried stuffed dumplings

SPUNTATURA DI MAIALE CON POLENTA   pork short ribs braised and served with cornmeal mush

TORTA DI POLENTA E FONTINA   cornmeal and cheese pudding

Eggs

CUSCINETTI PANDORATI   egg-fried bread stuffed with ham, anchovy, cheese, deep fried

FRICO DI FRIULI   pan-fried eggs with pork and cheese

FRITTATA   egg pancake *or* omelette (also see OMELETTES)

FRITTATA AI CARCIOFI   omelette with artichoke hearts

FRITTATA AI FUNGHI   mushroom omelette

FRITTATA AI TARTUFI   omelette made with truffles

FRITTATA AL BASILICO   omelette flavored with basil

FRITTATA AL FORMAGGIO   cheese omelette

FRITTATA ALLA GENOVESE   spinach omelette

FRITTATA ALLA MOZZARELLA E CROSTINI   omelette with cheese and bread cubes

FRITTATA ALLA TRENTINA   fluffy omelette filled with either a sweet or savory mixture

FRITTATA ALLE CIPOLLE   open-faced omelette with onions

FRITTATA CON ARSELLE   omelette with mussels

FRITTATA CON ZOCCOLI   omelette with bacon chunks

FRITTATA DI MELE   omelette with apples

FRITTATA DI PASTA   spaghetti omelette

FRITTATA DI PATATE   potato omelette

FRITTATA DI PATATINE FRITTE   open-faced omelette with pan-fried potatoes

FRITTATA DI PEPERONI E PATATE   pepper and potato omelette

FRITTATA DI PISELLI   omelette with onion, ham, peas, fennel

FRITTATA DI RICOTTA   omelette made with ricotta cheese
FRITTATA DI SPINACI AL FORNO   baked spinach omelette
FRITTATA SEMPLICE   plain omelette
FRITTATA ZUCCHINI   omelette with zucchini, chopped
   tomato, potato, rosemary
FRITTE ALLA PIEMONTESE   fried eggs on a bed of rice
   with grated cheese, tomatoes and sliced truffles
IMBROGLIATA D'UOVO AL POMODORO   scrambled
   eggs fried with bacon and tomato
LUGANEGA E UOVA SODE   eggs and sausages
MANZO SALMISTRATO CON UOVA AFFOGATE
   Italian corned beef hash with herbs, poached eggs,
   polenta, cheese
MOLLETTE CON FUNGHI E FORMAGGIO   soft-boiled
   eggs with grated cheese and mushrooms cooked in butter
OMELETTE   fried, whipped eggs (see FRITTATA)
OMELETTE ALLA CONTADINA   omelette with red
   onion, bacon, potatoes
OMELETTE ALLA PIEMONTESE   omelette made with
   truffles
OMELETTE CON VERDURE   omelette with fresh
   seasonal vegetables
OMELETTE DI GAMBERETTI   omelette made with shrimp
OMELETTE DI PATATE E MAIALE   omelette filled with
   diced potato and lean pork
OMELETTE DI RISO   omelette with rice, Gruyère cheese
   and salami
SFORMATO   baked mold
SFORMATO ALLA BESCIAMELLA   baked mold of egg
   whites, milk, cheese, meat sauce
UOVA   eggs
UOVA AFFOGATE   poached eggs
UOVA AFFOGATE AL POMODORO   poached eggs in
   tomato sauce
UOVA AFFOGATE AL VINO   eggs poached in wine
UOVA AFFOGATE COL RISO   poached eggs served with
   cheese and rice

UOVA AFFOGATE CON LE PUNTE DI ASPARAGI
 poached eggs with asparagus tips

UOVA AGLI SPINACI   omelette with spinach

UOVA AL BURRO   eggs fried in butter

UOVA AL FORMAGGIO   eggs with cheese

UOVA AL FORNO   baked eggs

UOVA AL GROVIERA   eggs made with Swiss or Gruyère

UOVA AL GUSCIO   soft-boiled eggs

UOVA AL LARDO   fried eggs with bacon

UOVA AL POMODORO   omelette with tomatoes

UOVA AL PROSCIUTTO   omelette with ham

UOVA AL PROSCIUTTO E PANNA   fried eggs with ham
 and Parmesan cheese

UOVA AL TEGAME   eggs cooked and served in individual
 pan

UOVA ALL'AMERICANA   fried eggs with bacon and
 tomato

UOVA ALLA CACCIATORA   eggs poached in a tomato
 sauce with herbs, onions and chopped chicken livers

UOVA ALLA CAMPAGNOLA   eggs with cooked vegetables, cheese

UOVA ALLA CAPRICCIOSA   poached eggs in fried
 bread with wine and bacon

UOVA ALLA CARDINALE   omelette with seafood,
 mushrooms

UOVA ALLA COCOTTE   shirred eggs *or* coddled eggs

UOVA ALLA COQUE   boiled eggs

UOVA ALLA FIORENTINA   fried eggs, served on a bed
 of spinach

UOVA ALLA PAESANA   omelette with vegetables and
 diced ham or bacon

UOVA ALLA PORTOGHESE   omelette with tomato sauce
 and paste

UOVA ALLA RUSSA   stuffed hard eggs with mayonnaise
 sauce

UOVA ALLA SARDA   hard-boiled eggs pan-fried then
 covered with bread crumbs, fried in garlic oil

UOVA ALLA SPAGNOLA   omelette with tomatoes, onions, peppers and garlic

UOVA ALLA TORINESE   eggs boiled, deviled, then deep fried

UOVA ALLE ERBE   fried eggs cooked with herbs

UOVA BARROTTE   very soft-boiled eggs

UOVA BOLLITTE   boiled eggs

UOVA COI CARCIOFI   poached eggs with artichoke hearts

UOVA COI FEGATINI DI POLLO   eggs with sautéed chicken livers

UOVA COI FRUTTI DI MARE   eggs made with seafood

UOVA COI FUNGHI   eggs with mushrooms

UOVA CON ASPARAGI   egg omelette with asparagus

UOVA CON CONFETTURA   jam-filled omelette

UOVA CON MARMELLATA   eggs prepared with preserves

UOVA CON UVA PASSA AL GUANCIALE   eggs fried with raisins and bacon

UOVA FARCITE   hard-cooked then stuffed eggs

UOVA FARCITE AL LIMONE   hard-boiled lemon-stuffed eggs

UOVA FARCITE AL PROSCIUTTO   hard-boiled ham-stuffed eggs

UOVA FRITTE   fried eggs

UOVA FRITTE CON LA FONTINA   fried eggs on melted cheese toast with anchovies

UOVA FRITTE CON LA MOZZARELLA   fried eggs with cheese

UOVA IN FRITTATA   eggs in an omelette form

UOVA MOLLI   soft-boiled eggs

UOVA MOZZARELLA   mozzarella cheese sandwich, dipped in egg batter and deep fried

UOVA RIPIENE   stuffed hard-boiled eggs

UOVA SEMPLICI   plain omelette

UOVA SODE   hard-boiled eggs

UOVA STRACCIATE   scrambled eggs

UOVA STRAPAZZATE   scrambled eggs

UOVA STRAPAZZATE COI PEPERONI   scrambled eggs with peppers

UOVA TRIPPATE ALLA ROMANA baked eggs cooked
to look like tripe
UOVA, PANCETTA AFFUMICATA E SALSICCE eggs,
smoked bacon and sausage
UOVO egg
UOVO IN CAMICIA poached egg

Fritters, Pancakes, Croquettes

BOMBOLETTE DI RICOTTA ricotta fritters
CASTAGNOLE FRITTE sweet lemon fritters
CREPES ALLA PIEMONTESE pancakes with anchovy
and truffle butter, glazed in brandy
CRESPOLINA pancake filled with veal, grated cheese,
baked in tomato sauce
CRESPOLINO spinach-filled pancake baked in cheese sauce
CROCCHETTE DI CERVELLA E ZUCCHINI FRITTI
croquettes of brains and zucchini, breaded and fried
FRITOLE spiced rum fritters
FRITTELLE fritters *or* croquettes (also see CROCCHETTA)
FRITTELLE ALLA VALTELLINA cheese fritters deep fried
FRITTELLE CON SCIROPPO D'ACERO pancakes with
butter and maple syrup
FRITTELLE DI CARCIOFI fritters made from ham,
cheese and cooked vegetables
FRITTELLE DI FRUTTA fried fruit fritters
FRITTELLE DI MITILI mussel fritters in batter
FRITTELLE DI PROSCIUTTO fritters of artichokes, fava
beans and peas, fennel
FRITTELLE DI RICOTTA DOLCE pan-fried ricotta cheese
sweet fritters
FRITTURA fritter
FRITTURA DI RICOTTA fried fritters of ricotta cheese
with almond macaroon flour
LACIADITT deep-fried apple fritters
PISCI OVO egg fritters with cheese, garlic, bread crumbs
RICOTTA FRITTA ricotta cheese fritters

SUPPLÌ   rice croquettes with cheese and meat sauce
SUPPLÌ AL TELEFONO   rice croquettes with mozzarella
TORTA FRITTA   fritters
TORTELLI   small fritters *or* fried cakes *or* stuffed pasta
ZEPPOLA   deep-fried fritter *or* doughnut
ZEPPOLE DI SAN GIUSEPPE   dessert fritters with cinnamon and sugar

Game

ALZAVOLA   teal
ANITRA   duck
ANITRA AL COGNAC   duck cooked with brandy, juniper berries and rosemary
ANITRA ALL'ARANCIA   oven roasted duck basted with orange juice
ANITRA ALL'AGRODOLCE   duck with a sweet-sour sauce
ANITRA ALLA SALSA D'ARANCIO   roast duck with orange sauce
ANITRA ALLE OLIVE   casserole of duck and olives
ANITRA ARROSTITA ALLA SICILIANA   roasted duck stuffed with pork, peppers and black olives, with Marsala
ANITRA ARROSTO ALLA GENOVESE   duck roasted in olive oil with herbs and fresh lemon juice
ANITRA CON SALSA DI CAPPERI   duck cooked in the oven with a sauce of Marsala, capers, white truffles
ANITRA IN SALMÌ   duck marinated in red wine with onion, herbs, garlic, anchovies, fried and then cooked in the marinade
ANITRA MUTA ALLA NOVARESE   duck stuffed with rice, meats, herbs, roasted
ANITRA SELVATICA   wild duck
ANITROCCOLO   duckling
BECCACCIA   woodcock
BECCACCIA ALLA ROMAGNOLA   stuffed and roasted woodcock
BECCACCIA FARCITA   stuffed and roasted woodcock

BECCACCIA IN SALMÌ   woodcock sautéed in oil and
butter with a sauce made of intestines

BECCACCINO   wild snipe bird

BECCAFICHI   small table birds

BECCAFICHI AL MARSALA   birds cooked in tomato,
anchovies, olives, garlic, Marsala, served on fried bread
with sauce

BISTECCHINE DI CINGHIALE   thin pan-fried wild boar
steaks in sweet and sour sauce

BOSCO   wild

CACCIAGIONE   game animals such as deer, also birds

CAMOSCIO   small wild deer

CAMOSCIO IN SALMÌ   deer meat cooked in sauce of
wine, olive oil, garlic, herbs and anchovies

CAPRIOLO   female deer

CAPRIOLO ALLA CASALINGA   home-style stew of wild
deer

CAPRIOLO IN SALMÌ   deer with wine, herbs and vegetables

CARNE DI PICCIONE   pigeon meat

CERVO   large, wild horned deer

CINGHIALE   wild boar

CINGHIALE ALLA CACCIATORA   boar with wine and
vegetables

CINGHIALE ARROSTO   roast wild boar

CINGHIALE IN AGRODOLCE ALLA ROMANA   boar
marinated with wine and spices, cooked in sweet-sour
sauce

CONIGLIO   rabbit

CONIGLIO AI CAPPERI   braised marinated rabbit with
wine, anchovies, onion, vinegar

CONIGLIO AL FORNO   rabbit baked in oven, with wine,
onion, broth

CONIGLIO AL MARSALA   rabbit cooked in Marsala with
onions, pimentos, tomatoes, eggplant

CONIGLIO ALL'AGRO   rabbit stewed in red wine and
lemon juice

CONIGLIO ALL'AGRODOLCE   sweet-sour rabbit

CONIGLIO ALLA BORGHESE   rabbit sautéed in white wine, herbs, onions and mushrooms

CONIGLIO ALLA BUONGUSTAIO   rabbit with vegetables and Marsala

CONIGLIO ALLA CACCIATORA   rabbit braised in wine, mushrooms, tomato and garlic

CONIGLIO ALLA CAMPAGNOLA   rabbit with garlic, rosemary and wine

CONIGLIO ALLA FRIULANA   rabbit with egg and lemon sauce

CONIGLIO ALLA LIVORNESE   rabbit casserole with tomatoes and anchovies

CONIGLIO ALLA MOLISANA   grilled rabbit and sausage chunks

CONIGLIO ALLA ROMAGNOLA   pieces of rabbit breaded, batter-dipped then fried in butter

CONIGLIO CON POLENTA   rabbit braised in sauce and served on cornmeal mush

CONIGLIO FARCITO AL FORNO   rabbit stuffed and roasted

CONIGLIO FRITTO   rabbit fried in bacon fat and oil, with sage and garlic

CONIGLIO FRITTO ALLA LOMBARDA   rabbit dipped in egg and chopped herbs, coated with bread crumbs and fried

CONIGLIO IN FRICASSEA   rabbit stew in wine sauce thickened with egg yolks, flavored with lemon

CONIGLIO IN PADELLA   rabbit sautéed in oil with bacon, tomatoes, garlic, wine and parsley

CONIGLIO IN SALMÌ   marinated and stewed rabbit

CONIGLIO IN SALSA CON UOVA   rabbit poached in sauce thickened with eggs and lemon juice

CONIGLIO IN SALSA PICCANTE   rabbit in spicy sauce with vegetables, wine, capers and anchovies

CONIGLIO IN UMIDO   rabbit stew

CONIGLIO IN UMIDO DI BERGAMO   rabbit stewed with basil, parsley, onion and vermouth

CONIGLIO RIPIENO AL FORNO   rabbit stuffed and roasted

CONIGLIO SELVATICO   wild rabbit

COSCIOTTO DI CONIGLIO   rabbit leg braised in gravy
COSCIOTTO DI DAINO   leg of venison usually roasted
CROSTONE DI QUAGLIE   quail roasted and served over
   cornmeal mush
DAINO   large wild horned deer
FAGIANO   pheasant
FAGIANO ALLA CREMA   pheasant cooked in butter and
   cream with lemon juice
FAGIANO ALLA MILANESE   pheasant sautéed with
   liver, pork, beef, onions, wine
FAGIANO ARROSTO TARTUFATO   pheasant stuffed
   with truffles and roasted
FAGIANO CON FUNGHI   pheasant sautéed with mushrooms
FAGIANO IN CASSERUOLA   pheasant cooked in butter
   and cognac
FAGIANO TARTUFATO   pheasant stuffed with truffles
   and roasted
FARAONA   guinea hen
FARAONA AL CARTOCCIO   guinea hen sautéed then
   baked with herbs and liver, in a sealed bag
FARAONA AL COCCIO   guinea hen baked in a clay case
FARAONA ALL'ARANCIA   oven roasted guinea hen
   basted with orange juice
FARAONA ALL'OLIVA   guinea hen braised in oil, herbs
   and olive
FARAONA ALLA CAMPAGNOLA   guinea fowl sautéed
   with wine and vegetables
FARAONA ALLA CRETA   guinea hen baked in a layer of clay
FARAONA ALLA FIAMMA   guinea hen roasted over
   open fire
FARAONA ALLA PANNA   guinea hen baked in the oven
   in a paper case with sage, juniper and rosemary and
   served with hot cream
FARAONA ALLA PIEMONTESE   guinea hen stuffed with
   herbs, juniper berries, bread crumbs, liver, wine and baked
FARAONA ALLA TEGLIA   guinea hen cooked in an open
   earthenware pan

FARAONA ALLO SPIEDO   guinea hen roasted on a spit
FARAONA ARROSTO   roasted guinea fowl
FARAONA CON SALSA AI CAPPERI   guinea fowl
  cooked with a caper sauce
FARAONA IN SALMÌ   guinea hen cooked in wine and
  vegetable sauce
FARAONA INCROSTATA   guinea fowl pie
FARAONA O FAGIANO ARROSTO   roast marinated
  guinea hen or pheasant
FARAONA RIPIENA   stuffed guinea fowl
GALLINELLA   water hen
GALLO CEDRONE   grouse
GERMANO   mallard
GRIVE   little thrushes stewed with myrtle leaves
LEPRE   hare
LEPRE AL BAROLO   hare stewed with red wine and
  vegetables
LEPRE AL DOLCE-FORTE   hare marinated in wine,
  onions, spices, with sauce of chocolate, candied fruits,
  raisins and nuts added after cooking
LEPRE ALL'AGRODOLCE   marinated hare, pan fried in
  wine, chocolate, herbs, onions
LEPRE ALLA CACCIATORA   hare with wine, sage,
  rosemary, garlic, olive oil and tomatoes
LEPRE ALLA CAMPAGNOLA   hare marinated in wine
  and herbs, cooked in casserole with wine
LEPRE ALLA TRENTINA   hare stewed in olive oil, garlic,
  onion and white wine, highly seasoned
LEPRE IN SALMÌ   stew made with marinated hare
LEPRE IN UMIDO   casserole of hare with mushrooms,
  vegetables, tomato, garlic and Marsala
LEPROTTO   young hare
MERLI   blackbirds
OCA ARROSTITA RIPIENA ALLA SALVIA E CIPOLLA
  goose roasted and stuffed with sage and onion
OCA ARROSTO AL FORNO   goose stuffed with sausage,
  herbs, chestnuts and bread crumbs and roasted

OCA ARROSTO RIPIENA   stuffed roast goose

OCA IN SALMÌ   goose cooked with wine, herbs, vegetables, mushrooms and truffles

PAGNOTTA CACCIATORE   game birds baked inside bread loaf

PALOMBA   wood pigeon

PALOMBACCE ALLO SPIEDO   wood pigeons roasted on a spit with various seasonings

PALOMBACCIO   wild pigeon

PAPPARDELLE ALL'ARETINA   duck cooked with red wine, tomatoes, herbs, served with wide ribbon pasta

PAPPARDELLE ALLA LEPRE   noodles with stew of hare giblets, well seasoned

PERNICE   partridge

PERNICE AL FORNO   roast partridge

PERNICE ALLA SARDA   partridge served cold with dressing of oil, vinegar, capers, parsley

PERNICE ARROSTO   partridge stuffed with bacon, juniper berries, mushrooms, roasted and served on fried bread

PERNICE IN SALMÌ   partridge cooked in vegetable and brandy sauce

PERNICI   partridges

PERNICI ALLE OLIVE   partridges pan fried with wine, ham, olives, oil, tomatoes, herbs

PERNICI IN SALSA D'ACETO   partridges pan fried in wine vinegar sauce

PETTO D'ANITRA   breast of duck

PICCIONE   pigeon, squab

PICCIONE ALLA DIAVOLA   grilled deviled squab

PICCIONE ALLA FIORENTINA   pigeon stuffed and braised in a wine, mushroom casserole

PICCIONE IN CASSERUOLA   pigeon braised in a wine, mushroom casserole

PICCIONE IN SALMÌ   pigeon stewed in wine vinegar sauce with oil, garlic, anchovy

PICCIONI SELVATICI   wood pigeons

PIVIERE   plover bird

POLENTA E OSEI   small roast birds served on polenta

POLENTA E UCCELLETTI   spit-roasted birds served on cornmeal

POLENTA E UCCELLI   small birds spit roasted with dumplings

PROSCIUTTO DI CINGHIALE   smoked wild boar

QUAGLIE   quails

QUAGLIE AI TARTUFI   quails sautéed with truffles

QUAGLIE AL MATTONE   quails roasted in a brick oven

QUAGLIE AL VINO BIANCO   quails stuffed with pine nuts and raisins, cooked in wine, cream, garlic and onion

QUAGLIE ALLA MONTANARA   quails braised in red wine

QUAGLIE ALLA PIEMONTESE   quails roasted, served with rice and truffles and Marsala and truffle-flavored cream sauce

QUAGLIE ALLO SPIEDO   quails roasted on a spit

QUAGLIE ARROSTO CON LA POLENTA   roasted quails with fried polenta

QUAGLIE COI PISELLI   quails roasted and served with peas and onions

QUAGLIE COL PURÉ DI PISELLI   quails in a casserole with pureed peas, ham and bacon

QUAGLIE COL RISO   quails with rice, ham, onion, bacon, grated cheese, cooked in a pan

QUAGLIE CON RISOTTO   quails with herbs, vegetables, wine

QUAGLIE IN CASSERUOLA   quails braised with herbs, mushrooms in sauce

SALMISTRATA   rabbit stew pickled in herb vinegar or wine and served cold

SELVAGGINA   game

STARNA   gray partridge

TORDO   thrush

TORRESANI   small pigeons, domesticated

UCCELLETTI   small birds

UCCELLETTI ALLA MAREMMANA   small birds cooked in oil with tomatoes, garlic, anchovy and olives, served on fried bread

ZUPPA CAODA   casserole made with pigeons, wine, cheese and baked

Meat

A PUNTINO   medium-cooked meat
A PUNTO   medium rare cooked meat
ABBACCHIO   milk-fed grilled lamb
ABBACCHIO AI CARCIOFI   braised lamb with artichokes
ABBACCHIO AL FORNO   oven roasted lamb chops
ABBACCHIO ALLA CACCIATORA   lamb with a dressing of olive oil, vinegar, sage, rosemary, garlic, anchovies
ABBACCHIO ALLA ROMANA   braised lamb Roman style
ABBACCHIO ALLO SPIEDO   lamb roasted on a spit
ABBACCHIO BRODETTATO   pieces of lamb cooked in a sauce of egg yolks flavored with lemon peel
ABRUZZESE   with red peppers and ham
AFFETTATO   sliced cold meat
AFFUMICATO   smoked
AGNELLO   lamb
AGNELLO AI FINOCCHIETTI   lamb cooked with fennel
AGNELLO AL FORNO   oven-roasted lamb, usually leg
AGNELLO AL FORNO CON PATATE E POMODORO   baked lamb with potato and tomato
AGNELLO ALL'ARETINA   roast lamb with rosemary, basted with oil and vinegar
AGNELLO ALL'ARRABBIATA   lamb cooked over a hot fire, basted with oil and vinegar
AGNELLO ALLA CACCIATORA   braised lamb with herbs, wine, garlic, vinegar and anchovy
AGNELLO ALLA PECORARA   lamb and onion casserole
AGNELLO ALLA TURCA   lamb stew
AGNELLO ARROSTO   roasted lamb, usually leg
AGNELLO CON CACIO E UOVA   lamb stew with wine, cheese, eggs
AGNELLO DORATO IN SALSA E UOVO   baked baby lamb chops casserole with ham, cheese and wine

AGNELLO IN FRICASSEA   pan-roasted lamb in white wine, with egg and lemon sauce

AGNELLO RUSTICO   baked leg of lamb with lemon juice and cheese

ALLA CACCIATORA   with mushrooms, herbs, shallots, wine, tomatoes, ham

ALLA FIAMMINGA   braised in beer, onion, mushrooms, herbs and broth

ALLA MILANESE   breaded, then fried

ALLA MONTANARA   made with different root vegetables, garlic, onion, oil, broth

ALLA PARMIGIANA   breaded and baked with Parmesan cheese

AMBURGHESE ALLA TIROLESE   hamburger grilled and served with onions

AMBURGO AL BURRO   hamburger fried in butter with sage

ANIMELLE   sweetbreads

ANIMELLE AL MARSALA   sweetbreads cooked in wine

ANIMELLE DI VITELLO   veal sweetbreads

ANNEGATI   slices of meat in white wine *or* Marsala wine

ARANCINE ALLA SICILIANA   rice balls stuffed with meat, breaded and fried

ARISTA   loin of pork

ARISTA AL FORNO   roast loin of pork

ARISTA ALLA FIORENTINA   loin of pork seasoned with garlic, cloves, rosemary, cooked slowly in oven with water

ARISTA DI MAIALE   pork loin, rubbed with herbs and garlic, roasted in oven or on spit

ARROSTETTI DI MAIALE   small pork roast

ARROSTI MISTI FREDDI   cold sliced roast meat

ARROSTICINI ALL'ABRUZZESE   skewered marinated grilled lamb cubes

ARROSTINO ANNEGATO AI FUNGHI   small veal roast covered with mushrooms

ARROSTINO DI MAIALE ALLA SALVIA   small pork roast basted in broth with herbs

ARROSTO   roast, usually of veal, cut into large portions and prepared with potatoes, cooked in a slow oven

ARROSTO ALLA GENOVESE   pot roast cooked in gravy of onion, wine, tomato paste

ARROSTO ALLA MONTANARA   pot roast cooked in gravy of onion, olive oil, tomato, herbs

ARROSTO DI MAIALE   roast of white pork seasoned with bay leaf and spices

ARROSTO DI MAIALE AL LATTE   roast pork cooked in milk

ARROSTO DI MAIALE UBRIACO   roast pork braised in red wine

ARROSTO DI VITELLO   roast veal, usually slices

ARROSTO IN PASTINE   roast of meat cooked in dough crust

ARROSTO MORTO AL FORNO   slowly roasted meat without gravy or sauce

ASCE DI VITELLO AI FERRI   veal hamburger grilled

BATTUTA   ground or chopped beef, as hamburger

BATTUTA AL PROSCIUTTO   ground beef mixed with ground ham

BEN COTTO   well-done

BIANCHETTE DI VITELLO   veal stew in herb mushroom cream sauce

BISTECCA   steak, usually beef

BISTECCA AL TARTUFO   grilled beef steak covered with grated truffle

BISTECCA ALLA BISMARK   steak pan fried in butter and served with fried egg on top

BISTECCA ALLA FIORENTINA   steak salted, coated with olive oil, charcoal broiled

BISTECCA ALLA PIZZAIOLA   beef or veal cutlet stewed in an open pan with tomato, olive oil, garlic and marjoram

BISTECCA ALLA SICILIANA   beefsteak pan fried in oil, garlic, tomatoes, olives, pickles and peppers

BISTECCA ARROSTO   roast loin of beef

BISTECCA DI AGNELLO   loin of lamb

BISTECCA DI MANZO   beefsteak

BISTECCA DI MANZO AI FERRI grilled beefsteak
BISTECCA DI VITELLO veal loin steak, grilled
BISTECCHINE ALLA GRIGLIA hamburgers
BISTECCHINE DI MANZO ALLA CACCIATORA thin
  beefsteaks fried with mushrooms, olive oil, red wine
  and tomatoes
BOCCONCINI diced meat with herbs
BOCCONCINI ALLA CACCIATORA beef chunks
  sautéed in oil, mushroom, herbs
BOCCONCINI ALLA FIORENTINA steak chunks
  sautéed in oil, garlic, onion, herbs
BOCCONCINI DI VITELLO AI SAPORI E FUNGHI
  herb-flavored bits of veal and mushrooms, braised
BOLLITO boiled, as meat *or* fish stew (also LESSATI)
BOLLITO DI MANZO boiled beef
BOLLITO RIFATTO ALLA MODA DEI PAPI grilled left-
  over boiled beef
BONDIOLA DI PARMA pork sausage from Parma
BOVE beef fillet
BRACIOLE rib steaks
BRACIOLE AI SASSI pan-fried steaks served with pan-
  fried potatoes
BRACIOLE ALLA FIORENTINA rib steaks that are
  salted, coated with olive oil and charcoal broiled
BRACIOLE ALLA PIZZAIOLA grilled steaks served with
  tomato, garlic and olive oil sauce
BRACIOLE ALLA TOSCANA grilled steaks and boiled
  potatoes served with sauce of wine, onion, olive oil
BRACIOLE DI ABBACCHIO ALLA SCOTTADITO small
  grilled lamb chops
BRACIOLE DI MAIALE pork chops
BRACIOLE DI VITELLO AL VINO E LIMONE veal
  chops braised with wine and lemon
BRACIOLETTE DI ABBACCHIO grilled lamb chops
BRACIOLINE DI AGNELLO baby lamb chops pan fried
  in wine

BRACIOLINE DI AGNELLO AI CARCIOFI   baby lamb chops and artichokes sautéed in wine

BRACIOLINE DI MAIALE AL VINO BIANCO   pork cutlets pan fried in white wine

BRACIOLINE SCOTTADITO   charcoal-grilled lamb chops

BRASATO   braised beef

BRASATO CON LENTICCHIE   braised beef with lentils

BRASATO DI MANZO   pot roast marinated in wine

BRASATO DI MANZO CON CIPOLLE   beef braised with onions

BRASATO DI MANZO CON SEDANO E CIPOLLE   beef braised with celery and onions

BRASATO DI VITELLO   veal roast marinated and braised in wine herb sauce

BRESAOLA AL LIMONE   salted, dried beef with lemon juice

BUDELLI DI MAIALE   entrails of pork

BUE   beef

BUE AL BAROLO   beef braised in red wine

CAPOCOLLO   smoked salt pork

CAPRETTO   kid, baby goat

CAPRETTO AI CARCIOFI   baby goat sautéed with wine, onion, artichokes, lemon, egg yolks and ham

CAPRETTO AL FORNO   roast goat, basted with herb broth

CAPRETTO AL VINO BIANCO   kid cooked in white wine

CAPRETTO ALLA PAESANA   baby goat roasted in casserole with potatoes, oil, cheese, onions

CAPRETTO ALLA PASQUALINA   oven-roasted baby goat basted with wine, olive oil, onion and broth

CAPRETTO ALLO SPIEDO   spit roasted baby goat

CAPRETTO RIPIENO AL FORNO   baby goat stuffed with herbs and cooked in the oven

CARATELLA   lamb pieces roasted on skewers

CARBONATA   beef stew in red wine

CARNE   meat

CARNE ARROSTO   roast meat

CARNE ARROSTO CON PROSCIUTTO E SPINACI   roast meat, ham and spinach

CARNE CARRARGIU   meat spit-roasted in the open air on wood with scented herbs

CARNE CON FEGATINI E TARTUFI   beef, chicken livers and truffles

CARNE CON FUNGHI SECCHI   beef and dried mushrooms

CARNE CRUDA   steak tartar, raw, finely ground meat and garlic, anchovy, oil

CARNE DI MANZO   roast beef

CARNE DI SUINO   pork meat

CARNE FREDDA ASSORTITA   roasted and boiled assorted cold meats

CARNE TRA DUE PIATTI   meat steamed between two plates

CARNE TRITATA   minced beef and ham

CARPACCIO   thinly sliced raw beef fillet, usually served with a piquant sauce

CARTOCCIO   roasted in a sealed bag

CASSERUOLA   casserole

CASSOEULA   pork feet, ears, lean meat sautéed in casserole with wine

CASTELLANA   thin veal cutlet, filled, folded then fried

CASTELLANA AL MARSALA   thin veal cutlet filled with ham, cheese, breaded and fried in wine

CASTELLANA AL PROSCIUTTO   thin veal cutlet filled with ham, breaded, fried in brown sauce

CASTELLANA TARTUFATA   veal cutlet filled with ham, cheese, breaded, fried in white wine

CASTRADINA   roast mutton

CASTRATO   castrated sheep *or* mutton

CASTRATO DI BRACIOLE   grilled or fried mutton chops *or* rib chops

CAZZOEULA   casserole of pork, cabbage and spices

CERVELLA   brains, usually veal

CERVELLA AI PISTACCHI   brains and pistachio nuts

CERVELLA AL BURRO   brains poached, floured, pan fried in butter

CERVELLA AL TEGAMINO   diced brains dipped in flour and egg batter, fried in butter

CERVELLA ALLA FINANZIERA   brains sliced, poached, served with brown mushroom sauce

CERVELLA ALLA SALVIA   brains sautéed with butter and sage

CERVELLA E ZUCCHINI   brains and zucchini breaded and pan fried

CERVELLA FRITTA CON CARCIOFI   brains and artichokes breaded and fried

CERVELLA FRITTA CON CARCIOFI E MOZZARELLA brains with artichokes and mozzarella, breaded and fried

CICCIA   meat

CICCIOLI   fried pork sausage

CIMA   cold, stuffed veal breast

CIMA ALLA GENOVESE   beef *or* veal stuffed with sweetbreads, pork, peas

CIMA DI MANZO   beef breast stuffed, cooked, sliced, served cold

CIMALINO DI MANZO   boiled stuffed beef breast and beans

CIPOLLE AL PROSCIUTTO E ROSMARINO   onions with ham and rosemary

CODA ALLA VACCINARA   pieces of oxtail stewed in tomato sauce, seasoned with celery

CODA DI BUE   oxtail

CODA DI BUE ALLA CAVOUR   oxtail stew

CODA DI VITELLO AL FORNO   veal tail braised then oven roasted

CONIGLIO   rabbit

CONIGLIO AI CAPPERI   braised marinated rabbit with wine, anchovy, onion, vinegar

CONIGLIO AL BUONGUSTAIO   rabbit with vegetables and Marsala

CONIGLIO AL FORNO   rabbit baked in oven, with wine, onion, broth

CONIGLIO AL MARSALA   rabbit cooked in Marsala with onions, pimentos, tomatoes, eggplant

CONIGLIO ALL'AGRO   rabbit stewed in red wine and lemon juice

CONIGLIO ALL'AGRODOLCE   sweet-sour rabbit

CONIGLIO ALLA BORGHESE   rabbit sautéed in white wine, herbs, onions and mushrooms

CONIGLIO ALLA CACCIATORA   rabbit braised in wine, mushrooms, tomato and garlic

CONIGLIO ALLA CAMPAGNOLA   rabbit with garlic, rosemary and wine

CONIGLIO ALLA FRIULANA   rabbit with egg and lemon sauce

CONIGLIO ALLA LIVORNESE   rabbit casserole with tomatoes and anchovies

CONIGLIO ALLA MOLISANA   grilled rabbit and sausage chunks

CONIGLIO ALLA ROMAGNOLA   pieces of rabbit breaded, batter-dipped then fried in butter

CONIGLIO CON POLENTA   rabbit braised in sauce and served on cornmeal mush

CONIGLIO FARCITO AL FORNO   rabbit stuffed and roasted

CONIGLIO FRITTO   rabbit fried in bacon fat and oil, with sage and garlic

CONIGLIO FRITTO ALLA LOMBARDA   rabbit dipped in egg and chopped herbs, coated with bread crumbs and fried

CONIGLIO IN FRICASSEA   rabbit stewed in wine sauce thickened with egg yolks, flavored with lemon

CONIGLIO IN PADELLA   rabbit sautéed in oil with bacon, tomatoes, garlic, wine and parsley

CONIGLIO IN SALMÌ   rabbit marinated in wine, cooked with chopped vegetables, oil, wine and herbs

CONIGLIO IN SALSA CON UOVA   rabbit poached in sauce thickened with eggs and lemon juice

CONIGLIO IN SALSA PICCANTE   rabbit in spicy sauce with vegetables, wine, capers and anchovies

CONIGLIO IN UMIDO   rabbit stew

CONIGLIO IN UMIDO DI BERGAMO   rabbit stewed with basil, parsley, onion and vermouth

CONIGLIO RIPIENO AL FORNO   stuffed and roasted rabbit
CONTROFILETTO DI VITELLO AI FERRI   veal loin steak
   grilled
CONTRONOCE DI VITELLO AL FORNO   oven roast
   veal bottom round
CONTRONOCE DI VITELLO ALLA GENOVESE   veal bot-
   tom round braised in wine, mushroom, vegetable broth
COPPA   kind of raw ham, usually smoked, sliced and
   served cold
COPPIETTE   small meatballs with ham, cheese, garlic,
   cheese, deep fried
CORATELLA   lamb's heart, lung, liver and spleen cooked
   in olive oil, seasoned with pepper and onion
CORATELLA DI CAPRETTO   lung and intestines of kid
CORDA   long strips of tripe, either roasted or stewed in
   tomato sauce, with peas
COSCIA   leg, thigh
COSCIA DI VITELLO AL FORNO   oven roast leg of veal
COSCIOTTO   leg
COSCIOTTO DI AGNELLO   leg of lamb, usually roasted
COSCIOTTO DI CONIGLIO   rabbit leg braised in gravy
COSCIOTTO DI PORCELLO AL FORNO   roast leg of
   young pig
COSTA   meat with bone in (see COSTOLETTA)
COSTA DI BUE ALLA FIORENTINA   bone-in steak,
   salted, coated with olive oil and charcoal broiled
COSTA DI BUE ALLA TIROLESE   bone-in steak, served
   with fried onions
COSTA DI BUE MAITRE D'   bone-in steak grilled with
   seasoned butter and lemon juice sauce
COSTA DI CAPRETTO ALLA BRACE   broiled baby goat
   chops
COSTA DI CAPRETTO ALLA MILANESE   pan-fried
   breaded baby goat chops
COSTA DI MAIALE   pork chop
COSTAGELLA   meat with bone in (see COSTOLETTA)
COSTALLATA   meat with bone in (see COSTOLETTA)

COSTARELLE PANUNTELLA pork chops grilled and
served over bread slices

COSTATA meat with bone in (see COSTOLETTA)

COSTATA AL FINOCCHIO pork chops pan fried with
wine and herbs

COSTATA ALLA FIORENTINA thick cut of beef grilled
over coal

COSTATA DI MANZO beef rib steak

COSTATA DI MANZO AL BAROLO marinated, boned
rib of beef in red wine

COSTATA DI MANZO DISOSSATO boned rib steak

COSTATA DI VITELLO veal chop bone in

COSTE meat with bone in

COSTE DI MAIALE CON CARCIOFI pork chops with
artichokes

COSTICINE DI MAIALE AI FERRI grilled marinated
spareribs

COSTICINE DI MAIALE ALLA TREVIGIANA pan-
roasted spareribs with garlic, sage and red wine

COSTOLA DI VITELLO veal rib with bone

COSTOLE DI AGNELLO ALLA MILANESE lamb chops
breaded and pan fried

COSTOLETTA veal *or* pork cutlet with bone or chop

COSTOLETTA AL PROSCIUTTO steak and ham slice
breaded, fried, then topped with melted cheese

COSTOLETTA AL SOAVE steak braised in white wine

COSTOLETTA ALLA BOLOGNESE breaded veal cutlet,
ham, cheese and tomato sauce

COSTOLETTA ALLA FIORENTINA grilled steak in oil,
garlic, onion, herb sauce

COSTOLETTA ALLA MAITRE D' steak grilled and
served with herb butter

COSTOLETTA ALLA MILANESE veal cutlet, batter
dipped in bread crumbs and cheese, pan fried in butter

COSTOLETTA ALLA PALERMITANA grilled, breaded
veal cutlets

COSTOLETTA ALLA PARMIGIANA   steak fried and covered with melted cheese

COSTOLETTA ALLA PETRONIANA   marinated veal chop, breaded and fried with onion, cream sauce and oven browned

COSTOLETTA ALLA PIZZAIOLA   steak partially fried then sautéed in tomato sauce with garlic, herbs and oregano

COSTOLETTA ALLA SALVIA   steak braised in wine served with grated cheese and sage

COSTOLETTA ALLA TIROLESE   steak grilled in and served with onions

COSTOLETTA ALLA VALDOSTANA   veal chops stuffed with cheese

COSTOLETTA ALLA ZINGARA   steak pan fried in wine, mushrooms, butter, basil and pieces of pickled tongue

COSTOLETTA CARPIONATA   veal chop floured, fried, served cold in herbal vinegar

COSTOLETTA DI AGNELLO CON PEPERONI   baby lamb chops baked with sweet peppers

COSTOLETTA DI MAIALE AL VINO   pork chops braised with Marsala and red wine

COSTOLETTA DI MAIALE ALLA MODENESE   pork chops, braised with sage and tomatoes

COSTOLETTA DI MAIALE CON FUNGHI   braised pork chops with mushrooms

COSTOLETTA DI VITELLO ALLA MILANESE   veal cutlets breaded and fried

COSTOLETTA DI VITELLO PROFUMATA ALL'AGLIO E ROSMARINO   veal chops sautéed with garlic and rosemary

COSTOLETTA FRITTA COI FUNGHI   fried steak with mushrooms

COSTOLETTA RIPIENA   veal steak stuffed with seasoned chopped meat, floured and pan fried

COSTOLETTA TRIFOLA   pan-fried steak served with truffles

COSTOLETTE DI ABBACCHIO ALLA GRIGLIA   grilled
lamb chops

COSTOLETTE DI MAIALE   pork chops

COSTOLETTE DI MAIALE ALLA MARCONI   pork chops
stuffed with cheese and ham, breaded and fried in oil

COTECHINO   boiled spiced pork sausage

COTICHE   pork skin preserved in lard

COTOLETTA   meat without bone (as cutlet see
COSTOLETTA)

COTOLETTA AL PROSCIUTTO   veal cutlet pan fried
with slice of ham or bacon

COTOLETTA ALLA BOLOGNESE   veal cutlet with slices
of ham and cheese, baked in oven and sprinkled with
white wine

COTOLETTA ALLA MILANESE   veal cutlet, dipped in
egg and bread crumbs, fried in olive oil

COTOLETTA ALLA VIENNESE   veal cutlet, dipped in
egg and bread crumbs, baked in olive oil

COTOLETTA DI VITELLO   veal steak without bone

COTOLETTE ALLA CALABRESE   thin slices of meat,
sautéed with olive oil, red peppers, garlic, tomato paste

CRAUTI CON SALUMI   pickled sauerkraut with sausage

CRESPOLINA   pancake filled with veal, grated cheese,
baked in tomato sauce

CROCCHETTA DI CARNE ARROSTITA   meatballs
roasted in skewer with pork fat and toast

CROCCHETTA DI CERVELLA E ZUCCHINI FRITTI
croquette of brains and zucchini, breaded and fried

CROCCHETTE DI PATATE ALLA ROMAGNOLA   potato
and ham croquettes

CULATELLI   spicy ham, specialty of Parma

CULATELLO   type of raw ham cured in white wine

CULATELLO DI ZIBELLO   loin of pork dried in warm air
and eaten raw

CUORE   heart

CUORE DI BUE   heart (from beef)

CUTTURIDDI   lamb stew flavored with rosemary

DAINO ALLA DIAVOLA   deer grilled with lots of
pepper, chili pepper, spicy

DAINO ALLA DORIA   deer highly spiced and grilled

ENTRECÔTE DI BUE   boneless beef steak

ENTRECÔTE   boneless beef *or* veal steak

ENTRECÔTE ALLA BISMARK   boneless steak fried in
butter and served with fried egg on top

ENTRECÔTE ALLA PIZZAIOLA   boneless steak fried in
oil with garlic and tomato sauce

ENTRECÔTE ALLA TIROLESE   boneless steak fried and
served with onions

FARSUMAGRU   breast of veal *or* beef, stuffed with spices
and hard-boiled eggs

FARSUMAGRU DI BRACIOLONE   beef *or* veal stuffed
with sausages, salami, cheeses, hard-boiled eggs

FAVATA   beans stewed in lard with pork sausage and spice

FEGATELLI ALLA FIORENTINA   pork liver breaded
with garlic, fennel, sage and oven roasted in olive oil

FEGATELLI DI MAIALE   pork liver

FEGATINI DI MAIALE   pigs' livers, seasoned and roasted
on a spit between two slices of bread

FEGATINI DI MAIALE   pork liver braised in wine and
onions with or without tomatoes

FEGATO   liver

FEGATO AL BURRO   liver, floured and pan fried in
butter

FEGATO ALL'AGRO DOLCE   liver, battered and fried,
sweet and sour

FEGATO ALLA FIORENTINA   liver, floured and cooked
in oil, garlic and tomatoes

FEGATO ALLA SALVIA   liver breaded and fried in butter
and sage

FEGATO ALLA TOSCANA   broiled pork liver and bread
chunks

FEGATO ALLA VENETA   liver sautéed in oil and onions

FEGATO ALLA VENEZIANA   calf's liver fried with onions

FEGATO DI VITELLO   calves' liver *or* veal liver

FEGATO DI VITELLO AL POMODORO   pan fried calves'
liver in tomato sauce

FEGATO DI VITELLO ALLA GRIGLIA   calves' liver
steak, charcoal grilled

FEGATO PICCANTE   calf's liver with vinegar

FESA   round steak cut from leg fillet of veal

FESA AL FORNO   veal leg fillet baked in oven

FESA AL VINO BIANCO   roast veal slices served in wine
sauce

FESA ARROSTO   veal leg fillet roasted in oven

FESA CON FUNGHI   veal leg fillet pot roast with mushrooms, peas, stock, herbs

FESA IN GELATINA   veal round steak in gelatin

FESA PRIMAVERILE   leg of veal larded with ham, carrot,
celery and bacon

FETTINE DI MANZO ALLA PIZZAIOLA   beef slices pan
fried with tomato, wine, garlic, oil

FETTINE DI MANZO FARCITE   pan-fried, stuffed thin
beefsteaks with cheese and ham

FILETTO   fillet (see COSTOLETTA)

FILETTO DI BUE AL BAROLO   beef fillet with red wine

FILETTO DI BUE ALLA BISMARK   boneless steak grilled,
served with fried egg

FILETTO DI BUE ALLA TARTARA   raw ground steak
served with egg, onion, anchovy

FILETTO DI VITELLO ALLA ROSSINI   butter-fried veal
steak topped with liver and red wine

FINOCCHIONA ALLA TOSCANA   pork salami flavored
with fennel

FOIOLO   tripe (stomach lining of cow or calf)

FOIOLO AL SUGO   tripe braised in onion, tomato and herbs

FOIOLO ALLA BOLOGNESE   tripe braised in tomato
sauce with wine, garlic, cheese

FOIOLO ALLA GENOVESE   tripe braised in tomato sauce
with wine, garlic, cheese

FOIOLO ALLA MILANESE   tripe braised in onion, herbs,
with wine, garlic, cheese

FRACOSTA ALLA GRIGLIA grilled rib steak

FRACOSTA DI BUE bone-in rib steak

FRICASSEA a white veal stew with mushrooms, sauce thickened with egg yolks

FRITTO ALLA ROMANA fried sweetbreads, artichokes and cauliflower

FRITTO STECCO veal, sweetbreads, brains and mushrooms dipped in egg yolk and bread crumbs and fried

FRITTURA DI VITELLO PICCATA veal cutlets breaded, battered and fried

GALANTINA DI PROSCIUTTO fine-chopped ham loaf in meat gelatine

GALANTINA IN GELATINA fine chopped meat loaf in meat gelatine

GAROFOLATO beef stew

GAROFOLATO AL SUGO IN UMIDO potted beef with wine, herbs, onions

GELATINA a meat jelly

GIRELLO round steak from the leg (also see FESA)

GIRELLO AL FORNO roast of veal round steak

GIRELLO AL MADERA roast of veal fried or braised in red wine

GIRELLO AL SOAVE roast of veal fried or braised in white wine

GIRELLO ALLA GENOVESE roast of veal served in cold olive oil, capers and anchovy

GIRELLO DI VITELLO veal fillet steak roasted

GNUMMARIELLI entrails of baby lamb, roasted on a spit

GOULASCH ALL'UNGHERESE chunks of veal *or* beef braised in paprika sauce

GRATINATA sprinkled with bread crumbs and cheese and oven-browned

GUANCIALE streaky bacon meat

GUAZZETTO meat stew with garlic, rosemary, tomatoes and pimentos

IN UMIDO stewed in broth with onions, carrots, tomatoes and herbs

INVOLTINI   stewed rolls of veal, stuffed with mince and spices

INVOLTINI AL COGNAC   stuffed veal rolls cooked in butter then flamed in brandy

INVOLTINI AL GROVIERA   veal rolls stuffed with Gruyère cheese sautéed in butter

INVOLTINI ALLA MILANESE   meat roll stuffed with chicken livers, cheese, wine

INVOLTINI DI BUE ALLA SICILIANA   beef rolls filled with parsley, ham, onion, nutmeg

INVOLTINI DI CAVOLO VERDE   meat filled cabbage leaves cooked in sauce

INVOLTINI DI FAGIOLONI   veal slices stuffed with ham and cheese, sautéed with beans

INVOLTINI DI MAIALE AL FORNO   stuffed baked pork rolls

LACCETT ALL'AGRODOLCE   sweetbreads in a sweet-sour sauce

LAME DI FEGATO   liver slices

LAMELLE DI FEGATO   very thin slices of liver sautéed in butter

LARDO   bacon

LARDO E FUNGHI   bacon and mushrooms

LASAGNE DI CARNEVALE   baked lasagne with sausage and meat sauce

LESSO   boiled meat

LINGUA   tongue

LINGUA AL POMODORO   boiled tongue slices served in tomato sauce

LINGUA AL PROSCIUTTO E MADERA   boiled tongue slices with ham served in wine sauce

LINGUA ALL'AGRODOLCE   tongue in a sweet-sour sauce

LINGUA ALL'ESCARLATE   boiled tongue sliced, served cold

LINGUA ALLA FIAMMINGA   tongue braised in beer with onion, mushrooms, herbs and broth

LINGUA ALLA PARMIGIANA   boiled tongue slices with Parmesan cheese melted atop

LINGUA DI VITELLO   veal *or* calf tongue boiled or corned

LINGUA DI VITELLO SALMISTRATA   marinated veal tongue

LINGUA IN SALSA VERDE   boiled tongue served cold in sauce of capers, anchovy, oil

LINGUA PICCANTE   spiced *or* pickled tongue

LINGUA SALMISTRATA   pickled beef tongue served cold

LOMBATA   loin

LOMBATA DI MAIALE   pork loin, can be roasted or fried

LOMBATA DI VITELLO   veal loin

LOMBATA DI VITELLO AL CARBONE   large grilled veal chop

LOMBATINE   flattened veal cutlets

LOMBATINE ALLA PARMIGIANA   flattened veal cutlets pan fried with ham, cheese

LONZA   loin (usually pork)

LUGANEGA   pork sausage made with Parmesan cheese

LUGANEGA E UOVA SODE   eggs and sausages

LUGANICA   long thin sausage

MAIALE   pork

MAIALE AL LATTE   pork cooked in milk

MAIALE ALLA PIZZAIOLA   pork slices braised in tomato, garlic, oil, capers

MAIALE ALLO SPIEDO   spit-roast pig

MAIALE CON SPINACI   pork and spinach

MAIALE PICCANTE   spicy pork

MAIALE UBRIACO   pork cooked in red wine

MANZO   beef

MANZO AL LIMONE   beef cooked in lemon juice

MANZO ALL'ACETO   pot roast with vinegar and capers

MANZO ALLA CERTOSINA   spicy pot roast

MANZO ALLA GENOVESE   beef braised with vegetables, wine, tomatoes

MANZO ALLA PIZZAIOLA   grilled steak served with sauce of garlic, oil, tomato and herbs

MANZO ARROSTO   roast beef

MANZO BATTUTO   ground beef either sautéed or fried

MANZO BOLLITO   boiled beef

MANZO BRASATO   beef pot roasted with wine

MANZO CON CIPOLLE   beef braised with onions, oil, butter and stock

MANZO LESSO   boiled beef

MANZO RIPIENO   stuffed beef

MANZO SALATO   corned beef

MANZO SALMISTRATO CON UOVA AFFOGATE
Italian corned beef hash with herbs, poached eggs, polenta, cheese

MANZO STUFATO AL BAROLO   marinated beef in red wine

MAZZAFEGATI   sausages of pigs' liver, seasoned with garlic, pepper, coriander, fried in olive oil

MEDAGLIONE   round fillet of beef *or* veal

MEDAGLIONE AL BAROLO   beef pieces braised in wine

MEDAGLIONE AL MADERA   beef steaks fried in red wine

MEDAGLIONE ALLA PROVINCIALE   beef pieces fried and served with brains, sweetbreads, broth and peas

MEDAGLIONE ALLA ZINGARA   beef steaks fried in sauce of onion, tomato and mushrooms

MEDAGLIONE PRIMAVERA   beef steaks fried with mushrooms, onions and tomato sauce

MESSICANI   stuffed veal scallops

MESSICANI ALLA MILANESE   veal rolls stuffed with meat, cheese, braised in wine sauce

MESSICANI ALLA VILLERECCIA   veal ribs stuffed with meat, cheese, braised in vegetable sauce

MESSICANI DI VITELLO   veal rolls stuffed with pork and cheese

MIDOLLO   bone marrow

MIGLIACCIO ALLA NAPOLETANA   baked casserole of cornmeal, sausage, cheeses

MODINO   small, round fillet slices, usually veal *or* beef

MODINO AI SASSI   small round fillet slices fried in wine and herbs

MODINO AL BURRO   small round fillet slices fried in butter

MODINO AL SOAVE small round fillet slices fried in wine and herbs

MODINO ALLA PANNA small round fillet slices fried in cream sauce with onions

MODINO ALLA PIZZAIOLA small round fillet slices fried with tomatoes, garlic, oil

MONTONE mutton

MORTADELLA pork sausage made of pork fat, peppercorns and pistachio nuts

MORTADELLA CAMPOTOSTO dry and spicy sausage, strong garlic flavor

MUSCOLETTI DI VITELLO AI FUNGHI veal shank stewed in wine, tomato, mushroom sauce

MUSCOLO ALLA FIORENTINA casserole of shin of beef, wine, vegetables and herbs

NOCE DI VITELLO roast *or* grilled sirloin of veal

NODINI DI VITELLO AL SUGHETTO CON ACCIUGHE veal chops sautéed with anchovy sauce

NODINO DI MAIALE ALLA GRIGLIA small grilled pork steaks

OLIVETTE small chunks of veal with olive-like appearance, cooked in white wine

OSSO bone

OSSO DI PROSCIUTTO CON FAGIOLI ham bone with white beans

OSSOBUCHI ALLA MILANESE veal shanks braised with tomatoes and wine

OSSOBUCO veal shank

OSSOBUCO AI FUNGHI veal shanks braised in mushroom gravy

OSSOBUCO AL VINO BIANCO veal shank braised in white wine, garlic and herbs

OSSOBUCO ALLA GREMOLADA veal shank breaded and fried with garlic, lemon, herb sauce

OSSOBUCO ALLA LOMBARDA veal shank braised then floured and butter fried, served with lemon juice

OSSOBUCO ALLA MILANESE   veal shank braised in
  wine, tomato sauce with lemon juice
OSSOBUCO CON PUREA   veal shank braised and served
  over pureed potatoes
PAILLARD   beef rib steak
PALLOTTOLINE   meatballs (see POLPETTA)
PANCETTA   bacon salted and spiced then rolled, eaten raw
PANCETTA AFFUMICATA   bacon and egg
PASTICCIO DI FEGATO   chopped liver with pistachio
  nuts
PASTICCIO DI MANZO AI FUNGHI   beef baked in
  pastry shell with gravy and mushrooms
PASTICCIO DI PATATE E SALSICCE   baked sausage and
  potato pie
PASTIZADA   beef pot roast
PASTIZADA ALLA VENETA   beef pot roast made with
  wine, onion, herbs
PATÉ   finely ground meat *or* liver paste served cold
PECORA   sheep
PERLA DI VITELLO   braised veal with diced ham,
  flavored with spices, herbs and onions
PEZZENTE   sausage of liver, lung and meat scraps, garlic,
  pepper, smoked
PIASTRA   grilled on steel sheet
PICCATA   thin veal scallop
PICCATA AL MADERA   veal scallops pan fried then
  braised in red wine
PICCATA AL MARSALA   thin veal scallops braised in
  Marsala sauce
PICCATA ALLA LOMBARDA   veal scallops pan fried in
  butter and lemon juice
PICCATA ALLEGRA   veal scallops pan fried in butter
  and lemon sauce
PICCATA CON CAPPERI   veal scallops pan fried in
  butter with capers and herbs
PICCATA DI FEGATO DI VITELLO AL LIMONE   sautéed
  calf's liver, thin-sliced with lemon juice

PICCATA DI VITELLO   pounded veal scallops or cutlets floured and sautéed in lemon and wine

PICCATA DORATA   veal scallops egg-dipped, pan fried in butter

PIEDE   foot

POLLO AL PROSCIUTTO   chicken and ham

POLMONE DI VITELLO   calves' lung

POLPETTA   meatball

POLPETTE AI CAPPERI   meatballs with capers

POLPETTE AL SUGO   meatballs stuffed with cheese, deep fried and served with tomato sauce

POLPETTE CASSARECCE   meatballs cooked and served in tomato sauce

POLPETTE COI FAGIOLI   meatballs served with boiled white beans

POLPETTE DI CARNE   meatballs in sauce with tomato, onion, cheese

POLPETTE DI MAIALE AL PITAGGIO   pan-fried pork meatballs with vegetables

POLPETTE DI MANZO   meatballs cooked in gravy

POLPETTE INVERNALI CON LA VERZA   meatballs with savoy cabbage

POLPETTINE   meat patties (see POLPETTA)

POLPETTONE   loaf of beef, veal, *or* vegetables

POLPETTONE IN BRODO   meat loaf in chicken broth

POLPETTONE SORPRESA veal loaf with cheese, onion, garlic, oil and tomato paste

PORCEDDU   suckling pig flavored with myrtle and roasted between hot stones in a hole in the ground, covered with earth

PORCELLO   very young pig

PORCHETTA   roast suckling pig

PORCHETTA AL FORNO   baked suckling pig

PORCHETTA DI MAIALE ARROSTO   roast suckling pig

PORTAFOGLIO   veal cutlet stuffed with chopped meat, ham, cheese, fried or sautéed

PROSCIUTTO   salted air-cured ham

PROSCIUTTO AFFUMICATO   cured, smoked ham

PROSCIUTTO AI TARTUFI E FUNGHI   ham with white
sauce, truffles and mushrooms

PROSCIUTTO AL MADERA   cooked ham in wine sauce

PROSCIUTTO COI FICHI   ham with ripe figs

PROSCIUTTO COI FUNGHI   ham, with cheese and
mushrooms

PROSCIUTTO COI FUNGHI COLTIVATI   ham with
button mushrooms

PROSCIUTTO CON LINGUA E TARTUFI   ham with
tongue and truffles

PROSCIUTTO COTTO   cured, smoked ham which is cooked

PROSCIUTTO CRUDO   salt-cured ham which is air-dried

PROSCIUTTO DI LANGHIRANO   ham from the province
of Parma

PROSCIUTTO DI MONTAGNA   ham from a mountain
district

PROSCIUTTO DI PARMA   cured ham from Parma

PROSCIUTTO E POMODORO   ham and tomatoes

PUNTA DI VITELLO ARROSTO   roast breast of veal

PUNTA DI VITELLO RIPIENA   stuffed veal breast
usually roasted

RAGÙ DI AGNELLO   braised lamb with tomatoes, basil
and black olives

RICOTTA CON SALSICCE   cottage cheese with sausages

RICOTTA CON SPINACI E CERVELLA   cottage cheese
with spinach and brains

RIFREDDO MISTO   assorted cold roast meat

RISO AL CAVROMAN   rice with mutton, onion, tomato,
cheese

RISO E LUGANEGA   rice and sausage

ROGNONCINI D'AGNELLO SALTATI CON CIPOLLA
sautéed lamb kidneys with onion

ROGNONE   kidney

ROGNONE AI FUNGHI TRIFOLATI   kidneys braised
with broth, garlic, mushroom and truffles

ROGNONE AL MADERA   kidneys braised in red wine

ROGNONE DI VITELLO ALLA GRIGLIA   pan-fried veal kidneys

ROLLATINE DI VITELLO   rolled and stuffed breast of veal

ROLLE DI FILETTO   rolled fillet of beef pot roasted with wine

ROSBIF   roast beef

ROTOLO   stuffed meat roll

ROTOLO DI VITELLO E SPINACI   veal and spinach roll, stuffed with ham

SALAME   salami

SALAME ALL'UNGHERESE   Hungarian salami of pork and beef

SALAME ALLA CACCIATORA   hard, dried salami

SALAME ALLA FINOCCHIONA   salami from Tuscany, flavored with fennel seed

SALAME ALLA GENOVESE   salami with a mix of pork, veal and pork fat

SALAME DI FABRIANO   salami with a mixture of pork and veal, from Marches

SALAME DI FELINO   pure pork salami from village of Felino near Parma

SALMÌ   stew cooked in earthen pot

SALSICCE   sausages eaten newly made and fried, or dry and seasoned

SALSICCE AL SUGO   fried pork sausage braised in meat sauce

SALSICCE AL VINO ROSSO E FUNGHI SECCHI   fried sausages with red wine and dried wild mushrooms

SALSICCE ARROSTO   pork sausages grilled over open fire

SALSICCE COL CAVOLO NERO   sausages with red cabbage

SALSICCE CON CIPOLLE   sausages with smothered onions

SALSICCE CON MELANZANE   sausages with eggplant

SALSICCE CON UOVA   sausages with eggs

SALSICCE DI FEGATO   sausages of pigs' liver, with garlic, salt and pepper, pinch of orange peel, eaten fried after they have been dried

SALSICCE FRITTE   fried pork sausage

SALSICCIA   sausage (see SALSICCE)

SALTIMBOCCA   slices of veal and prosciutto ham
sautéed in wine

SALTIMBOCCA ALLA GENOVESE   veal and ham rolls
sautéed in Marsala wine

SALTIMBOCCA ALLA ROMANA   veal cutlet flavored
with ham and sage, sautéed

SALTIMBOCCA ALLA SORRENTINA   thin veal slices
baked with ham and cheese slices and tomato sauce

SALUMI   sausages served sliced cold

SALUMI NOSTRANI   local salami

SANATO   milk fed calf (veal)

SCALOPPA, SCALOPPINA   veal slice (see SCALOPPINE)

SCALOPPINE   thin veal slices

SCALOPPINE AI FUNGHI   pan-fried veal slices, then
grilled in mushroom cream sauce

SCALOPPINE AL BURRO   veal slices floured and pan
fried in butter

SCALOPPINE AL FORMAGGIO   veal slices fried,
covered with cheese and baked

SCALOPPINE AL LIMONE   veal slices marinated and
sautéed in oil with lemon juice

SCALOPPINE AL MADERA   veal slices sautéed in butter
and red wine

SCALOPPINE AL MARSALA   veal slices sautéed in
Marsala wine

SCALOPPINE AL MARSALA ARRICCHITE   veal slices
with Marsala wine and cream

SCALOPPINE AL POMODORO   veal slices sautéed in
herb, tomato sauce

SCALOPPINE AL POMODORO E FUNGHI   veal slices
sautéed in herb, mushroom, tomato sauce

SCALOPPINE AL VINO BIANCO   veal slices sautéed in
butter and white wine

SCALOPPINE ALL'ARANCIO   veal slices sautéed in
butter, oil and orange juice

SCALOPPINE ALLA BISMARK   veal slices fried and
topped with fried egg

SCALOPPINE ALLA BOLOGNESE   veal slices breaded and fried with ham and cheese and meat sauce

SCALOPPINE ALLA BOSCAIOLA   veal slices sautéed, then broiled with onion, mushrooms and tomato

SCALOPPINE ALLA CACCIATORA   veal slices floured, pan fried in tomato, mushrooms, herb sauce

SCALOPPINE ALLA CAMPAGNOLA   veal slices sautéed then broiled with onion, mushrooms, tomato, carrot

SCALOPPINE ALLA CAPRICCIOSA   veal slices sautéed in mushroom sauce with ham, herbs, melted cheese

SCALOPPINE ALLA CONTADINA   veal slices sautéed in tomato sauce with onion, cheese, capers, olives

SCALOPPINE ALLA LOMBARDA   veal slices marinated and sautéed in oil with lemon juice and parsley

SCALOPPINE ALLA MILANESE   veal slices floured, breaded and fried with grated cheese

SCALOPPINE ALLA PANNA   veal slices sautéed in white cream sauce

SCALOPPINE ALLA PANNA E FUNGHI   veal slices sautéed in white cream sauce with mushrooms

SCALOPPINE ALLA PARMIGIANA   breaded, fried with grated cheese then baked with cheese on top

SCALOPPINE ALLA PIZZAIOLA   veal slices sautéed in garlic, tomato, oil and herb sauce

SCALOPPINE ALLA SORRENTINA   veal slices pan fried then baked with mozzarella cheese and tomato sauce

SCALOPPINE ALLA VALDOSTANA   veal slices stuffed with Fontina cheese, breaded and fried

SCALOPPINE ALLA VIENNESE   veal slices breaded, topped with lemon and anchovies then fried

SCALOPPINE ALLA ZINGARA   veal slices sautéed in butter and red wine, mushrooms and herbs

SCALOPPINE AMMANTATE   veal slices with mozzarella

SCALOPPINE CON GLI ASPARAGI AL CARTOCCIO veal slices and asparagus, Fontina cheese, Marsala sauce baked in foil pouch

SCALOPPINE CON PISELLI   veal slices sautéed in butter
and covered with peas
SCALOPPINE CREMATE   veal slices sautéed in white
cream sauce with cognac
SCALOPPINE DI MAIALE AL MARSALA   pork fillet pan
fried in wine
SCALOPPINE DI VITELLO   boneless thin slice of veal
SCALOPPINE PICCANTI   veal slices braised with butter
and brandy, capers and anchovy
SCALOPPINE PICCATE   veal slices sautéed in butter and
served with pan juices
SCANELLO   round steak
SCANELLO DI VITELLO   veal leg fillet braised in onion
and vinegar and sugar-glazed
SCOTTADITO   veal cutlets
SELLA DI DAINO   saddle of venison usually roasted
SGUAZZETO   braised lamb stew
SGUAZZETO ALLA BECHERA   stew made of various meats
SOAVE DI LEPRE   kid stewed in red wine
SOPPRESSATA   large sausages of a flattened oval shape,
sometimes preserved in oil
SOTTO FILETTO   loin steak
SOTTO FILETTO FARCITO   loin steak stuffed with
seasoned meat and roasted
SOTTO NOCE   veal top round *or* roast veal cutlet
SOTTONOCE DI VITELLO   veal leg fillet
SPALLA   shoulder
SPALLA DI VITELLO AL FORNO   veal shoulder usually
roasted
SPALLA DI VITELLO BRASATA   braised shoulder of veal
with white wine
SPEZZATINO   meat *or* fowl stew
SPEZZATINO AL PROSCIUTTO   veal chunks braised in
herb, tomato and wine sauce
SPEZZATINO ALLA CONTADINA   veal chunks braised
with oil, onion, tomato, herbs, anchovy and cheese

SPEZZATINO ALLA PAESANA   veal chunks braised
with oil, onion, tomato, mushrooms, herbs and cheese
SPEZZATINO D'AGNELLO O CAPRETTO   lamb *or* kid
stew with Marsala wine
SPEZZATINO DI MAIALE AL POMODORO   pork
stewed with tomatoes and onions
SPEZZATINO DI STUFATO E PISELLI   beef stew with peas
SPEZZATO   veal chunks braised in herb, onion and wine
sauce (also see SPEZZATINO)
SPEZZATO D'AGNELLO AL PEPERONE E PROSCIUTTO
lamb stew with white wine, ham and pepper
SPEZZATO DI MUSCOLO   beef stewed slowly with
tomatoes and onion
SPEZZATO DI VITELLO   veal stew made in tomato,
wine, herb sauce
SPIEDINI   pieces of meat grilled or roasted on a skewer
(usually basted)
SPIEDINI ALL'UCCELLETTO   skewered veal and sausage
with sage and white wine
SPIEDINI DI AGNELLO   lamb brochette, grilled on skewers
SPIEDINI DI CAPRETTO   baby goat meat roasted on skewers
SPUNTATURA   short ribs of beef
SPUNTATURA DI MAIALE CON POLENTA   pork short
ribs braised and served with cornmeal mush
STAGIONATA   long-aged meat
STRACOTTO   meat stew, slowly cooked for several hours
STRACOTTO ALLA TOSCANA   veal stew cooked in
wine, herbs and tomato sauce
STRACOTTO DI BUE AL BAROLO   beef braised in red wine
STRACOTTO DI BUE CON PEPERONATA   beef braised
with bell peppers
STUFATINO   meat stew
STUFATINO ALLA SICILIANA   beef stew with onions in
thick sauce
STUFATINO D'AGNELLO ALL'ACETO   lamb stew with
vinegar and green beans

STUFATINO DI MAIALE ALLA BOSCAIOLA   braised
pork with wild mushrooms and juniper berries

STUFATINO DI MANZO COI PISELLI   beef stew with
red wine and peas

STUFATINO DI VITELLO ALL'ANTICA   veal stew

STUFATO   stewing beef cooked slowly in sauce of
tomatoes and other vegetables

SVIZZERINA DI VITELLO   grilled veal hamburger

TENNERONI DI VITELLO CON PISELLI   veal braised in
wine with broth and peas

TESTA DI VITELLO   calf's head

TESTARELLE D'ABBACCHIO   lambs' heads seasoned
with rosemary, basted with olive oil, browned in oven

TESTARELLE DI AGNELLO   roast lambs' heads, flavored
with honey

TETTINI DI VITELLO ALLA PIZZAIOLA   veal slices
fried in garlic, herb oil and tomato sauce

TIMBALLO DI INVERNO   pie filled with mozzarella,
ham, pork, chicken livers, breast of chicken

TIMBALLO DI TAGLIATELLE   baked or meat-stuffed
pasta casserole

TINCO   knuckle of veal, shin of beef

TORDI MATTI   veal cut into pieces and cooked on a skewer

TORNEDÓ ALLA ROSSINI   fillet steak fried in butter
with ham and mushrooms

TOURNEDOS   beef *or* veal steak from tenderloin fillet

TOURNEDOS AL BAROLO   fillet steak fried in red wine

TOURNEDOS AL COGNAC   fillet steak fried in ham,
mushrooms and cognac

TOURNEDOS AL MADERA   fillet steak fried in butter
and Madeira red wine

TOURNEDOS ALLA BISMARK   fillet steak fried and
served with fried egg atop

TOURNEDOS ALLA BORDOLESE   fillet steak fried in
butter, wine and marrow sauce

TOURNEDOS ALLA FINANZIERA   sweetbreads sautéed
with marrow, wine and veal slices

TRACCIOLE DI AGNELLO   lamb and vegetable chunks roasted on a skewer

TRANCIA DI VITELLO   roast veal slice

TRANCIA DI VITELLO AI FUNGHI   roast veal slice with mushrooms

TRIPPA   stomach lining, tripe

TRIPPA AL SUGO   tripe sautéed in a meat mushroom sauce

TRIPPA ALLA BOLOGNESE   tripe braised in onion, garlic, lard, grated cheese and broiled

TRIPPA ALLA GENOVESE   tripe in meat and tomato sauce, flavored with marjoram and served with grated cheese

TRIPPA ALLA LUCCHESE   tripe with onion, butter, cheese and cinnamon

TRIPPA ALLA MILANESE   tripe stewed with onions, leek, carrots, tomatoes, beans and spices

TRIPPA ALLA PARMIGIANA   tripe with herbs, vegetables, tomato sauce, Parmesan cheese

TRIPPA ALLA ROMANA   tripe in sweet and sour sauce with grated cheese

TRIPPA ALLA SENESE   tripe with local sausage and flavored with saffron

TRIPPA COI FAGIOLI   tripe and beans

TRIPPA CON OSTRICHE   tripe and oysters in white wine sauce

TRIPPA MARCHIGIANA   tripe sautéed with onion, cabbage, potato, vegetables

UCCELLETTI ALLA GOLOSA   gourmet veal dish with omelette, mozzarella, tomato sauce, wine

UCCELLETTI DI CAMPAGNA   thin beef and ham slices rolled, skewered with bread slices and grilled

VALDOSTANA   ham and Fontina cheese

VALIGETTA   stuffed braised *or* roasted veal breast

VENTRESCA   boiled pork belly served cold with white beans

VERZADA   pork sausages sautéed in onion and cabbage

VITELLO   veal

VITELLO AI FUNGHI   veal cooked with mushrooms

VITELLO AL FORNO   veal roast

VITELLO AL PORTAFOGLIO   stuffed veal cutlet braised in sauce

VITELLO AL VINO ROSSO   veal stewed in red wine

VITELLO ALL'ASSISIANA   veal larded with ham and cooked with vegetables, herbs, white wine and milk

VITELLO ALL'UCCELLETTO   roast veal flavored with sage

VITELLO ALLA MARENGO   veal simmered with wine, tomatoes, garlic, onions, mushrooms

VITELLO ALLE MELANZANE   pan-fried veal and eggplant

VITELLO ARROSTO   roast veal, usually leg

VITELLO ARROSTO AL SOAVE   roast veal in white wine

VITELLO DI BATTUTA   veal cutlet pounded thin and grilled

VITELLO IN GELATINA ALLA MILANESE   calf's foot cooked in wine, sliced, gelatine added, served cold

VITELLO MAGRO   veal loin slices

VITELLO TONNATO   thin veal slices served cold, after sautéed with tuna, anchovies, olive oil, wine

VITELLONE   young steer (best beef for steaks)

WURSTEL   boiled sausage

WURSTEL AL SUGO DI CARNE   sausage and brown sauce

WURSTEL COI CRAUTI   boiled sausage with sauerkraut

ZAMPE DI MAIALE   pigs' feet boiled in broth

ZAMPONE DI MODENA   pigs' foot stuffed with minced and spiced pork

ZUCCHINE IMBOTTITE DI CARNE   zucchini stuffed with meat

Pasta

AGNELOTTI   small ravioli made with egg, stuffed with minced meat, chopped vegetables, boiled and served with meat sauce

AGNOLOTTI ALLA PIEMONTESE   pasta filled with meat, spinach, cheese and eggs

AGNOLOTTI D'AGNELLO CON SALSA AL FINOCCHIO lamb-filled ravioli with fennel sauce

AGNOLOTTI DI CARNE   pasta filled with meat

AL DENTE   pasta *or* noodles served firm by undercooking

ALLA CARBONARA   pasta with smoked ham or bacon, cheese, eggs and olive oil

ALLA MARCONI   pasta stuffed with ham and cheese, breaded and fried in olive oil

ANELLI   small rings of pasta

BARDELE MARAI   special green noodle with butter, pepper and cheese sauce

BAVETTE   small flat noodle pasta

BAVETTE AI BROCCOLI   bavette pasta with broccoli

BAVETTE ALLA TRASTEVERINA   small flat pasta with tuna and mushrooms

BIGOLI   spaghetti-like pasta

BIGOLI ALL'ANATRA   spaghetti-like pasta with duck sauce

BIGOLI CON CARNE E POMODORO ALLA VENETA   round solid pasta with meat and tomatoes

BIGOLI CON SALSA   round solid noodles with anchovy or sardine sauce

BUCATINI   pasta, like a thick spaghetti

BUCATINI AL CAVOLFIORE   pasta like a thick spaghetti with cauliflower

BUCATINI ALLA BOSCAIOLA   thick spaghetti with eggplant

BUCATINI ALLE ACCIUGHE   thick spaghetti with anchovies

CACIO E PEPE   pasta served with pepper and string cheese

CALCIONI   small ravioli made with egg, stuffed with meat and browned in oven

CALCIUNI   fried ravioli (pasta)

CALCIUNI DEL MOLISE   fried ravioli stuffed with chestnuts

CANNELI   tubes of pasta

CANNELLONI   tubular pasta stuffed with meat, cheese or vegetables

CANNELLONI ALLA BARBAROUX   tubular pasta with chopped ham, veal, cheese and white sauce

CANNELLONI ALLA LAZIALE   tubular pasta with meat and onion filling, baked in tomato sauce

CANNELLONI ALLA NAPOLETANA   tubular pasta with cheese and anchovy filling and tomato herb sauce

CANNELLONI ALLA PARTENOPEA   tubular pasta stuffed
with ricotta cheese and ham, baked in tomato sauce
CANNELLONI ALLA ROMAGNOLA   tubular pasta stuffed
with meat mixture, baked in garlic and tomato sauce
CANNELLONI RIPIENI ALLA TOSCANA   pasta tubes with
a stuffing of meat, chicken livers, eggs, cheese and wine
CANNOLICCHI   pasta of small curved noodle with hole
CANNOLICCHI CON FAGIOLI FRESCHI   pasta served
with white beans in tomato sauce
CANNOLO   short pasta tubes as macaroni
CAPELLINI   very thin solid pasta often called Angel Hair
CAPELLINI AL POMODORO NATURALE   angel hair
pasta with chopped fresh tomatoes, basil, garlic
CAPPELLETTI   small ravioli, filled with cottage cheese,
minced turkey, Parmesan cheese, egg and spices
CAPPELLETTI ALLA ROMANA   ravioli stuffed with
cheese, pork, chicken and served with meat sauce
CAPPELLETTI CON SALSA ALLA BOLOGNESE   small
ravioli with meat and tomato sauce
CAPPELLETTI DI PESCE AL SUGO DI GAMBERETTI
ravioli with fish stuffing and shrimp sauce
CAPPELLETTI DI ROMAGNA   ravioli stuffed with cheese
CAPPELLETTI DI ZUCCA   ravioli stuffed with pumpkin
CASONCELLI   meat-stuffed pasta like macaroni
CASONSEI DI BERGAMO   meat, herb and cheese stuffed
ravioli
CON CREMA DI CECI   pasta served with chick-peas
CONCHIGLIE   shells of pasta
CONCHIGLIE CON BACON, PISELLI E RICOTTA   pasta
shells with bacon, peas and ricotta cheese
CULINGIONES   pasta stuffed with spinach and cheese
CUSCINETTI   pasta dumplings stuffed with jam
DIAVOLO   spicy tomato sauce
FARFALLETTE   pasta shaped like butterflies
FETTUCCINE   long, thin, narrow noodles
FETTUCCINE AL DOPPIO BURRO   fettuccine noodles
with double butter

FETTUCCINE ALLA GOLOSA   fettuccine with creamy ham and mushroom sauce

FETTUCCINE ALLA PAPALINA   fettuccine with butter, ham, mushrooms and Parmesan cheese

FETTUCCINE ALLA RICOTTA   thin noodles with cheese

FETTUCCINE CON SALSA   fettuccine in tomato cheese sauce

FETTUCCINE CON ZUCCHINE FRITTE   fettuccine noodles with fried zucchini

FETTUCCINE VERDI   green noodles made with spinach

FETTUCCINE VERDI ALLA BORAGGINE   green noodles with black butter

FETTUCCINE VERDI CON FUNGHI FRESCHI   green noodles with fresh mushrooms

FOCACCETTE FRITTE   cheese-filled pasta fritters

FRITTATA DI PASTA   spaghetti omelette

FUSILLI   pasta made as solid spiral coils

FUSILLI AI VEGETALI   corkscrew pasta, fresh vegetables, herbs

FUSILLI AL RAGÙ   macaroni in the form of long thin tubes, boiled and served with meat sauce and grated cheese

GNOCCHI AL FORNO   potato-stuffed pasta baked in sauce

GNOCCHI ALLA GENOVESE   potato-stuffed pasta served in basil, garlic, pine nut, pecorino cheese sauce

GNOCCHI TENERI AL LATTE   pasta stuffed with cheese and baked

GRATINATA   sprinkled with bread crumbs and cheese and oven-browned

INCASCIATA   lasagna-type pasta with meat sauce, eggs and cheese

INSALATA DI SPAGHETTI   cold spaghetti with anchovies, olives, olive oil

LAGANELLE   pasta of small stuffed lasagne

LASAGNE   pasta of broad noodles with tomato, meat sauce baked in oven

LASAGNE AI CARCIOFI   broad ribbon noodles with artichokes

LASAGNE AI FUNGHI E PROSCIUTTO   broad ribbon
noodles with mushrooms and ham

LASAGNE AL FORNO   thin layers of macaroni dough
alternating with others of ragout, butter, cheese and
baked in oven

LASAGNE ALL'ANATRA   pasta sheets layered with duck
ragout, bechamel sauce, baked in oven

LASAGNE ALLA BOLOGNESE   baked pasta with meat
sauce, mushrooms, cheese, bechamel sauce

LASAGNE ALLE OLIVE NERE, MALANZANE E
PEPERONI   lasagne with black olives, eggplant and
peppers

LASAGNE CON RICOTTA   baked pasta with tomato
paste, olive oil, wine, cheese, pork sausage

LASAGNE DI CARNEVALE   baked pasta with sausage
and meat sauce

LASAGNE IMBOTTITE   timbale of macaroni dough with
egg, in alternate layers with ragout, cheese, meatballs,
baked in oven

LASAGNE VERDI CON SALSA ALLA BOLOGNESE
green lasagne pasta with tomato, meat

LINGUINE   flat noodles

LINGUINE GHIOTTE   pasta with zucchini and sausage

MACCHERONI   macaroni

MACCHERONI AI CARCIOFI   macaroni with artichokes

MACCHERONI AI GAMBERI   macaroni with shelled
prawns mixed in with tomatoes

MACCHERONI AL FORNO   pie made of macaroni, filled
with buffalo cheese and meatballs, then put in oven

MACCHERONI ALLA BOSCAIOLA   macaroni with
mushrooms

MACCHERONI ALLA CALABRESE   macaroni served with
garlic, hot pepper, cheese, tomatoes, ham, chili pepper

MACCHERONI ALLA CARRETTIERA   macaroni with
sauce of capers, olives, garlic, spices, olive oil and ginger

MACCHERONI ALLA CHITARRA   macaroni spread over
an object resembling a "guitar" and cut into square strips

MACCHERONI ALLA CIOCIARA   macaroni with a sauce of bacon, ham and sausage

MACCHERONI ALLA TRAINIERA   macaroni with sauce of capers, olives, garlic, spices, olive oil and ginger

MACCHERONI CON ALICE FRESCHI   macaroni with fresh anchovy

MACCHERONI CON PISELLI E PEPERONI   macaroni with peas and peppers

MACCHERONI CON RICOTTA   macaroni in a sauce or cream made of cottage cheese

MACCHERONI CON SAFFI   macaroni with asparagus, cream and ham

MACCHERONI CON SARDE   macaroni in a sauce containing pine seeds, fennel, olive oil, chopped sardines

MACCHERONI GRATINATI AL PROSCIUTTO   macaroni with ham, bread crumbs and cheese

MACCHERONI NERI   macaroni with a sauce of garlic, oil and hot red peppers

MALFATTINI   very small egg pasta pieces boiled and served with cheese

MALTAGLIATI   small pasta tubes

MANICOTTI   pasta wide ribbons filled with ricotta cheese, meat, herbs, tomato sauce, baked

MEZZELUNE ALLE ERBE AMARE   half-moon ravioli, ricotta, bitter herbs, brown butter, sage

MINUICCHI   pasta of small stuffed pockets

ORECCHIETTE   pasta of semolina made into small shells

ORECCHIETTE AL POMODORO   pasta shells with sauce of tomato, garlic, oil, onion, basil, cheese, meat

PAGLIA E FIENO   called straw and hay, egg pasta and spinach pasta

PAGLIA E FIENO CON GAMBERETTI   spinach and egg linguine, marinated, grilled shrimp, garlic

PANZAROTTI   fried or baked meat-filled dough envelopes

PANZEROTTI   ravioli filled with buffalo cheese, anchovies, eggs and butter, first fried then browned in oven

PANZONI   pasta pillows stuffed with cheese, walnuts, basil, garlic

PAPPARDELLE   long, broad noodles

PAPPARDELLE AI CANTUNZEIN   yellow and green broad noodles with sweet peppers and sausage

PAPPARDELLE ALL'ANATRA   long broad noodles with duck

PAPPARDELLE ALLA LEPRE   noodles with stew of hare giblets, well-seasoned

PASSATELLI   pasta mixed with egg, cheese, bread crumbs, cooked in broth

PASSATELLI ALLA BOLOGNESE   pasta made with eggs, cheese, bread crumbs in cooked broth

PASTA   dough made in various shapes

PASTA - AGNOLOTTI   square pasta, filled with a savory meat stuffing

PASTA - ALL'UOVO   egg noodles

PASTA - BAVETTE   pasta one size larger than linguine

PASTA - BAVETTINE   next smallest of ribbon-like pasta

PASTA - BOMBOLOTTI   short smooth cylinders of pasta

PASTA - BUCATINI   smallest tubular pasta

PASTA - CANNELLONI   pasta tubes filled with a savory meat stuffing

PASTA - CAPELLINI   very small cylindrical pasta

PASTA - CAPPELLETTI   discs of stuffed pasta, twisted into a small tricorn hat shape

PASTA - CONCHIGLIE   pasta shaped like seashells

PASTA - DENTI DI ELEFANTE   short and tubular pasta with a ribbed exterior

PASTA - FARFALLE   pasta like butterflies

PASTA - FEDELI, FEDELINI   cylindrical pasta, smaller than spaghetti

PASTA - FETTUCCINE   flat ribbon-like form of egg pasta

PASTA - FIOCCHETTI   small bows of pasta

PASTA - FISCHIETTI   smallest tubular pasta

PASTA - FUSILLI   twisted ribbon-like pasta

PASTA - LASAGNE SECCHE   largest of the flat ribbon-like pasta

PASTA - LINGUE DI PASSERO smallest of flat ribbon-like pasta

PASTA - LINGUINE pasta one size larger than bavettine

PASTA - LUMACHE pasta shaped like snail shells

PASTA - MACCHERONCINI small tubular pasta

PASTA - MACCHERONI macaroni

PASTA - MACCHERONI CHITTARA flat ribbon-like forms of egg pasta

PASTA - MALTAGLIATI short and tubular pasta with a smooth exterior

PASTA - MEZZI RIGATONI short and tubular pasta with a ribbed exterior

PASTA - MEZZI ZITI large macaroni

PASTA - MILLE RIGHE pasta curved, elbow-like, and ribbed

PASTA - MILLE RIGHE GRANDI same as MILLE RIGHE, but larger

PASTA - PAPPARDELLE flat ribbon-like forms of pasta uovo (with egg)

PASTA - PENNE short and tubular pasta with a smooth exterior

PASTA - PERCIATELLI small tubular pasta

PASTA - RAVIOLI pasta squares stuffed with spinach and ricotta

PASTA - RIGATONI biggest of the short tubular pasta

PASTA - ROTOLI giant stuffed pasta tubes

PASTA - SECCA hard pasta

PASTA - SPAGHETTI cylindrical pasta, usually hard wheat

PASTA - SPAGHETTINI cylindrical pasta, smaller than spaghetti

PASTA - TAGLIATELLE flat ribbon-like form of egg pasta

PASTA - TAGLIERINI flat ribbon-like form of egg pasta

PASTA - TAGLIOLINI pasta one size larger than bavette

PASTA - TORTELLINI round stuffed pasta

PASTA - TORTIGLIONI twisted ribbon-like pasta

PASTA - TRENETTE, LASAGNETTE pasta larger than TAGLIOLINI

PASTA - VERDE spinach and egg pasta

PASTA - VERMICELLI   pasta like spaghetti but bigger

PASTA - ZITI   very large macaroni

PASTA - ZITONI   largest of all macaroni

PASTA AL FORNO   partially cooked pasta, mixed with other ingredients and baked

PASTA ALLA FINOCCHIELLA   pasta boiled in fennel water served with cheese

PASTA AMMUDDICATA   pasta served with bread crumbs, anchovies, oil, chili

PASTA ASCIUTTA   any pasta not eaten in a broth or soup

PASTA ASCIUTTA ALLA CALABRESE   spaghetti or macaroni served with thick tomato sauce with ginger

PASTA CON SARDE   pasta with fennel, sardines, anchovy, onions, oil, pepper, raisins

PASTA CON SARDE ALLA PALERMITANA   pasta with sardines, anchovies, raisins, saffron, fennel

PASTA DEL GIORNO   pasta of the day

PASTA-E FASOI COL PISTELO DI PARSUTO   pasta with beans, cheese and ham bone

PASTA FREDDA   cold pasta salad

PASTA GIALLA   pasta made with egg

PASTA IN BRODO   pasta in a soup

PASTA 'NCACIATA   pasta with cheese, eggplant, tomato, salami, hard eggs, garlic, oil

PASTA NONNA   pasta with spinach and ham

PASTA RIPIENA   pasta stuffed, then cooked

PASTICCIO   pie *or* baked type of pasta like lasagne

PASTICCIO ALLA FERRARESE   pasta tubes with meat, mushroom sauce and bechamel sauce, oven baked

PASTICCIO DI LASAGNE   lasagne with mozzarella, Bolognese sauce and mushrooms

PASTICCIO DI MACCHERONI   macaroni and chicken liver

PASTICCIO DI MACCHERONI E PICCIONI   macaroni and pigeon pie

PASTINA   small pasta in various shapes

PASTINA IN BRODO   small pasta cooked and served in soup

PENNE   short pasta tubes

PENNE AL SUGO DI CAVOLFIORE   pasta with cauliflower, garlic and oil

PENNE ALL'ARRABBIATA   short, thick pasta with red hot sauce

PENNE ALLA RUSTICA   pasta tubes, fresh tomato sauce, pancetta, oregano

PENNE CON SPINACI E RICOTTA   pasta tubes with ricotta cheese and spinach sauce

PENNE CONTADINE ALLA GROSSETANA   pasta tubes with mushrooms and tomatoes

PICCAGGE AL PESTO E RICOTTA   broad ribbon noodles with ricotta cheese and pesto

PINCIGRASSI   dish made of layers of macaroni dough, separated by layers of ragout, cheese, bechamel and tiny meatballs, browned in oven

PISELLI CON PASTA   pasta with peas

PIZZOCCHERI   buckwheat noodles with Swiss chard and potatoes

RAVIOLI   pillow-shaped pasta stuffed with meat, cheese, vegetables, boiled, served with sauce

RAVIOLI ALLA BOLOGNESE   pillow-shaped pasta served in a tomato meat sauce

RAVIOLI ALLA GENOVESE   pillow-shaped pasta served in a tomato meat sauce

RAVIOLI ALLA PIEMONTESE   pillow-shaped pasta with beef and brown sauce

RAVIOLI ALLA ROMANA   pasta pillows stuffed with ricotta cheese served in an herbal meat sauce

RAVIOLI DI RICOTTA E SPINACI   pasta pillows with ricotta cheese and spinach

RAVIOLI DI SAN GIUSEPPE   baked pasta pillows stuffed with jam

RAVIOLI DI RICOTTA   pockets of macaroni dough filled with cottage cheese, boiled and served with tomato sauce and grated cheese

RECCHIATELLE   macaroni in the form of little ears, served with a chopped green vegetable sauté and garnished with cottage cheese

RIGATONI   pasta of large tube shape, in short pieces

RIGATONI AI PEPERONI   pasta tubes with sweet peppers and tomato sauce

RIGATONI AL PROSCIUTTO   pasta tubes with ham

RIGATONI ALLA CARBONARA   pasta tubes with bacon, cheese, garlic, eggs, oil

RIGATONI ALLA NAPOLETANA CON PEPERONI FRESCHI   rigatoni with roasted sweet peppers

SFOGLIA   homemade egg pasta

SFORMATO DI BUCATINI   pasta boiled then baked with meat or cream sauce

SFORMATO DI CAPELLINI   mold of capellini with ham and mozzarella cheese

SFORMATO DI TORTELLINI   baked pasta casserole

SOUFFLÉ DI TAGLIATELLE   pasta soufflé

SPAGHETTI   spaghetti, long strings of pasta

SPAGHETTI AI CANESTRELLI   thin spaghetti with scallops

SPAGHETTI AI CARCIOFI   thin spaghetti with artichokes

SPAGHETTI AI FRUTTI DI MARE   spaghetti with seafood

SPAGHETTI AI TARTUFI NERI   spaghetti with flaked black truffles

SPAGHETTI AL CACIO E PEPE   spaghetti with strong goat cheese and pepper

SPAGHETTI AL GUANCIALE   spaghetti with bacon

SPAGHETTI AL POMODORO   spaghetti with tomato sauce and oil

SPAGHETTI AL POMODORO E BASILICO   spaghetti with fresh tomatoes and basil leaves

SPAGHETTI AL POMODORO E GRASSO DI PROSCIUTTO   spaghetti with tomato and the fat of ham

SPAGHETTI AL POMODORO E ORIGANO   spaghetti with tomato and oregano

SPAGHETTI AL POMODORO E SCALOGNO   spaghetti with tomatoes and shallots

SPAGHETTI AL SUGO DI CIPOLLE   spaghetti with onion sauce

SPAGHETTI AL SUGO DI PESCE   spaghetti with fish-head sauce

SPAGHETTI AL TARTUFO NERO   spaghetti with black truffle

SPAGHETTI AL TONNO   spaghetti with tuna

SPAGHETTI AL TONNO E FUNGHI SECCHI   spaghetti with tuna and dried mushrooms

SPAGHETTI ALL'AGLIO E OLIO   spaghetti with olive oil, fried garlic and ginger

SPAGHETTI ALL'AGLIO, OLIO E ORIGANO   spaghetti with garlic, oil and oregano

SPAGHETTI ALL'AGLIO, OLIO E PEPERONCINO   spaghetti with garlic, oil and hot peppers

SPAGHETTI ALL'AMATRICIANA   spaghetti with sauce of olive oil, bacon and tomato, seasoned with peppers *or* ginger, served with goat cheese

SPAGHETTI ALLA CAPRESE   spaghetti with sauce of tomato, anchovy, tuna, olives and cheese

SPAGHETTI ALLA CARBONARA   spaghetti with bacon, onion, wine, egg and cheese sauce

SPAGHETTI ALLA NURSINA   spaghetti with black truffles

SPAGHETTI ALLA PANNA ACIDA   spaghetti with sour cream

SPAGHETTI ALLA PUTTANESCA   spaghetti with sauce of tomato, garlic, anchovy, capers, cheese, olives

SPAGHETTI ALLA SICILIANA   spaghetti with eggplant and ricotta cheese

SPAGHETTI ALLA SIRACUSANA   thin spaghetti, eggplant, tomatoes, anchovies, olives

SPAGHETTI ALLE UOVA E FORMAGGIO   thin spaghetti with eggs and cheese

SPAGHETTI AROMATICI   spaghetti with anchovy sauce

SPAGHETTI COI WURSTEL   spaghetti with frankfurter type sausage

SPAGHETTI CON CIPOLLE   spaghetti with onions
SPAGHETTI CON CONDIMENTO VEGETALE CRUDO
   spaghetti with raw tomatoes and basil
SPAGHETTI CON MELANZANE   spaghetti with
   eggplants, oil, garlic, cheese
SPAGHETTI CON MOZZARELLA   thin spaghetti with
   mozzarella cheese
SPAGHETTI CON OLIVE E CAPPERI   spaghetti with
   olives and capers
SPAGHETTI CON PEPERONI E MELANZANE   spaghetti
   with peppers and eggplant
SPAGHETTI CON PISELLI   spaghetti with peas
SPAGHETTI CON POLLO, MELANZANE E SALSA ALLA
   BOLOGNESE   spaghetti with chicken, eggplant and
   meat sauce
SPAGHETTI CON SALSA ALLA BOLOGNESE   spaghetti
   with meat and tomato sauce
SPAGHETTI CON VONGOLE   spaghetti with mussels
SPAGHETTI CON VONGOLE, POLPETTE E
   GAMBERETTI   spaghetti with clams, squid, shrimp
SPAGHETTI ESTIVI FREDDI   cold spaghetti with
   spearmint, olives, anchovy, mushrooms, olive oil
SPAGHETTI VERDI   thin spaghetti made with spinach
SPAGHETTINI   thin spaghetti (see SPAGHETTI)
STELLETTE   star-shaped pasta
STRASCINATI   shell-shaped fresh pasta with different sauces
STRISCE   wide ribbon-style pasta
STRISCE E CECI   wide ribbon-style pasta with chick-peas
TAGLIATELLE   flat noodles
TAGLIATELLE AI QUATTRO FORMAGGI   white *or*
   green pasta with four cheeses
TAGLIATELLE ALLA BOLOGNESE   flat noodle pasta
   with tomato meat sauce
TAGLIATELLE ALLA GENOVESE   flat spinach noodles
   with mushroom sauce
TAGLIATELLE ALLA SALSA D'UOVO   flat noodle pasta
   with egg sauce

TAGLIATELLE VERDI ALLA GENOVESE spinach
noodle pasta with sauce of basil, olive oil, garlic, cheese

TAGLIATELLE VERDI CON SALSA ALLA BOLOGNESE
E CREMA spinach noodle pasta with sauce of tomato,
meat, onion, olive oil

TAGLIERINI narrow flat noodles made with egg dough

TAGLIOLINI thin flat noodles

TAGLIOLINI ALL'OLIO, AGLIO E ROSMARINO
noodles with oil, garlic and rosemary

TAGLIOLINI ALLA BEBÉ noodles with chicken, mushrooms and truffles

TAGLIOLINI BERNARDO noodles with tuna

TIMBALLO baked pasta casserole with sauce

TIMBALLO DI LASAGNE ALLA MODENESE baked
lasagne with meat and bechamel sauce

TIMBALLO DI MACCHERONI E POLLO baked macaroni and chicken pie

TIMBALLO DI RIGATONI RIPIENI baked stuffed pasta
casserole

TIMBALLO DI SPAGHETTI E PESCE baked spaghetti
and fish pie

TIMBALLO DI TAGLIATELLE baked, meat-stuffed pasta
casserole

TONNARELLI square homemade noodles

TONNARELLI AI FUNGHI square noodles with mushroom sauce

TONNARELLI AL ROSMARINO square noodles with
butter and rosemary

TORTELLI small fritters *or* fried cakes *or* stuffed pasta

TORTELLI ALLE ERBETTE pasta stuffed with cheese,
spinach, boiled

TORTELLI DI ZUCCA ravioli made with pumpkin
cheese stuffing

TORTELLINI squares of dough stuffed with pork, turkey,
veal, beef marrow, cheese

TORTELLINI ALLA BOLOGNESE dough squares with
tomato meat sauce

TORTELLINI ALLA MONTOVANA   squares of dough
    stuffed with ham, veal, pork, chicken and Parmesan
    cheese, boiled
TORTELLINI ALLA PANNA   stuffed pasta with cream sauce
TORTELLINI IN BRODO   stuffed pasta with ham, turkey,
    cheese, boiled in soup
TORTELLINI VERDI   stuffed spinach pasta
TORTELLONE   half round stuffed pasta
TORTINO DI CRESPELLE   crepes stuffed with tomatoes,
    ham and cheese
TRENETTE   flat ribbon-shaped noodles
TRENETTE AL PESTO   flat pasta with basil sauce
TUBETTI   small tube-shaped pasta often used in salads
TURCINIELLI   macaroni in the form of little spirals, boiled
    and served with meat or tomato sauce and grated cheese
VERMICELLI   very thin long pasta strands
VERMICELLI AI CAPPERI   noodles with caper sauce of
    capers, anchovy, black olives, garlic, sharp cheese
VERMICELLI AI PEPERONI, OLIVE E CAPPERI   pasta
    noodles with peppers, olives and capers
VERMICELLI AL SALAME   pasta noodles with salami
VERMICELLI ALL'AGRO   pasta noodles with lemon and oil
VERMICELLI ALLA SICILIANA   pasta noodles served
    with eggplant, oil, garlic, cheese, olives, anchovies, capers
VERMICELLI ALLE VONGOLE   thin spaghetti, clams,
    spicy fresh tomato sauce, herbs
VINCISGRASSI   pastry filled with meatballs, ragout and
    bechamel sauce
ZITE ALLA NAPOLETANA   macaroni with meat gravy
ZITI   large macaroni
ZITONI   very long macaroni

Pizza, Calzone

CALZONCINO MEZZADRO   turnover filled with
    scrambled eggs, sausage, onions, potatoes, Parmesan
    cheese

CALZONE   pizza dough envelope baked, filled with ham, cheese and herbs

CALZONE ALLA NAPOLETANA   pizza dough envelope containing buffalo cheese, anchovies and tomato

CALZONE ALLA PUGLIESE   folded pizza dough filled with capers, olives, onions, anchovies

FOCACCIA ALLA MORTADELLA E PEPERONI   pizza bread, pork sausage, roasted peppers

LIBRETTI   pizza folded double enclosing toppings then baked

PIZZA   flat, baked open pie, bread dough bottom, variety of toppings

PIZZA AI CECINIELLE   baked pizza with small fish

PIZZA AI FUNGHI   baked pizza with mushrooms

PIZZA AL FORMAGGIO   cheese pizza

PIZZA ALL'AGLIO E OLIO   baked pizza with garlic and olive oil

PIZZA ALL'AGLIO, OLIO E POMODORO   baked pizza with garlic, olive oil and tomatoes

PIZZA ALLA CALABRESE   pizza dough sandwich enclosing tuna, anchovies, olives, capers, then baked

PIZZA ALLA MARINARA   pizza with tomato, garlic, olive oil

PIZZA ALLA NAPOLETANA   light, leavened dough onto which is spread olive oil, buffalo cheese, anchovies, marjoram and tomato sauce, baked in oven, served very hot

PIZZA ALLA ROMANA   baked pizza with cheese, basil, oil

PIZZA ALLA SICILIANA   baked pizza with tomatoes, anchovy, capers, olives

PIZZA ALLE COZZE   baked pizza with mussels

PIZZA ALLE QUATTRO STAGIONI   baked pizza in 4 sections with shrimp, anchovy, squid, tomatoes, cheese

PIZZA ALLE VONGOLE   baked pizza with clams

PIZZA BIANCA ALLA ROMANA   pizza with mozzarella, olive oil, anchovies and Parmesan cheese

PIZZA CON LUGANEGA   pizza with tomato sauce, mozzarella, sausage, roasted peppers, oregano

PIZZA D'UOVA E CIPOLLE   pizza with onions, hard eggs

PIZZA DI PASQUA   bread dough without yeast (Easter Cake)

PIZZA DI SAN VITO   baked pizza with tomato, onion, sardines, caciocavallo cheese, oil

PIZZA DI SCAROLA   escarole pie

PIZZA FINOCCHIONA   pizza topped with tomato sauce, mozzarella, fennel salami, roasted peppers, oregano

PIZZA INCHIUSA   pizza dough sandwich enclosing pork renderings then baked

PIZZA LIEVITATA CON LE VERDURE   baked vegetable pizza with garlic, capers, olive oil

PIZZA MARGHERITA   pizza with tomato, mozzarella, olive oil and Parmesan cheese

PIZZA RUSTICA   pizza pie made of macaroni dough filled with green vegetables, cottage cheese, sausage, baked in oven

PIZZETTA   small pizza

PIZZETTA AL GORGONZOLA   baked cheese biscuits

PIZZETTA ALLA PAPALINA   pizza topped with eggs, bacon, asparagus

SCACCIATA   pizza dough sandwich enclosing cheese, anchovies, ham, onion, tomato, olives

SFINCIUNI   stuffed pizza, sealed edges, sandwich form (see PIZZA)

Poultry

ALA   wing

ALLA CACCIATORA   with mushrooms, herbs, shallots, wine, tomatoes, ham

ALLA DORIA   highly spiced and grilled

ALLA DUCHESSA   chicken livers sautéed in melted butter, cheese

ALLA PARMIGIANA   breaded and baked with Parmesan cheese

ALLODOLA   lark

ANATRA   duck

ANATRA ALLE OLIVE   duck sautéed in oil, herbs, olives

ANATRA ARROSTO   roast duck

ANATRA CON SALSA PICCANTE   duck stuffed with veal, sausage and cheese, baked in wine vinegar sauce

ANATRA RIPIENA   duck, stuffed with veal, sausage, cheese, baked

ANATRA SELVATICA   wild duck roasted and basted with wine and herbs

ANITRA   duck

ANITRA AL COGNAC   duck cooked with brandy, juniper berries and rosemary

ANITRA ALL'AGRODOLCE   duck with a sweet-sour sauce

ANITRA ALL'ARANCIA   oven-roasted duck basted with orange juice

ANITRA ALLA SALSA D'ARANCIO   roast duck with orange sauce

ANITRA ALLE OLIVE   casserole of duck and olives

ANITRA ARROSTITA ALLA SICILIANA   roasted duck stuffed with pork, peppers and black olives, with Marsala wine

ANITRA ARROSTO ALLA GENOVESE   duck roasted in olive oil with herbs and fresh lemon juice

ANITRA CON SALSA DI CAPPERI   duck cooked in the oven with a sauce of Marsala, capers, white truffles

ANITRA IN SALMÌ   duck marinated in red wine with onion, herbs, garlic, anchovies, fried and then cooked in the marinade

ANITRA MUTA ALLA NOVARESE   duck stuffed with rice, meats, herbs, roasted

ANITRA SELVATICA   wild duck

ANITROCCOLO   duckling

BOLLITO DI GALLINA   boiled chicken

BUDINO DI POLLO   chicken mousse

CAPPONCELLO AL FORNO   roast capon

CAPPONE   capon

CAPPONE RIPIENO   capon stuffed with veal, ham, eggs, cheese, bread crumbs

COSTOLETTINE   chicken breasts (also see POLLO)

COSTOLETTINE DI POLLO CON POMODORI E FUNGHI
  chicken breasts braised in tomato mushroom sauce
CROCCHETTE DI POLLO   fried chicken croquettes
CROCHETTE DI POLLO   chicken croquettes, usually fried
CROSTINI MARCHESE   toast with chicken liver
DINDO   turkey
FAGOTTINI DI POLLO E FUNGHI   chicken livers with
  mushrooms
FAGOTTINI DI RICOTTA E MOZZARELLA   chicken
  livers with ricotta and mozzarella cheese
FEGATELLI DI POLLO AL MARSALA   chicken livers
  with Marsala wine
FEGATINI   chicken livers
FEGATINI DI POLLO   sautéed chicken livers
FEGATINI DI POLLO AI CARCIOFI   chicken livers, arti-
  chokes, chopped ham, cooked in butter with chopped
  parsley and lemon juice
FEGATINI DI POLLO AL POMODORO   chicken livers
  and tomatoes
FEGATINI DI POLLO ALLA SALVIA   chicken livers with sage
FEGATINI DI POLLO CON FUNGHI FRESCHI   chicken
  livers with ham, mushrooms
FEGATINI DI POLLO CON SALSA ALLA BOLOGNESE
  chicken livers and Bolognese sauce
FEGATO DI OCA   goose liver
FEGATO DI VOLATILI   various fowl livers
FILETTI DI TACCHINO   slices of turkey breast with ham
  and cheese, baked in oven and sprinkled with white wine
FILETTO DI TACCHINO   turkey breast meat
FILETTO DI TACCHINO AL MARSALA   turkey breast
  sautéed in wine
FOIE GRAS DI POLLO   chicken liver pâté
FRATTAGLIE   chicken giblets
FRICASSEA DI POLLO   pieces of chicken poached in a
  cream sauce with onions and rosemary
FRICASSEA DI POLLO ALLA MARCHIGIANA   sautéed
  chicken with egg and lemon sauce

GALANTINA DI POLLO   fine chopped chicken loaf in meat gelatine

GALLINA   hen

GALLINA AL MIRTO   hen with myrtle leaves

GALLINACCIO BRODETTATO   turkey cock stewed with wine, vegetables, herbs and served with a cream sauce thickened with egg yolks

GALLINELLA   water hen

GIAMBONETTE   boned chicken leg, stuffed with chicken, ham, cheese and fried

GRATINATA   sprinkled with bread crumbs and cheese and oven-browned

IN UMIDO   stewed in broth with onions, carrots, tomatoes and herbs

INVOLTINI DI POLLO E PROSCIUTTO   chicken and ham slices, floured and pan fried in wine

OCA   goose

OCA ARROSTITA RIPIENA ALLA SALVIA E CIPOLLA goose roasted and stuffed with sage and onion

OCA ARROSTO AL FORNO   goose stuffed with sausage, herbs, chestnuts and bread crumbs and roasted in the oven

OCA ARROSTO RIPIENA   stuffed roast goose

OCA IN SALMÌ   goose cooked with wine, herbs, vegetables, mushrooms and truffles

PAETA   young turkey

PAETA ARROSTO CON MELAGRANE   roast turkey with pomegranates

PAIATA   hen turkey

PAIATA MALGARAGNO   turkey roasted and basted with drippings

PAPPARDELLE ALL'ARETINA   duck cooked with red wine, tomatoes, herbs, served with wide ribbon pasta

PASTICCIO DI MACCHERONI E PICCIONI   macaroni and pigeon pie

PASTICCIO DI TACCHINO   turkey with a cream sauce in pastry

PATÉ D'OCA   fine ground goose liver loaf sliced and served cold

PATÉ DI FEGATO   fine liver paste usually served cold

PATÉ DI POLLO TARTUFATO   fine chicken liver with truffles

PETTICINI   breast of chicken (see PETTO POLLO)

PETTO   breast

PETTO D'ANITRA   breast of duck

PETTO DI POLLO   chicken breast

PETTO DI POLLO AI FUNGHI   chicken breast braised in butter with mushrooms

PETTO DI POLLO AL BURRO   chicken breast floured, fried in butter, then oven-braised

PETTO DI POLLO AL MARSALA   breast of chicken fried in butter, flavored with Marsala and grated Parmesan cheese

PETTO DI POLLO AL PROSCIUTTO   chicken breast pan fried with ham and cheese covered and broiled

PETTO DI POLLO AL VINO BIANCO   chicken breast floured pan fried in wine and butter sauce

PETTO DI POLLO ALLA BOLOGNESE   chicken breast floured pan fried with ham, cheese, butter

PETTO DI POLLO ALLA FIORENTINA   breast of chicken fried in butter

PETTO DI POLLO ALLA GRIGLIA   grilled breast of chicken

PETTO DI POLLO ALLA MILANESE   chicken breast floured, egg battered, breaded and pan fried

PETTO DI POLLO ALLA PANNA   chicken breast braised in cream sauce with wine and herbs

PETTO DI POLLO ALLA PANNA E FUNGHI   chicken breast braised in wine, cream sauce with mushrooms and lemon juice

PETTO DI POLLO ALLA PARIGINA   chicken breast braised in cream sauce with mushrooms

PETTO DI POLLO ALLA PRINCESSA   chicken breast pan fried and served with fried egg

PETTO DI POLLO ALLA SOVRANA breast of chicken with artichokes and a cream sauce

PETTO DI POLLO ALLA VALDOSTANA breast of chicken cooked with slices of cheese, white truffles, white wine and brandy

PETTO DI POLLO DORATO chicken breast braised in oil

PETTO DI POLLO TONNATO chicken breast, tuna sauce with lemon and capers

PETTO DI TACCHINO breast of turkey

PETTO DI TACCHINO ALLA NAPOLETANA turkey breast baked with cheese and tomatoes

POLASTRO IN TEGLIA chicken casserole with onion, wine, tomato, mushrooms

POLLAME fowl

POLLASTRA hen

POLLASTRO chicken (also see POLLO)

POLLO chicken (also see PETTO DI POLLO)

POLLO AI FUNGHI pieces of chicken sautéed in butter with mushrooms and tomato sauce

POLLO AI PEPERONI chicken cooked with pimentos, tomatoes, white wine, herbs and onions

POLLO AI SOTT'ACETI roasted chicken served with vinegar, pickles and onion

POLLO AI TARTUFI chicken and truffles

POLLO AL CHIANTI chicken braised in red wine, onion and herbs

POLLO AL COCCIO chicken baked in a clay case

POLLO AL DIAVOLO grilled chicken

POLLO AL FORNO baked *or* roast chicken

POLLO AL GIAMBONETTE boned chicken stuffed with ham, bacon, garlic, cheese, herbs, then fried

POLLO AL GIRARROSTO chicken roasted on a spit

POLLO AL LATTE chicken cooked in milk

POLLO AL LIMONE chicken cooked in lemon juice

POLLO AL MARCUGO chicken fried in oil and butter with tomato sauce and mushrooms

POLLO AL POMODORO chicken and tomato

POLLO AL POTACCHIO   chicken sautéed in wine, onion, garlic, tomato sauce, with chili powder

POLLO AL PROSCIUTTO   chicken and ham

POLLO AL ROSMARINO   chicken roasted with rosemary and other spices

POLLO AL TARTUFO E COGNAC   chicken with brandy, truffle and cream

POLLO AL TEGAME CON LIMONE   pan-roasted chicken with lemon juice

POLLO AL VINO BIANCO   chicken in white wine

POLLO AL VINO ROSSO   chicken in red wine

POLLO ALL'ABRUZZESE   chicken sautéed with onion, tomato, peppers

POLLO ALL'ARANCIO   chicken roasted *or* braised in orange juice

POLLO ALL'ARRABBIATA   chicken sautéed in wine, tomatoes, chili powder

POLLO ALL'INDIANA   chicken with spices and curry powder

POLLO ALLA CACCIATORA   chicken with tomatoes and hot peppers

POLLO ALLA DIAVOLA   chicken roasted and sprinkled with lemon juice

POLLO ALLA FINANZIERA   stew made of chicken giblets, with sweetbreads, mushrooms and truffles, cooked in a thick meat or tomato sauce

POLLO ALLA FIORENTINA   chicken with mushrooms, olive oil, bacon, onion, white wine, tomatoes

POLLO ALLA GHIOTTONA   pieces of chicken sautéed in butter with white wine, milk and tomatoes

POLLO ALLA LIVORNESE   chicken poached in a casserole with broth, butter, parsley and lemon juice

POLLO ALLA MACERATESE   chicken sautéed in broth with lemon, egg yolks

POLLO ALLA MARENGO   chicken sautéed in brown mushroom sauce with truffles

POLLO ALLA MARESCIALLA   boneless fried chicken, pan fried in butter

POLLO ALLA MONTANARA   chicken braised in olive oil with garlic, onion, brandy and broth

POLLO ALLA NAPOLETANA   chicken jointed and cooked slowly with mushrooms, onions, garlic, tomato and wine

POLLO ALLA PADOVANA   chicken roasted on the spit and highly spiced

POLLO ALLA PORCHETTA   chicken stuffed with ham, garlic and fennel

POLLO ALLA ROMANA   chicken sautéed in pork and bacon fat with garlic, wine and tomato paste

POLLO ALLA SICILIANA   chicken sautéed in onion, butter with vegetables and Marsala wine

POLLO ALLA ZINGARA   chicken baked in a clay case

POLLO ALLO SPIEDO   chicken broiled on a spit

POLLO ARROSTITO ALLA GENOVESE   chicken stuffed with its giblets, onion, celery, herbs, bread crumbs, butter and roasted

POLLO ARROSTO   roasted chicken

POLLO BOLLITO   boiled chicken

POLLO FARCITO TARTUFATO   roasted chicken stuffed with spinach, ham, cheese, truffles

POLLO FRITTO ALLA FIORENTINA   chicken fried in olive oil with lemon pieces added

POLLO FRITTO ALLA TOSCANA   fried egg batter-dipped chicken with lemon juice added

POLLO IMBOTTITO   stuffed and roasted chicken

POLLO IN BELLAVISTA   roasted chicken served on fried bread with cooked vegetables

POLLO IN BIANCO   pieces of chicken sautéed with onions, celery, herbs

POLLO IN CASSERUOLA   chicken cooked in a casserole

POLLO IN PADELLA ALLE ERBETTE   chicken fried with herbs

POLLO IN SALSA PICCANTE   pieces of chicken cooked with oil, garlic, white wine, vinegar, black olives and chopped anchovy

POLLO IN SUPREMA GELATINA   chicken breast in aspic jelly

POLLO IN TEGLIA   chicken baked in a shallow earthenware pan

POLLO IN UMIDO   chicken stewed in broth with onion, tomato, carrot and herbs

POLLO IN UMIDO COL CAVOLO NERO   chicken fricassee with red cabbage

POLLO LESSO   chicken boiled in vegetable broth

POLLO NOVELLO   spring chicken

POLLO PICCANTE   spicy chicken

POLLO RIPIENO   stuffed boned chicken

POLLO RUSPANTE   chicken farm-grown *or* free-ranging

POLLO SCHIACCIATO   chicken grilled with bacon

POLPETTONE DI POLLO E VITELLO   chopped chicken and veal roll

POLPETTONE DI TACCHINO   turkey meatballs with cheese, breaded and fried

RIGAGLIE   giblets

RIGAGLIE DI POLLO   chicken giblets and livers sautéed with herbs

RISO ALLA SBIRRAGLIA   rice with chicken broth, chopped chicken, wine, cheese

RISOTTO ALLA SBIRRAGLIA   chicken and rice dish, with herbs, vegetables, sausage and wine

ROTOLO DI TACCHINO   turkey meat boned and rolled

ROTTAMI DI POLLO IN PADELLA   chicken cut up and sautéed

SPEZZATINO   meat *or* fowl stew

SPEZZATINO DI POLLO   chicken chunks braised in herbal tomato sauce

SPEZZATINO DI POLLO   small pieces of chicken sautéed in oil with pimentos, onion, mushrooms and tomatoes

SPEZZATINO DI POLLO PICCANTE   chicken fricassee with tomatoes, peppers and capers

SPEZZATO DI POLLO CON LE MELANZANE   chicken braised in wine, tomatoes, herbs, eggplants

SPEZZATO DI TACCHINO   turkey braised with olives
SPIEDINI ALLA PISTOIESE   skewered little birds with
bread, bacon, sage, juniper berries, bay leaf
STECCHINI ALLA BOLOGNESE   chicken livers, truffles,
cheese, sweetbread, tongue on skewers, coated with a white
wine sauce, egg and bread crumbs and fried in butter
STUFATO DI TACCHINO AL VINO BIANCO   stew with
wine, mushrooms, vegetables and herbs
TACCHINO   turkey
TACCHINO AL PROSCIUTTO   turkey breast fried,
topped with ham and Parmesan cheese and broiled
TACCHINO ALLA BOSCAIOLA   turkey breast in
mushroom, tongue, ham and herb sauce
TACCHINO ALLA CANZANESE   turkey seasoned with
bay leaf, rosemary, sage, pepper, served cold with gelatin
TACCHINO ALLA TETRAZZINI   cut-up turkey with
creamed mushroom sauce and pasta, covered with
grated cheese and bread crumbs and baked
TACCHINO ARROSTO   roasted turkey
TACCHINO ARROSTO RIPIENO   roast stuffed turkey
TACCHINO ARROSTO RIPIENO DI CASTAGNE   roast
turkey with chestnut stuffing
TACCHINO ARROSTO TARTUFATO   roasted turkey with
Marsala, butter and truffles
TACCHINO BOLLITO   turkey boiled with vegetables and
served cold
TACCHINO CON MAIONESE   cold turkey with mayonnaise
TACCHINO CON SALSA REALE   turkey breast in cream
sauce with cognac
TACCHINO IN CARPIONE   turkey marinated in wine,
herbs, oil and vinegar after cooking
TACCHINO NOSTRANO ARROSTO   turkey local grown
and roasted
TACCHINO RIPIENO   stuffed turkey
TACCHINO RIPIENO ALLA LOMBARDA   turkey stuffed
with veal, beef, sausage, apple, prunes chestnuts, cheese
and herbs

TIMBALLO DI INVERNO   pie filled with mozzarella, ham, pork, chicken livers, breast of chicken
TIMBALLO DI MACCHERONI E POLLO   baked macaroni and chicken pie
TORRESANI   small pigeons, domesticated

Rice

ARANCINE ALLA SICILIANA   rice balls stuffed with meat, breaded and fried
BOMBA DI RISO   rice pudding
CROCCHETTA DI RISO   rice croquette with cheese center, deep-fried
CROCHETTE DI RISO   rice croquettes
INSALATA DI RISO   cold rice with vegetables and seafood, mayonnaise sauce
MIGNESTRIS DE RIS VERT   rice cooked with spinach and other vegetables
PANISCIA ALLA NOVARESE   rice cooked with vegetables and red wine added to vegetable soup
PANISSA   rice and bean dish with bacon, onion and tomato
RISI   rice (also see RISO and RISOTTO)
RISI E BISI   rice and peas cooked in broth with onions
RISO   boiled rice with various ingredients
RISO AI QUATTRO FORMAGGI   rice with four different cheeses
RISO AL BURRO   rice with butter, onions and broth
RISO AL CAVROMAN   rice with mutton, onion, tomato, cheese
RISO AL LIMONE   rice with eggs and lemon
RISO AL SALTO   rice pan fried with grated cheese
RISO AL SUGO   rice with meat sauce, tomatoes, herbs
RISO AL VERDE   rice with sage and chopped spinach
RISO ALL'ANITRA   rice cooked in sauce of chopped duck meat and giblets
RISO ALL'UOVO E LIMONE   egg and lemon juice beaten up and mixed into the rice

RISO ALLA BOLOGNESE   rice with meat sauce, tomatoes, garlic, broth

RISO ALLA CAMPAGNOLA   rice with tomatoes, onion, bacon, mushrooms

RISO ALLA CAPPUCCINA   rice with anchovies, onion, butter and oil

RISO ALLA CERTOSINA   rice with fish stock and served with shrimp and fish

RISO ALLA FINANZIERA   rice with meat sauce, brandy, bacon, chicken livers and broth

RISO ALLA GENOVESE   rice with onion, mushroom, tomatoes

RISO ALLA MARINARA   rice with onion, clams, tomatoes, butter, garlic

RISO ALLA MILANESE   rice with wine and saffron

RISO ALLA PARMIGIANA   rice with onion, mushrooms, livers, sausage, meat sauce

RISO ALLA PESCATORA   rice cooked in fish broth with pieces of fish

RISO ALLA PIEMONTESE   rice boiled in meat broth with cheese and butter

RISO ALLA SARACENA   rice with finely-chopped shellfish

RISO ALLA SBIRRAGLIA   rice with chicken broth, chopped chicken, wine, cheese

RISO ALLA TOSCANA   rice sautéed with liver, vegetables, wine, cheese, tomato paste

RISO ALLA VALENCIANA   rice with pork, sausage, clams, tomato, pepper, onion, garlic

RISO ALLA VALTELLINESE   rice with cabbage, beans, cheese

RISO ALLA VENETA   rice sautéed with mussels, garlic, onion, fish broth

RISO ARANCINO ALLA SICILIANA   large rice ball stuffed with meat and fried

RISO ARROSTO ALLA GENOVESE   casserole of rice, sausage, peas, artichokes, mushrooms, cheese and onion, browned in oven

RISO BISATI   rice cooked with eel and herb olive oil

RISO COI CECI   broth of rice and chick-peas, flavored
with tomatoes and spice

RISO COI FINOCCHI   rice with fennel, onion, cheese

RISO COI FUNGHI   rice with butter and mushrooms

RISO COI GAMBERI   rice with sauce of shrimp, garlic,
olive oil, pepper and tomato

RISO COI PEOCI ALLA VENETA   rice with butter, olive
oil, mussels and broth

RISO COI PISELLI   rice with peas, onion, meat, butter

RISO COI ROGNONCINI TRIFOLATI   rice cooked in broth
with butter and oil, chopped vegetables, kidneys and cheese

RISO COI TARTUFI   rice with ham, cheese and truffles

RISO COL POMODORO   rice with tomatoes

RISO CON ASPARAGI   rice cooked with asparagus, onion
and butter

RISO CON CAPAROZZOLI   rice with shellfish, garlic, wine

RISO CON RIGAGLIE   rice with giblets, veal, white wine,
tomato

RISO CON SALSICCE   rice with sausage

RISO CON SCAMPI   shrimp pan fried with rice and wine

RISO CON SEDANI   with celery

RISO CON SEPPIE   rice cooked with cuttlefish, olive oil,
wine, tomato, garlic

RISO CON VERZA   rice with savoy cabbage

RISO CON VONGOLE   rice with clams, onion, olive oil, broth

RISO CON ZUCCA   rice with pumpkin, onion, oil, grated
cheese

RISO CON ZUCCHINE   rice with zucchini, onion, cheese

RISO DI MARE   with oil, onion, seafood, wine, broth

RISO DI SARTÙ   bread crumb crust filled with rice, sauce,
livers, meatballs, cheese

RISO E FAGIOLI   rice with butter and beans

RISO E LUGANEGA   rice and sausage

RISO GRECO   rice cooked in broth with vegetables,
sausage, lemon juice

RISO IN BIANCO   white rice with butter

RISO IN BIANCO COI FEGATINI   rice cooked with white wine, chicken livers

RISO IN BIANCO COI TARTUFI BIANCHI   boiled rice and white truffles, served with grated Parmesan cheese and butter

RISO IN CAGNONE   rice with butter, cheese, garlic

RISO IN TAZZA   rice served in a cup

RISO MANTECATO   rice cooked in butter and milk

RISO PRIMAVERA   rice with spring vegetables

RISOTTO   cooked rice (see RISO)

RISOTTO ALLA CERTOSINA   rice with a sauce of peas, crayfish tails or prawns and mushrooms

RISOTTO ALLA CHIOGGIOTTA   fish rice

RISOTTO ALLA GENOVESE   rice with a meat sauce containing wine, herbs and vegetables

RISOTTO ALLA MARINARA   rice with seafood

RISOTTO ALLA MILANESE   rice cooked in consommé, mixed with butter, saffron, chicken giblets, beef marrow, mushrooms and Parmesan cheese

RISOTTO ALLA MONZESE   rice with sausage meat, tomato and Marsala wine

RISOTTO ALLA PAESANA   thick soup of rice with beans, cabbage, salami, bacon

RISOTTO ALLA PARMIGIANA   rice cooked in beef broth with chicken livers, sausage, mushrooms, herbs, bacon and vegetables

RISOTTO ALLA PESCATORA   rice with fish

RISOTTO ALLA SBIRRAGLIA   chicken and rice dish, with herbs, vegetables, sausage and wine

RISOTTO COI CARCIOFI   rice with hearts of baby artichokes cut up and cooked with rice

RISOTTO COI FEGATINI   rice with chicken livers

RISOTTO COI FRUTTI DI MARE   rice with shellfish

RISOTTO COI FUNGHI   rice with mushrooms and chopped onions

RISOTTO COI GAMBERI   rice with prawns

RISOTTO COI TARTUFI   rice with truffles

RISOTTO CON LUMACHE   rice with snails in a highly
   flavored sauce
RISOTTO CON SCAMPI   rice with prawns, butter and cheese
RISOTTO CON SECOLE   rice with small pieces of beef or veal
RISOTTO CON TELLINE   rice with clams and a tomato
   sauce with peppers
RISOTTO CON VONGOLE   rice cooked in sauce of oil,
   parsley, tomato, garlic and clams
RISOTTO CON ZUCCA   rice with small pieces of pumpkin
RISOTTO DI MAGRO   rice with anything but meat
RISOTTO IN BIANCO   rice cooked with water and white
   wine instead of broth
RISOTTO IN CAGNONE   rice flavored with sage and
   garlic, butter and cheese
SARTÙ   rice casserole filled with chicken giblets, minced veal,
   tomato, mushrooms and buffalo cheese, cooked in oven
SARTÙ ALLA NAPOLETANA   baked rice mold with
   sausages, livers, peas, meat, cheese, bacon
SUPPLÌ   rice croquettes with cheese and meat sauce
SUPPLÌ AL RAGÙ   croquettes made of rice and meat
   sauce, dipped in bread crumbs and fried in olive oil
SUPPLÌ AL TELEFONO   rice croquettes with mozzarella cheese
TIMBALLO DI RISO   baked rice casserole

Salads

ACETOSELLA   sorrel, succulent acid leaves used in salads
ALLA TOSCANA   tomatoes, celery, and herbs
BROCCOLETTI DI RAPA   turnip greens
CAPONATA   chopped eggplant, cooked in open pan with
   sauce of tomatoes, onion and herbs
CAPPON MAGRO   boiled vegetable and pickled fish salad
CARDOONS   thistle-like plant, leaves and stalks eaten as
   celery (see CARDI)
CATALOGNA   green salad leaf
CETRIOLI   cucumbers
CETRIOLI ALL'ACETO   pickled cucumbers

CETRIOLINI   small pickles
CICORIA   endive, chicory
CIPOLLINE NOVELLE   green onions (scallions)
CONDIGLIONE   mixed salad
INDIVI   chicory, endive
INDIVI BELGA   Belgium endive
INDIVI CRUDA   endive braised with garlic
INSALATA   salad
INSALATA AI TARTUFI   green salad with truffles
INSALATA ALL'AMERICANA   shrimp, salad greens with
   mayonnaise
INSALATA ALLA SICILIANA   salad of tomato, bean,
   mushroom, peas with mayonnaise dressing
INSALATA CAPRICCIOSA   salad of diced raw vegetables
   with sauce or mayonnaise (sometimes with ham)
INSALATA CONDIGLIONE   mixed salad
INSALATA CRUDITA   salad of mixed raw vegetables
   with sauce or mayonnaise
INSALATA DI ARANCIA   orange and cucumber salad
INSALATA DI ARINGHE   herring salad
INSALATA DI BORLOTTI E RADICCHIO   cranberry,
   beans and endive salad
INSALATA DI CAMPO   lettuce salad
INSALATA DI CARNI   chopped-up meat salad with cold
   cooked vegetables and hard-boiled eggs
INSALATA DI CAVOLFIORE   cauliflower salad
INSALATA DI CECI   chick-pea salad
INSALATA DI CIME DI RAPE ROSSE   red beet tops salad
INSALATA DI COMPOSTA COTTA   salad of cold cooked
   vegetables with sauce or mayonnaise
INSALATA DI FINNOCHIO   salad of fennel
INSALATA DI FONTINA   salad of cooked peppers, olives
   and cheese with cream sauce
INSALATA DI FRUTTI DI MARE   seafood salad, dressing
   of oil, lemon juice, mustard, garlic
INSALATA DI GAMBERETTI   shrimp salad in
   mayonnaise sauce

INSALATA DI LATTUGA E GORGONZOLA   romaine
lettuce with gorgonzola cheese and walnuts
INSALATA DI LENTICCHIE   lentil salad
INSALATA DI PATATE   potato salad
INSALATA DI PESCE   seafood salad with oil and lemon sauce
INSALATA DI POLLO   chicken salad with mayonnaise sauce
INSALATA DI POLLO ARROSTO   salad of roast chicken,
mixed greens, chopped bacon, croutons, Parmesan
cheese, vinaigrette
INSALATA DI RISO   salad of cold rice with vegetables
and seafood, mayonnaise sauce
INSALATA DI SEDANI   cold salad of celery and truffles
with mayonnaise
INSALATA DI SPINACI E TACCHINO   salad of spinach,
tomato, bacon, roasted turkey, vinaigrette
INSALATA DI TONNO   tuna fish salad
INSALATA DI VERDURA   salad of green vegetables
INSALATA DI VERDURA COTTA   salad of cooked green
vegetables
INSALATA DI VERZA CRUDA   raw savoy cabbage salad
INSALATA MASCHERATA   mixed salad with mayonnaise
INSALATA MISTA   salad of mixed raw vegetables with
sauce or mayonnaise
INSALATA NOSTRANA   local *or* home grown salad
INSALATA PANZELLA   salad of fresh tomatoes, cucum-
bers, onions, bread, vinaigrette
INSALATA RUSSA   salad of diced cooked vegetables,
hard eggs in mayonnaise dressing
INSALATA VIENNESE   salad of tuna, eggs, onions,
cooked beans
LATTUGA   lettuce
LATTUGA ROMANA   romaine lettuce
OLIO D'OLIVA   olive oil
PANZANELLA   tomatoes, cucumbers, green onions,
bread, vinaigrette
PASTA FREDDA   cold pasta salad
PEPERONCINI   pickled, small green peppers

RADICCHIO   chicory, lettuce with bitter taste
RADICCHIO ROSSO   wild chickory *or* curly endive (red)
RADICI   radishes
RAPA ROSSA   white turnip with some red color
RAPE ROSSE AL FORNO   baked red beets *or* turnips
SALMONE RIPIENO ALL'ANETO   salmon filled with
  onions and fresh dill, baked, served cold
SCAROLA   escarole lettuce
SEDANO   celery

Sauces

ACCIUGHE FRESCHE   sauce of fresh anchovies
AGLIATA   garlic sauce; garlic mashed with bread crumbs
  and olive oil
AGLIO, OLIO E ACCIUGHE   garlic, oil and anchovies
AGLIO, OLIO E POMODORO   garlic, oil and tomato
AGLIO, OLIO E SAETTINE   garlic, oil and ground hot
  peppers
AGRO   dressing of lemon juice and oil
AI QUATTRO FORMAGGI   sauce made with four
  cheeses; Parmesan, Gruyère, provolone dolce, Pontina,
  sometimes with anchovies
AL PURGATORIO   sautéed in oil with tomatoes, parsley,
  garlic and peppers
ALL'AMATRICIANA   sauce of fresh tomatoes, chopped
  bacon, onion and garlic
ALL'OLIO E ACCIUGHE   sauce of olive oil, anchovies
  and garlic
ALL'OLIO E LIMONE   oil and lemon juice dressing
ALLA BOLOGNESE   with tomatoes, meat or ham, cheese
ALLA CARBONARA   pasta with smoked ham or bacon,
  cheese, eggs and olive oil
ALLA CAVALLEGGERA   with eggs and walnuts
ALLA GENOVESE   sauce with basil and other herbs, pine
  kernels, garlic and oil
ALLA LUCCHESE   with ricotta and chicken livers

ALLA MARINARA   cooked in olive oil, garlic, capers, olives

ALLA NAPOLETANA   made with cheese, tomatoes, herbs and sometimes anchovies

ALLA PAPALINA   chopped ham, mushrooms, cheese and butter

ALLA PUTTANESCA   sauce of tomatoes, black olives, hot peppers, garlic, oil, chopped parsley

ALLA ROMANA   sautéed in pork and bacon fat with wine, garlic and tomato paste

ALLA SICILIANA   with eggplant and provolone cheese

ALLA SIRACUSANA   sauce of tomatoes, eggplant, pimento, capers, olives, anchovies, with garlic and oregano

BAGNA CAUDA   hot sauce for dipping raw vegetables with anchovies, wine, garlic

BESCIAMELLA   white sauce

BESCIAMELLA CON FORMAGGIO E UOVA   white sauce, cheese and egg

BIGOLI CON SALSA   round solid noodles with anchovy or sardine sauce

BOSCAIOLA   tomatoes, mushrooms, oil, garlic, basil, butter and cheese

CACIO E PEPE   pasta served with pepper and string cheese

CALABRESE   tomato sauce flavored with ginger

CAMPAGNA   sauce of minced beef and cottage cheese

CARNE CON MELANZANE   meat sauce and eggplant

CARRETTIERA   sauce of tuna fish and mushrooms

CIOCIARA   sauce of fat bacon, ham and sausage

CIUPPIN   thick fish stew *or* sauce

CREMA PASTICCERA   custard cream sauce

DIAVOLO   spicy tomato sauce

DOPPIO FORMAGGIO   sauce with more than the usual amount of cheese

FILETTI DI SOGLIOLA   sauce made with fillets of sole

FINANCIERE SAUCE   bechamel sauce with Marsala wine and cheese

FINTA ZUPPA DI PESCE   fish soup sauce with olive oil, garlic, tomatoes, anchovies

FONDUTA   sauce of melted Fontina cheese, egg yolks, butter and milk flavored with white truffles

FUNGHI CON PISELLI   sauce of mushrooms, bacon and green peas

GRANERESI   sauce of pounded walnuts, cream cheese and garlic

GREMOLADA   sauce of lemon, oil, garlic, sage, parsley, served over cooked meat

LO STRACOTTO   overcooked meat sauce

MACCHERONI NERI   macaroni with a sauce of garlic, oil and hot red peppers

MAIONESE   mayonnaise

MOLLICA   sauce with bread crumbs and anchovies fried in oil

NOVELLI   tomato sauce with anchovies and herbs

OSTRICA   mushroom sauce

PANNA ACIDA ALLE ERBE AROMATICHE   sour cream and herbs

PEARA   peppery sauce for boiled meats

PESTO   sauce of basil leaves, garlic, cheese, pine kernels and marjoram

PESTO ALLA GENOVESE   sauce with basil, garlic, pine nuts, cheese and olive oil

PEVERADA DI TREVISO   sauce of pork sausage, chicken livers, onion, white wine, pickles, pepper

PINZIMONIO   raw vegetable dressing of oil, salt and pepper

PIZZAIOLA   tomato sauce with garlic, hot peppers, olive oil and parsley

POMAROLA   mild tomato sauce with onions, carrots, basil and olive oil

POMODORO CON RICOTTA   tomato and ricotta

RAGÙ   meat sauce for pasta (also called BOLOGNESE)

RAGÙ ALLA NAPOLETANA   thick meat and tomato sauce

RAGÙ DI AGNELLO COI PEPERONI   thick lamb meat sauce with peppers

SALAMINI   sauce of tomatoes and fresh sausage

SALMORIGLIO   sauce of olive oil, lemon juice, parsley, oregano, salt

SALSA   sauce

SALSA ABRUZZESE   sauce with oil, garlic and bell peppers

SALSA AI CAPPERI   tomato-based caper sauce

SALSA AI FRUTTI DI MARE   olive oil, tomatoes and seafood

SALSA AI FUNGHI   mushroom sauce

SALSA AL BURRO   melted butter and herb sauce

SALSA AL BURRO E AL PARMIGIANO   melted butter
with grated Parmesan cheese

SALSA AL COGNAC   brandy sauce

SALSA AL FORMAGGIO   cheese sauce

SALSA AL PROSCIUTTO   sauce with tomato, herb and ham

SALSA AL RAGÙ   sauce with ground meat, bacon, garlic,
tomato, olive oil

SALSA AL SARMORIGLIO   sauce served hot for meat or
cooked vegetables with oil, lemon, oregano, tabasco

SALSA AL SUGO   sauce of ground meat, bacon, garlic,
tomato, olive oil, like Bolognese

SALSA AL TONNO   sauce of tuna, garlic, olive oil, capers,
anchovies

SALSA ALL'AGLIO E OLIO   sauce of olive oil in which
garlic was cooked

SALSA ALL'AMATRICIANA   sauce with oil, garlic,
tomato, onion, peppers

SALSA ALL'ARRABBIATA   sauce with tomato, pepper,
bacon, sausage

SALSA ALL'OLIO DI MANDORLE E LIMONE   sauce for
boiled fish with almonds, garlic, lemon, olive oil

SALSA ALL'UOVO   sauce with eggs, mozzarella and
anchovies

SALSA ALLA BOLOGNESE   sauce of ground meat, bacon,
garlic, tomatoes, olive oil

SALSA ALLA BOSCAIOLA   sauce of tuna, anchovy,
tomato, olive oil, mushroom, garlic

SALSA ALLA BUCANIERA   sauce with clams, octopus,
tomato, olive oil, mushroom, garlic

SALSA ALLA CACCIATORA   sauce with tomato, meat,
white wine, mushrooms

SALSA ALLA CAMPAGNOLA   sauce with mushrooms, olive oil, garlic, seasoning

SALSA ALLA CARBONARA   sauce with olive oil, butter, garlic, diced bacon

SALSA ALLA CARRETTIERA   sauce with tuna, garlic, mushrooms, olive oil, meat sauce

SALSA ALLA CIOCIARA   sauce of meat, butter, Parmesan cheese

SALSA ALLA CONTADINA   sauce of butter, tomato paste, mushrooms, Parmesan cheese

SALSA ALLA CREMA   sauce of butter, milk, flour, egg yolks, cheese

SALSA ALLA DIAVOLA   sauce of tomato, meat, peppers

SALSA ALLA FINANZIERA   sauce of giblets, bacon, onion and broth

SALSA ALLA FIORENTINA   sauce with tomato, meat, herbs, peas

SALSA ALLA GENOVESE   sauce with basil leaves, garlic, olive oil, pine nuts, pecorino cheese

SALSA ALLA GHIOTTONA   sauce of meat, onion, chicken livers, wine, mushrooms

SALSA ALLA LEPRE   tomato hare sauce with garlic, herbs, olive oil

SALSA ALLA MARINARA   sauce with capers, olive oil, garlic, olives

SALSA ALLA NAPOLETANA   sauce with tomatoes, cheese, herbs, garlic

SALSA ALLA NORCINA   sauce with melted mozzarella cheese, butter, sausage, peas

SALSA ALLA PANNA   sauce with cream and grated cheese

SALSA ALLA PIEMONTESE   mild brown meat sauce

SALSA ALLA PIRATA   sauce with tomatoes, anchovies, capers, olives

SALSA ALLA PIZZAIOLA   meat sauce with garlic, tomato, olive oil, oregano

SALSA ALLA POSILLIPO   tomato, herb sauce, usually with seafood

SALSA ALLA PROVENZALE   sauce with onion, oil, tomato, mushrooms, olives

SALSA ALLA RICOTTA ROMANA   sauce with tomato, garlic and ricotta cheese

SALSA ALLA ROMANA   meat sauce with butter, cheese, seasonings

SALSA ALLA TARTARA   sauce with hard egg yolks, oil, mustard, herbs

SALSA ALLE ACCIUGHE   sauce of anchovies, garlic, olive oil

SALSA ALLE ALICI   anchovy sauce

SALSA ALLE MELANZANE   eggplant sauce with olive oil, meat, spices

SALSA ALLE NOCI   sauce with walnuts, cream, basil, garlic, Parmesan cheese

SALSA BESCIAMELLA   sauce of butter, flour and milk

SALSA BIANCA   white sauce

SALSA COI FEGATINI DI POLLO   chicken liver sauce

SALSA CON COZZE   olive oil, mussels, garlic sauce

SALSA CON SALSICCIA   sauce with sausage meat

SALSA CON SARDE   sauce with olive oil, onion, sardines, anchovy, fennel, pine nuts

SALSA CON ZUCCHINE ALLA FRIULANA   sauce with zucchini, tomatoes, peppers, olive oil

SALSA D'UMIDO DI RIGAGLIE   sauce with chicken livers and beef gravy

SALSA DELLA CASA   special house *or* restaurant sauce

SALSA DI CARNE   sauce with tomato, butter, Parmesan and brown meat sauce (same as SUGO or BOLOGNESE)

SALSA DI CARNE E FEGATINI   sauce with brown meat sauce and chicken livers

SALSA DI CIPOLLA   sauce with onions sautéed in butter and tomato paste

SALSA DI MAGRO   sauce of mushrooms, pesto, anchovy, olive oil, onion

SALSA DI MANZO E FUNGHI   meat sauce with mushrooms

SALSA DI PESCE   sauce with olive oil, anchovy, lemon, for fish

SALSA DI POMODORO   sauce of tomatoes, olive oil and herbs

SALSA DI POMODORO ALLA NAPOLETANA   tomato sauce with oil, garlic base

SALSA DI POMODORO FRESCO   fresh tomato sauce

SALSA DI ROGNONE   sauce of chopped kidneys, herbs and spices in a tomato sauce

SALSA FINTA   tomato sauce with onion, garlic, meat stock, oil, herbs

SALSA PER INSALATE AL VINO BIANCO   white wine salad sauce

SALSA PER VERDURE LESSATE   thin sauce of egg and lemon

SALSA PEVERADA   hot sauce of chicken liver, anchovy, sausage, wine, lemon

SALSA PICCANTE   spicy (sharp) sauce

SALSA POMMAROLA   tomato sauce for pasta

SALSA SEMPLICE AI CAPPERI   sauce with capers, lemon juice, oil, tabasco

SALSA VERDE   sauce with green pesto

SALSA VERDE ALLA MILANESE   anchovy, parsley, oil, garlic sauce

SALSA VERDE ALLA PIEMONTESE   sauce with anchovies, egg yolk, parsley, garlic, capers and bread crumbs

SALSA VERDE PICCANTE   uncooked spicy green sauce

SALSETTA DI PEPERONI   uncooked sweet pepper sauce

SPOLETINA   truffles and anchovies added to a tomato sauce

SUGO   sauce *or* gravy (see SALSA)

SUGO DI CARNE   brown meat sauce

SUGO DI MARE   seafood sauce

SUGO DI RICOTTA   ricotta cheese sauce with ground meat, tomatoes, olive oil

TAORMINA   sauce of bacon, black olives, anchovies, garlic and mushrooms

TARTUFI FRESCHI   fresh white truffles with butter

TONNATO   tuna sauce of garlic, oil, tomato, capers, anchovy
TRAINIERA   sauce with olives, capers, garlic and ginger
TRASTEVERINA   tomato sauce with white wine,
    chopped bacon and chicken livers
TRIESTINA   meat sauce with chopped ham, butter and cream
UMBRIA   sauce of anchovies, oil and garlic flavored with
    tomatoes and truffles
VILLEROY   white sauce thickened with egg yolk, flavored
    with Parmesan, truffles, tongue, pieces of cooked ham
VONGOLE   clam or mussel sauce, tomatoes, garlic and
    pimento

Seafood

ACCIUGHE   anchovies
ACCIUGHE AL LIMONE   fresh anchovies with lemon
    sauce, oil, breaded
ACCIUGHE AL POMODORO   anchovies, tomato and
    bread crumbs
ACCIUGHE E FUNGHI   anchovies and mushrooms
ACCIUGHE RIPIENE   deep-fried anchovies stuffed with
    cheese and bread crumbs
ACCIUGHE TARTUFATE   anchovies prepared with garlic
    and truffles
ACQUADELLA   small fish used for deep frying
AFFOGATO   fish poached in white wine and herbs
AFFUMICATO   smoked
AGONI   shad-type fish
AGONI AL BURRO E SALVIA   freshwater shad cooked in
    butter with sage flavoring
AGONI SECCATI ALLA GRATICOLA   grilled, dried shad fish
ALICI   salt-cured anchovies
ALICI AL LIMONE   fresh anchovies baked with olive oil
    and lemon juice
ALLA DORIA   highly spiced and grilled
ALLA LIVORNESE   seafood braised in olive oil, garlic,
    onion, tomato and herbs

ANELLETTI GRATINATI   rings of cuttlefish, dipped in bread crumbs, oil, salt, pepper, garlic and parsley, baked in oven

ANGUILLA   eel

ANGUILLA ALLA FIORENTINA   eel browned in oil then baked with wine and garlic

ANGUILLA ALLA VENEZIANA   eel braised with tuna and lemon

ANGUILLA CARPIONATA   eel fried and left to soak in vinegar, flavored with garlic, bay leaf and sage

ANGUILLA DEL LAGO MONTICCHIO   eels from Lake Monticchio, roasted over coals or fried, dipped into vinegar and seasoned with garlic, sage and rosemary

ANGUILLA IN UMIDO   eel braised in oil with onion and tomato paste

ANGUILLA STUFATA   baked stuffed eels

ANGUILLE DI CALDARO   eels from Lake Caldaro, grilled or marinated

ANTIPASTI DI MOLLUSCHI   plate of assorted shellfish

ANTIPASTO DI MARE   seafood appetizer

ANTIPASTO DI PESCE   fish appetizer

ARAGOSTA   spiny lobster

ARAGOSTA ALLA MAIONESE   lobster boiled or roasted with mayonnaise

ARINGA   herring

ARINGA AI CETRIOLI E BARBABIETOLE   herring in thick cream, cucumber, beets

ARINGA ALLA CALABRESE   fresh herring braised in garlic oil, mashed and spread on toast

ARSELLA   kind of mussel

ARSELLE   clams

ASTACO   lobster (also ASTICE)

ASTICE   lobster

BABBALUCI   snails in olive oil with tomatoes and onions

BACCALÀ   dried codfish

BACCALÀ AGLIATA   dried salt cod with garlic sauce

BACCALÀ AL POMODORO   braised codfish cooked with tomatoes and herbs

BACCALÀ ALLA LIVORNESE   stewed codfish with tomatoes and sliced potatoes

BACCALÀ ALLA MILANESE   pan-fried, dried cod fritters

BACCALÀ ALLA NAPOLETANA   pan-fried salt cod baked with sauce of garlic, oil, capers, tomatoes

BACCALÀ ALLE OLIVE VERDI   salt cod baked with oil, pickles, tomato, onion, green olives

BACCALÀ ALLA VICENTINA   dried codfish cooked in milk, flavored with onion, garlic, anchovies

BACCALÀ CON POLENTA   braised codfish served atop cornmeal mush (polenta)

BACCALÀ FRITTO   fried *or* deep-fried, dried codfish

BACCALÀ MANTECATO   dried codfish, boiled, then beaten in milk to make a smooth cream

BIANCHETTI   just hatched anchovies *or* sardines boiled, served cold

BIANCHETTI FRITTI   fried small sardines

BISATO   eel

BISATO IN TEGLIA   stewed eel

BISATO SULL' ARA   baked eel

BOCCONCINI DI PESCE SPADA FRITTO   fried swordfish

BOLLITO   boiled, as meat *or* fish stew (also LESSATI)

BONITO   small tuna fish

BOTARGUE   smoked *or* dried tuna *or* mullet roe, served with oil and lemon

BOTTARGA   hard roe of tuna fish, eaten with olive oil and lemon or lightly baked

BOTTARGA DI TONNO   tuna roe, grilled or boiled and served with oil and lemon

BRANZINO   sea bass

BRANZINO AL VINO BIANCO   marinated sea bass baked in white wine

BRANZINO ALLA FIAMMA   sea bass braised in wine then flamed with brandy

BRANZINO ALLA RIVIERASCA COI CARCIOFI   baked striped bass with artichokes

BRANZINO BOLLITO sea bass poached in wine, herbs, onion
BRODETTO fish stew with onion, garlic, parsley, tomatoes
BRODETTO DI CHIETI squid and fish broth
BRODETTO DI PESCE single fish cooked fish-soup style
BRODETTO VASTESE fish-stew soup
BURANELLA mixed seafood antipasto
BURRIDA fish casserole *or* soup stew
BUTTARIGA tuna *or* mullet roe
CACCIUCCO ALLA LIVORNESE spicy fish soup made
  with red wine
CALAMARETTI FRITTI baby squid, lightly floured
CALAMARETTI RIPIENI broiled stuffed squid
CALAMARETTI RIPIENI AI FUNGHI SECCHI stuffed
  squid with dried wild mushrooms
CALAMARETTO young squid (see CALAMARI,
  CALAMARETTI, CALAMARO)
CALAMARI squid
CALAMARI ALLA LUCIANA squid stewed in olive oil,
  herbs and garlic
CALAMARI ALLE ERBE squid cooked in olive oil, herbs
  and garlic
CALAMARI FRITTI fried squid
CALAMARO squid (see CALAMARI)
CALAMITO grey mullet fish
CANESTRELLI DI MARE small clams, scallops
CANESTRELLI TRIFOLATI sautéed scallops with garlic
  and parsley
CANNOCCHIE shrimp-type shellfish
CANOCCHIE prawn-type crustacean
CAPARAZZOLI like baby clams
CAPITONE fat eel roasted in large rounds, or fried and
  flavored with vinegar, garlic and spices
CAPITONE MARINATO pickled eel
CARPA carp
CARPIONATA carp marinated in herb oil then fried
CARPIONE carp fish

CARPIONE AL VINO   carp, pan fried in wine, onion, vinegar
CARPIONE FRITTO   fish fried in oil then marinated in
   vinegar, served cold
CARTOCCIO   roasted in a sealed bag
CASSERUOLA   casserole
CASSOLA   highly spiced, very tasty fish stew
CAVEDANO   chub
CAVIALE   caviar
CECHINE   eels
CEFALO   gray mullet fish
CERNIA   grouper type fish
CICALA AL SALMORIGLIO   broiled lobster tails with
   olive oil, lemon juice and oregano
CIPOLLATA DI TONNO   tuna fish fried with sliced onions
CIRIOLE   little eels
CIUPPIN   thick fish stew *or* sauce
COSCE DI RANA   frogs' legs
COZZE   mussels
COZZE ALLA MARINARA   mussel stew with garlic,
   pepper or ginger and gravy, in which there is some of
   the sea water taken up with the mussels themselves
COZZE CON RISO   mussels pan fried with tomatoes, rice,
   garlic, oil
COZZE E VONGOLE   baby clams and mussels
COZZE FRITTE   mussels breaded and deep-fried
COZZE GRATINATE   mussels with half of their shell
   removed, covered in oil, parsley, garlic and bread
   crumbs, then browned in oven
COZZE IMPEPATE   mussels highly flavored with pepper
COZZE PELOSE   mussels with hairy shells
CROSTACEO   shellfish
CROSTINI ALLA NAPOLETANA   small toast with
   anchovies and melted cheese
DATTERI DI MARE   mussels *or* small clams
DATTERI MARINATI   little shellfish in sauce of olive oil,
   vinegar, sage and garlic
DENTICE   a flat Mediterranean fish

FILETTI DI BACCALÀ   thin strips of fish dipped in batter of flour and water, fried in boiling oil

FILETTO   fillet (see COSTOLETTO)

FILETTO DI BACCALÀ FRITTO   fried fillets of salt codfish

FILETTO DI PESCE ALLA MILANESE   fish breaded with egg batter and fried

FRITTELLE DI MITILI   mussel fritters in batter

FRITTO ALLA NAPOLETANA   fried fish, vegetables and cheese

FRITTO DI PESCE SPADA   swordfish pan fried in oil and lemon juice

FRITTO MISTO   fry of fish, cottage cheese, cauliflower, potatoes and sweetbreads

FRITTO MISTO DI PESCE   fried fish such as sole, octopus, shrimp, mullet and cod

FRUTTI DI MARE   small shellfish

GAMBERETTI   very small shrimp

GAMBERETTI ALLA GRIGLIA   shrimps broiled in lemon juice

GAMBERI   shrimp (also SCAMPI)

GAMBERI AI FERRI E CANNOCCHIE   grilled shrimp, marinated in olive oil, salt and black pepper

GAMBERI ALLA PANNA   shrimps sautéed in cream

GAMBERI DI FIUME   freshwater crayfish

GAMBERI DORATI   shrimp fried in batter containing yeast

GAMBERO   crayfish, crawfish *or* prawns (see GAMBERI)

GAMBERONI   large prawns

GIANCHETTI   tiny white boneless fish for antipasti

GRANCEOLA   sea crab

GRANCEOLA ALLA VENEZIANA   sea crab boiled in lemon juice, oil

GRANCHIO   crab (see GRANCEOLA)

GRATINATA   sprinkled with bread crumbs and cheese and oven-browned

IN BIANCO   poached in white wine, herbs and onions (usually fish)

IN UMIDO   stewed in broth with onions, carrots, tomatoes and herbs

INSALATA DI ARINGHE   herring salad

INSALATA DI FRUTTI DI MARE   seafood salad, dressing of oil, lemon juice, mustard, garlic

INSALATA DI GAMBERETTI   shrimp salad in mayonnaise sauce

INSALATA DI TONNO   tuna fish salad

LAMPREDA   sea eel

LATTERINI   sand smelts fish

LUCCIO   pike-type fish

LUCCIO ALLA MARINARA   pike sautéed in onion, carrot, herb and wine

LUCIANA   fish braised with oil, garlic, peppers, tomato and wine

LUMACHE   boiled snails cooked in sauce of tomatoes and ginger

LUMACHE ALLA BORGOGNONA   snails stuffed with garlic and parsley butter

LUMACHE ALLA BOURGUIGNONNE   snails cooked in garlic butter

LUMACHE ALLA MILANESE   snails sautéed in garlic, oil, butter, anchovies, onions

LUMACHE ALLA PARIGINA   snails cooked in garlic butter

LUMACHE ALLA ROMANA   snails cooked in tomato, anchovy and garlic

LUMACHE ALLA VALDOSTANA   snails braised in oil, garlic, mushrooms, tomato and herbs

LUPO DI MARE   sea perch

MACCARELLO   mackerel-type fish

MARSIONI   small Adriatic fish

MAZZACUOGNI/MAZZANCOLLE   very large prawns

MAZZANCOLLE   large prawns

MERLANO   whiting-type fish

MERLUZZO   codfish

MISSOLTITT   shad fish which are dried with bay leaves

MISTO NAVE   mixed seafood antipasto

MITILI   mussels

MOLECCHE   soft-shell crabs

MONZETTE   snails (see LUMACHE)

MORMORA   flounder-type fish

MOSCARDINI   small squid

MOSCARDINO   small squid

MUSCOLI   mussel-type shellfish

MUSCOLI ARROSTO   mussels in half shell, breaded with
  ham and cheese and baked

MUSCOLI GRATINATI   mussels in half shell braised in
  wine and white sauce

NASELLO   whiting-type fish

NASELLO BIANCO   codfish *or* whiting poached in wine
  and herbs

NASELLO BOLLITO   codfish *or* whiting stewed in herbs,
  onion, olive oil

NAVE   fish *or* seafood

OCCHIATE   flat sea bream-type fish

OMBRINA   fish

ORATA   fish (like pompano)

ORATA AL CARTOCCIO   bream-type fish baked in bag
  with mussels, shrimp, mushrooms

ORATE AL LIMONE E MAGGIORANA   pan-roasted
  porgies with marjoram and lemon

OSTREGHE   (Venetian) oysters

OSTRICHE   oysters

OSTRICHE ALLA TARANTINA   baked fresh oysters

PAGARO   pompano-type fish

PALOMBO CON PISELLI   halibut with peas

PEOCI   mussels

PERSICO   lake perch

PESCATRICE   angler fish

PESCE   fish

PESCE AI DUE PIATTI   fish steamed between two plates

PESCE AI FINOCCHI   fish with fennel

PESCE AI FINOCCHI FRESCHI   sea bass with fresh fennel

PESCE AL CARTOCCIO   marinated fish baked in a bag
  with seafood or anchovy sauce

PESCE AL FORNO   fish baked with potatoes and cheese

PESCE AL FORNO PICCANTE   baked marinated spiced
swordfish *or* tuna steak

PESCE AL TAGLIO IN SALSA   turbot fish with white
wine and anchovy sauce

PESCE ALLA GRATELLA   grilled fish

PESCE AMMOLICATO   small fish browned with bread
crumbs

PESCE FRESCO   fresh fish

PESCE IN CARPIONE   fried fish marinated with onions
in vinegar

PESCE IN UMIDO   fish stew with tomato, onion, garlic,
oil, herbs

PESCE MARINATO   marinated fish stew

PESCE PASSERA   flounder

PESCE PERSICO ALLA SALVIA   perch fillets pan fried in
oil and herbs

PESCE RIPIENO AL FORNO   fish stuffed with mushrooms, egg, anchovy, crumbs and baked

PESCE SPADA   swordfish

PESCE SPADA AL FORNO   swordfish baked in tomato
sauce

PESCE SPADA AL LIMONE   swordfish steaks made with
lemon and capers

PESCE SPADA AL SALMORIGLIO   swordfish with sauce
of olive oil, lemon, oregano

PESCE TURCHINO AL FORNO CON PATATE   baked
bluefish with potatoes, garlic, oil, parsley

PESCI   fish

PETTO DI POLLO ALL'ARANCIA   chicken breast
sautéed in brown sauce with orange juice

POLPETTONE DI TONNO E SPINACI   tuna and spinach
loaf

POLPO   octopus *or* small squid

POLPO AL PURGATORIO   octopus cooked in oil, tomato,
parsley, garlic and pepper

POLPO ALLA LUCANA   cuttlefish slowly cooked in
sauce of olive oil, parsley and ginger

POMODORI AL TONNO   tomatoes with tuna fish, olive oil and vinegar

POSILLIPO   seafood served in a tomato herb sauce

RAGNO   sea bass *or* sea perch

RANE   frogs or frogs' legs

RANE AL GUAZZETTO   stewed frogs' legs made with wine

RANE DORATE   skinned frogs' legs dipped in egg and fried in olive oil

RANE FRITTE   fried frogs' legs

RANOCCHI   frogs (also see RANE)

RAZZA   ray fish

REGINA   large carp

RICCI   sea urchins

RICCI DI MARE   sea urchins, served raw with lemon

RIGHINI   sweet water sunfish

RISO ALLA CERTOSINA   rice with fish stock and served with shrimp and fish

RISO CON CAPAROZZOLI   rice with shellfish, garlic, wine

RISO CON SCAMPI   shrimp pan fried with rice and wine

ROMBO   turbot, fish

SALMÌ   stew cooked in earthen pot

SALMONE   salmon fish

SALMONE AFFUMICATO   smoked salmon

SALMONE DI STIMPIRATA   salmon fried with olive oil, onions, celery, capers

SALMONE RIPIENO ALL'ANETO   salmon filled with onions and fresh dill, baked, served cold

SALMONE SCOZZESE   Scotch salmon

SAN PIETRO   porgy type of fish

SAN PIETRO ALLA MUGNAIA   fish filets floured, pan fried in butter and lemon

SARAGNO   porgy type of fish

SARAGO   ocean sunfish

SARDE   sardines

SARDE AL BECCAFICCU   stuffed, baked sardines

SARDE AL FINOCCHIO   fresh sardines baked in tomato wine sauce

SARDE AL VINO BIANCO sardines baked with wine, anchovies

SARDE ALL'OLIO E ORIGANO sardines baked in olive oil and oregano

SARDE ALLA BRACE grilled sardines

SARDE IN CARPIONE fried marinated sardines

SARDE IN TORTIERA baked sardines with garlic, oil, lemon

SARDE RIPIENE stuffed sardines

SARDELLE sardines

SARDELLINE young sardines

SARDINA small sardine (also see SARDE)

SCAMPI shrimp *or* prawns (also see GAMBERI)

SCAMPI ALL'AMERICANA prawns sautéed in tomato sauce, wine, onion sauce

SCAMPI ARROSTO shrimp marinated then baked in tomato sauce

SCAMPI DORATI breaded and deep-fried shrimp

SCAMPI E PEOCETI shrimp cooked with capers, mussels, butter, brandy, tomato, cream

SCAMPI FRITTI breaded and deep-friedshrimp

SCAMPI ALLA VENEZIANA shrimp boiled and served cold with lemon juice

SCAPECE pickled, fried fish in white vinegar, seasoned with saffron

SCAVECCIO eel in Tuscany

SCORFANO Mediterranean scorpion fish

SCUNGILLI ALLA MARINARA conch-like seafood sautéed in tomatoes, wine, peppers

SEPPIA cuttlefish, squid

SEPPIA ALLA VENETA squid marinated in garlic, oil, white wine and squid ink

SEPPIA IN UMIDO stewed squid

SFIRENA sea pike

SFOGIE sole

SFORMATO FREDDO DI TONNO E PATATE cold tuna and potato mold

SGOMBRO   mackerel

SGOMBRO ALLA MARINARA   mackerel sautéed in tomatoes, wine, peppers

SOGLIOLA   sole fish

SOGLIOLA AI FERRI   grilled sole

SOGLIOLA AL GRATIN   sole baked in cream sauce with mushrooms, shallots, garlic

SOGLIOLA ALL'ARLECCHINO   sole poached in cream sauce with onions, tomatoes, garlic and squash

SOGLIOLA ALLA MUGNAIA   sole floured and pan fried in butter and oil served with lemon sauce

SOGLIOLA ALLA PARTENOPEA   sole poached in wine and served on pasta with cheese and white sauce

SOGLIOLA ARROSTO   sole baked in olive oil, herbs and white wine

SOGLIOLA DORATA   breaded and fried sole

SOGLIOLA FRITTA   breaded and deep-fried sole

SOGLIOLA MARGHERITA   sole poached in wine and herbs and served with hollandaise sauce

SPANNOCCHI   large prawns

SPARNOCCHIE   large shrimp-like shellfish

SPIEDINI DI MARE   pieces of fish and seafood skewered and roasted

SPIEDINI DI PESCE   swordfish *or* tuna broiled on skewers

SPIEDINO DI CALAMARI   squid marinated then grilled

SPIEDINO DI SCAMPI   sole broiled on skewers

SPIGOLA   sea bass

SPIGOLA CON SALSA E CAPPERI   striped bass with tomato caper sauce

SQUADRO   monk fish

STOCCAFISSO   dried cod

STOCCAFISSO ALL'ANCONETANA   dried unsalted cod, cooked with onion, tomato, garlic, oil, anchovies and milk

STOCCAFISSO IN UMIDO   dry salt cod stewed in tomatoes and herbs

STORIONE   sturgeon

STORIONE AFFUMICATO   smoked sturgeon fish

STORIONE ALLA MILANESE   sturgeon breaded and
  fried in butter and oil
TARTARUGA   turtle
TARTUFI DI MARE   cockles *or* small clams with truffles
TELLINE   small shellfish
TIMBALLO DI SPAGHETTI E PESCE   baked spaghetti
  and fish pie
TINCA CARPIONATA   fried fish marinated in wine,
  vinegar, sage, garlic and onion
TINCHE   fish, like bass
TINCHE MARINATE   bass marinated then pan fried
TONNO   tuna
TONNO AL RAGÙ   pan-fried tuna fish with wine,
  tomato, onion, garlic
TONNO ALL'AGRODOLCE ALLA TRAPANESE   sweet
  and sour tuna steaks sautéed in vinegar, wine and sugar
TONNO E ACCIUGHE   tuna and anchovies
TONNO SOTT'OLIO   tuna fish in oil
TORTA ALLE ALICI   baked anchovy pie
TOTANI   young squid
TOTANI E PATATE IN TEGAME ALLA GENOVESE   squid
  and potatoes, sautéed in olive oil, garlic, tomatoes and herbs
TRIGLIA   red mullet fish
TRIGLIA AL CARTOCCIO   mullet fish grilled in oiled paper
TRIGLIA ALL'ANCONETANA   mullet fish marinated
  then baked with ham
TRIGLIA ALLA CALABRESE   mullet fish baked with
  olive oil, lemon juice, oregano
TRIGLIA ALLA LIGURE   mullet fish sautéed in tomato,
  wine, anchovy
TRIGLIA ALLA LIVORNESE   mullet fish pan fried with
  tomato sauce, onion, garlic
TRIGLIA ALLA SICILIANA   mullet fish broiled in wine,
  meat gravy, orange and lemon juice
TRIPPA ALLA FIORENTINA   tripe stewed in meat sauce
  with tomatoes

TROTA   trout

TROTA AFFUMICATA   smoked trout

TROTA AL BURRO   trout pan fried in butter

TROTA AL MARSALA   trout cooked in Marsala wine

TROTA AL POMODORO   trout casserole with tomatoes and garlic

TROTA ALLA BRACE   trout grilled or broiled with garlic oil

TROTA ALLA PIEMONTESE   trout pan fried in vinegar, oil and herbs

TROTA ALLE MANDORLE   stuffed trout, seasoned, baked in cream and topped with almonds

TROTA ARROSTO   trout marinated and baked in herb oil and white wine

TROTA BOLLITA   trout poached in white wine and herbs

TROTA IN BLU   trout boiled and served with mayonnaise

TROTA SALMONATA   salmon trout

TROTE ARROSTITE   spiced trout baked on an open fire or in the oven, sometimes steamed and served with oil, lemon or mayonnaise

TROTELLA   large lake trout (see TROTA)

TROTELLE AL POMODORO   trout with parsley, oil and tomato paste

UMIDO DI GAMBERI E POMODORI PICCANTI   stewed shrimp with tomatoes and hot peppers

VENTRESCA DI TONNO   belly of tuna fish often canned with oil

VONGOLA   small clam

ZIMINO   fish stew

ZUPPA ALLA MARINARA   stew of fish, with garlic, parsley and tomatoes, served with pieces of toasted, fried bread

ZUPPA DI PESCE   fish stew

ZUPPA DI PESCE ALLA POZZUOLI   fish stew soup

ZUPPA DI PESCE E GAMBERI   creamy fish soup with shrimps and saffron

Soup

ACQUA ALLA FIORENTINA   mushroom and tomato soup

ACQUA COTTA ALLA FIORENTINA   soup of bread and vegetables, sometimes with eggs and cheese

ANOLINI   rolls of egg paste stuffed with bread crumbs, cooked and eaten in beef and chicken broth

BRODETTO DI CHIETI   squid and fish broth

BRODETTO DI POLLO   chicken broth

BRODETTO MISTO   chicken, beef and vegetable broth

BRODETTO PASQUALE   broth of meat, vegetables, herbs, thickened with egg yolks, served with grated cheese

BRODETTO VASTESE   fish stew soup

BRODO   bouillon, broth, soup, consommé

BRODO ALLA GIARDINIERA   broth with rice and vegetables

BRODO CON ROMBETTI ALLA GIARDINIERA   clear broth served with squares of cheese and vegetable-flavored custard

BRODO DI BUE   concentrated beef broth

BRODO DI MANZO   beef broth

BRODO DI POLLO   chicken bouillon *or* stock

BRODO IN TAZZA   broth served in a cup

BRODO VEGETALE   vegetable bouillon *or* stock

BURRIDA   fish casserole *or* soup stew

BUSECCA   thick tripe and vegetable soup

CACCIUCCO ALLA LIVORNESE   spicy fish soup made with red wine

CACIUCCO CON CECI   chick-pea soup

CAVOLATA   pork and cauliflower soup

CELESTINA   clear soup with little stars of pasta

CONSOMMÉ   broth *or* clear soup (also see CREMA, MINISTRA, MINISTRONE, ZUPPA)

CONSOMMÉ ALLA MADRILENA   jellied beef broth flavored with tomato juice

CONSOMMÉ ALLE MILLE FANTI   consommé with egg shreds

CONSOMMÉ BENSO   chicken broth gelatine with white
   truffles
CONSOMMÉ CALDO O FREDDO IN TAZZA   hot *or* cold
   consommé served in a cup
CONSOMMÉ CON PASSATELLI   consommé with pasta
   pieces
CONSOMMÉ CON PASTINA   consommé with very small
   pasta pieces added
CONSOMMÉ DI TARTARUGA   clear turtle soup
CONSOMMÉ DOPPIO   double strength consommé soup
CONSOMMÉ GELLÉ   jellied beef broth
CONSOMMÉ JULIENNE   consommé with small pieces of
   vegetable
CONSOMMÉ REALE   consommé with pastry garnish
CONSOMMÉ RISTRETTO   consommé cooked down for
   added strength
CREMA   cream soup *or* custard
CREMA DI ASPARAGI   cream of asparagus soup
CREMA DI FAGIOLI   cream of haricot bean soup
CREMA DI FUNGHI   cream of mushroom soup
CREMA DI GALLINA   cream of chicken soup
CREMA DI ORZO   cream of barley soup
CREMA DI PISELLI   cream of green pea soup
CREMA DI POLLO   cream of chicken soup
CREMA DI POMODORO   cream of tomato soup
CREMA DI PORRI   cream of leek soup
CREMA DI RISO E ASPARAGI   cream of rice and
   asparagus soup
CREMA DI SEDANI   cream of celery soup
CREMA DI SPINACI   cream of spinach soup
CREMA DI VERDURE   cream of vegetable soup
CUSCUSU   fish soup with macaroni
CUSCUSU DI TRAPANI   fish stew soup with semolina
   flakes
FARINATE   soup made with flour
FREGULA   soup with semolina and saffron dumplings
INCAVOLATA   bean and red cabbage soup

MINESTRA   soup (also see MINISTRINA AND
MINISTRONE, ZUPPA, CONSOMMÉ)
MINESTRA CON PASSATELLI   consommé with meat
dumplings
MINESTRA DI CASTAGNE   chestnut soup
MINESTRA DI CECI   soup made with chick-peas
MINESTRA DI ERBE MARITATA   soup with chopped
meat and greens
MINESTRA DI FAGIOLI   thick bean soup
MINESTRA DI FUNGHI   cream of mushroom soup
MINESTRA DI LENTICCHIE E BIETE   lentil soup with
chard
MINESTRA DI PASTA E CECI   soup with pasta and
chick-peas
MINESTRA DI PASTA GRATTATA   soup with grated
pasta and cheese
MINESTRA DI PISELLI FRESCHI E CARCIOFI   soup of
fresh peas and artichokes
MINESTRA DI POMODORO   tomato soup
MINESTRA DI RISO E FAGIOLI   rice and bean soup
MINESTRA DI RISO E SCAROLA   rice and escarole soup
MINESTRA DI SEDANI   thick celery rice soup
MINESTRA DI TRIPPA   tripe soup
MINESTRA IN BRODO   pasta *or* rice cooked in broth
MINESTRA PARADISO   soup of meat stock, eggs, bread
crumbs and cheese
MINESTRINA DI BROCCOLI E MANFRIGUL   broccoli
and barley soup
MINESTRINA DI MANZO   thin clear beef broth
MINESTRINA DI POLLO   thin clear chicken broth
MINESTRINA DOPPIA   double strength clear broth
MINESTRONE   thick vegetable broth with pieces of
macaroni, seasoned with herbs and spices
MINESTRONE AL PESTO   vegetable soup with mush-
rooms, garlic, cheese and pesto
MINESTRONE ALL'ABBRUZZESE   very thick soup of
beans, vegetables, meat, lentil and cheese

MINESTRONE ALL'ITALIANA vegetable soup with chopped ham

MINESTRONE ALLA FIORENTINA vegetable soup with white beans

MINESTRONE ALLA GENOVESE vegetable soup with spinach, basil, macaroni

MINESTRONE ALLA MILANESE vegetable soup with rice, bacon, garlic and herbs

MINESTRONE ALLA NOVARESE hearty vegetable soup

MINESTRONE ALLA TOSCANA vegetable soup with white beans, chopped ham, rosemary

MINESTRONE DI ASTI vegetable soup with beans, pork, cheese

MINESTRONE DI FAGIOLI bean soup with tomatoes and celery

MINESTRONE DI PASTA vegetable soup with pasta included

MINESTRONE DI RISO vegetable soup with rice included

MINESTRONE ESTIVO vegetable stew soup made without water

MINESTRONE SEMIFREDDO vegetable soup with rice served cold

MINESTRONE VERDE vegetable soup with green beans

NOCCIOLINI DI VITELLO IN BRODO broth with veal meatballs

PANATA bread soup with grated cheese and egg

PANCOTTO bread slices soaked in "soup" of tomatoes, bay leaves, garlic, oil, chili

PANISCIA ALLA NOVARESE rice cooked with vegetables and red wine added to vegetable soup

PAPAROT spinach soup

PAPPA AL POMODORO tomato soup with bread, herbs, olive oil

PASSATELLI DI CARNE IN BRODO meat dumpling soup

PASSATO DI LEGUMI puree of vegetables

PASSATO DI LENTICCHIE puree of lentils

PASSATO DI PISELLI puree of split peas

PASSATO DI VERDURA   mashed vegetable soup, with croutons

PASTA E FAGIOLI   broth of beans, with onions, bacon and tomatoes, sprinkled with grated cheese

PASTA E FASOI   soup of beans and pork rind with pieces of pasta

PASTA IN BRODO   pasta in a soup

PASTINA IN BRODO   pasta cooked and served in soup

PESCE DI BRODETTO   single fish cooked fish-soup style

POLPETTE IN BRODO   meatball and pasta soup

PREBOGGION AL PESTO   greens and rice soup with basil sauce

RIBOLLITA   bean soup with leeks, onion, garlic, cheese, oil, herbs, on bread, baked

RISO E LATTE   rice and milk soup flavored with cheese

RISOTTO ALLA PAESANA   thick soup of rice with beans, cabbage, salami, bacon

RISTRETTO   consommé

SA CASSOLA   fish soup of Sardinia

SOFFIONCINI IN BRODO   light dumplings in broth

SOPA   soup (see ZUPPA, MINESTRA, MINESTRONE, CONSOMMÉ)

SPINACI E RISO IN BRODO   spinach and rice soup

STRACCIATELLA   thin batter of eggs, flour, grated Parmesan cheese, lemon rind, poured into boiling meat broth

STRACCIATELLA ALLA ROMANA   chicken broth with shirred egg, cheese and lemon juice

STROZZAPRETI   spinach and cheese paste boiled, sliced and later added to soup

SUCCU TUNNU   soup with semolina and saffron dumplings

VELLUTATA DI CARCIOFI   cream of artichoke thickened with egg yolk

VELLUTATA DI POLLO   cream of chicken thickened with egg yolk

ZUPPA   soup (also see MINISTRINA, MINISTRONE, CONSOMMÉ)

ZUPPA AL COLTIVATORE   thick vegetable soup with chopped bacon

ZUPPA ALLA CERTOSINA   broth from fish, onion, olive oil, tomato, egg and cheese

ZUPPA ALLA CONTADINA   thick vegetable soup with garlic, wine and rice

ZUPPA ALLA PAESANA   peasant vegetable soup with anchovy, herbs and cheese

ZUPPA ALLA PAVESE CON L'UOVO   consommé in which floats an egg yolk, sprinkled with Parmesan cheese, on a little raft of toast

ZUPPA ALLA SARDA   soup of meat stock with eggs and cheese added then served over toast

ZUPPA DEI POVERI ALLA RUGOLA   tart salad green and potato soup

ZUPPA DI ANGUILLE   eel soup with onions, vegetables, wine vinegar

ZUPPA DI BACCALÀ   soup with salt cod, wine, tomato, potato, herbs

ZUPPA DI CALAMARI E CARCIOFI   squid and artichoke soup

ZUPPA DI CASTAGNE   chestnut soup

ZUPPA DI CECI   chick-pea soup

ZUPPA DI CIPOLLE   onion soup

ZUPPA DI CODA DI BUE   oxtail soup

ZUPPA DI COZZE   mussel soup *or* chowder

ZUPPA DI DATTERI   fish soup

ZUPPA DI DATTERI ALLA VIAREGGINA   mussel soup heavily seasoned with olive oil, tomatoes, pepper and garlic

ZUPPA DI FAGIOLI   bean soup

ZUPPA DI FARINA ABBRUSTOLITA   light soup in which hard grain flour, slightly toasted, is cooked in place of the more usual greens or semolina

ZUPPA DI FONTINA   bread and cheese soup

ZUPPA DI FRUTTI DI MARE   all shellfish soup

ZUPPA DI LATTUGHE RIPIENE   stuffed lettuce soup

ZUPPA DI ORTAGGI   vegetable soup of mostly greens
ZUPPA DI PESCE   fish stew
ZUPPA DI PESCE ALLA POZZUOLI   fish stew soup
ZUPPA DI PESCE E GAMBERI   creamy fish soup with
   shrimps and saffron
ZUPPA DI PISELLI E VONGOLE   pea and clam soup
ZUPPA DI POLLO   chicken soup
ZUPPA DI RISO E CAVOLO RAPA   rice and kohlrabi
   cabbage soup
ZUPPA DI RISO E CAVOLO STUFATO   rice and
   smothered cabbage soup
ZUPPA DI SEDANO   celery soup
ZUPPA DI TRIPPA   soup with strips of tripe, chopped
   potato and tomato, flavored with bacon, onion and
   celery
ZUPPA DI VERDURA   soup of vegetables and greens
ZUPPA PRIMAVERA   fresh spring vegetable soup
ZUPPA SANTA   puree of potato, sorrel and herbs

Spices, Condiments, Herbs

ALLORO   bay leaf
ANICE   aniseed, licorice-flavored
BASILICO   basil
CANNELLA   cinnamon
CHIODO DI GAROFANO   clove
GINEPRO   juniper berry
LAURO   bay leaf
MAGGIORANA   marjoram, a mint-flavored herb
MENTA   mint
MOSTARDA   sweet-sour pickle
NOCE MOSCATA   nutmeg
OLIO D'OLIVA   olive oil
ORIGANO   oregano
PEPATO   peppered
PEPE   pepper
PREZZEMOLO   parsley

ROSMARINO   rosemary
SENAPE   mustard
TIMO   thyme
VANIGLIA   vanilla

Vegetables

AGLIO   garlic
ALLA CAMPAGNOLA   with vegetables
ALLA LAZIALE   with onions
ALLA PAESANA   made with bacon, potatoes, carrots, squash and other root vegetables
ALLA PARMIGIANA   breaded and baked with Parmesan cheese
ALLA VENEZIANA   onions *or* shallots, white wine and mint
ANTIPASTO AI FUNGHI   appetizer of marinated mushrooms
ASPARAGI   asparagus
ASPARAGI AI FUNGHI PASSATI AL BURRO   asparagus and mushrooms sautéed in butter
ASPARAGI ALLA BISMARK   boiled asparagus with butter sauce and fried egg
ASPARAGI ALLA MILANESE   asparagus baked with cheese, butter and eggs
ASPARAGI ALLA MILANESE CON LE UOVA   boiled asparagus with grated cheese, butter sauce and fried egg
ASPARAGI ALLA PARMIGIANA   boiled asparagus with grated cheese, butter sauce and fried egg
ASPARAGI CON SALSA TARTARA   asparagus in seasoned egg and oil sauce
BACCELLI   raw, broad beans
BARBABIETOLA   beet root
BIETOLE   Swiss chard
BIETOLE IN PADELLA   Swiss chard pan fried in butter or oil
BISI   peas (in Venetian dialect)

BORLOTTI red kidney beans

BROCCOLETTI DI RAPA turnip greens

BROCCOLETTI FRITTI fried flowering broccoli

BROCCOLETTI STRASCINATI broccoli sautéed with pork fat and garlic

BROCCOLI AL CRUDO broccoli sautéed in wine and garlic

BROCCOLI AL PROSCIUTTO boiled broccoli sautéed with ham

BROCCOLI ALL'OLIO E LIMONE broccoli fried with oil and lemon

BROCCOLI ALLA ROMANA broccoli cooked in oil, garlic and wine

BROCCOLI ALLA SICILIANA broccoli sautéed in wine, oil, onion, olives

BROCCOLI STUFATI AL VINO ROSSO broccoli smothered in red wine

CAPONATA chopped eggplant, cooked in open pan with sauce of tomatoes, onion and herbs

CAPPELLE DI FUNGHI RIPIENE baked stuffed mushroom caps

CAPPERI capers

CARCIOFI artichokes

CARCIOFI AI FUNGHI artichokes stuffed with mushrooms, bread crumbs, onion and herbs

CARCIOFI AL FORNO artichokes baked in a covered pan with olive oil, garlic and parsley

CARCIOFI AL TEGAME young artichokes pan fried in oil

CARCIOFI AL VINO BIANCO artichokes stewed in oil, white wine and herbs

CARCIOFI ALLA CONTADINA artichokes stuffed with bread crumbs, garlic, anchovies, capers, stewed in oil

CARCIOFI ALLA FIORENTINA artichoke hearts with a cheese sauce, mushrooms and cauliflower

CARCIOFI ALLA GIUDA artichokes fried in olive oil and flattened out in frying pan, served crisp

CARCIOFI ALLA ROMANA artichokes stuffed with garlic and mint, cooked with oil over slow fire

CARCIOFI ALLA VENEZIANA   artichokes stewed in oil and white wine

CARCIOFI ARROSTITI   roasted artichokes with garlic, olive oil and parsley

CARCIOFI BOLLITI   hot or cold boiled artichokes served with a dressing

CARCIOFI CON MAIONESE   artichoke hearts with mayonnaise

CARCIOFI DORATI   artichokes dipped in egg and flour and fried

CARCIOFI E PISELLI   artichokes and peas

CARCIOFI FRITTI   fried artichokes

CARCIOFI IN PINZIMONIO   artichokes eaten raw with olive oil, herb sauce

CARCIOFI RIPIENI   cheese-stuffed artichokes

CARCIOFINO   small artichoke (see CARCIOFI)

CARCIOFO   artichoke (see CARCIOFI)

CARDI   celery-like vegetable usually blanched, stalks and leaves eaten like celery

CARDI AL GRATIN   whitish-green thistle-like plant, with cheese

CARDI ALLA FIORENTINA   celery-like plant boiled for a short time then sautéed

CARDI ALLA PERUGINA   chopped chards boiled and dipped into a flour batter, fried in oil

CARDOONS   thistle-like plant, leaves and stalks eaten as celery (see CARDI)

CAROTA   carrot

CAROTE AL MARSALA   carrots cooked with Marsala wine

CAROTE ALLA VICHY   carrots cooked in butter and water, sugar-coated

CAROTE CON CAPPERI   carrots with capers

CASSERUOLA   casserole

CAVOLFIORE   cauliflower

CAVOLFIORE AL POMODORO   cauliflower with tomato

CAVOLFIORE ALLA BESCIAMELLA   boiled cauliflower covered with white sauce, cheese and baked

CAVOLFIORE ALLA MILANESE   cauliflower breaded with cheese, fried

CAVOLFIORE DORATO   cauliflower, batter coated and fried

CAVOLFIORE FRITTO IN PASTELLA AL PARMIGIANO fried cauliflower with Parmesan cheese batter

CAVOLINO   brussel sprouts

CAVOLO   cabbage

CAVOLO ROSSO   red cabbage

CAVOLO STUFATO ALLA VENEZIANA   stuffed green cabbage

CAVOLO VERDE   green cabbage

CECI   chick-peas

CERFOGIO   parsley

CIAMBOTTA   vegetable stew

CICORIA   endive, chicory

CIPOLLE   onions

CIPOLLE AL POMODORO   onions stewed with tomatoes

CIPOLLE AL PROSCIUTTO E ROSMARINO   onions with ham and rosemary

CIPOLLE ALL'AGRODOLCE   onions cooked in sweet and sour tomato sauce

CIPOLLE CON PISELLI   button onions and peas

CIPOLLE DI NAPOLI   onions baked with oil and Marsala wine

CIPOLLE GLASSATE   onions sugar coated and cooked in herb broth

CIPOLLINA   pearl onion

CIPOLLINE D'IVREA   pearl onions sautéed in herb wine

CIPOLLINE STUFATE E TOPINAMBUR   braised scallions and Jerusalem artichokes

CONTORNI   vegetables, side dishes

CONTORNO DI CIPOLLE E FUNGHI   garnish of onions and mushrooms

COSTE DI BIETE SALTATE   sautéed Swiss chard stalks

COURGETTES   zucchini

CRAUTI   sauerkraut

CRAUTI CON SALUMI   pickled sauerkraut with sausage

CRESCIONE   watercress

CROCCHETTA   potato *or* rice croquette

CROCCHETTE DI PATATE   potato croquettes

CROCCHETTE DI PATATE ALLA ROMAGNOLA   potato and ham croquette

CUORE DI SEDANO   celery heart

CUORI DI CARCIOFI   artichoke hearts

ERBAZZONE   spinach pie with onions, ham, cheese, garlic

ERBETTE   boiled Swiss chard

ERBETTE SALTATE   sautéed greens

FAGIOLI   beans

FAGIOLI AL FORNO   baked white beans with tomatoes

FAGIOLI AL FORNO CON FUNGHI   baked white beans with tomatoes and mushrooms

FAGIOLI ALL'UCCELLETTO   white beans boiled with tomato sauce, garlic and herbs

FAGIOLI ALLA FIORENTINA   boiled white beans with olive oil

FAGIOLI CON COTICHE   beans cooked in tomato sauce with pork

FAGIOLI E CAVOLI ALLA GALLORESE   beans and cabbage

FAGIOLI FRESCHI   fresh kidney beans

FAGIOLI FRESCHI AL POMODORO   fresh beans cooked with tomato, onion and ham

FAGIOLI IN FIASCO   beans cooked in wine bottle over open fire

FAGIOLI LESSATI AL FORNO   beans first boiled then baked

FAGIOLI ROSSI   red kidney beans

FAGIOLI SGRANATI FRESCHI   fresh shelled and boiled beans

FAGIOLI TOSCANI   white beans boiled with olive oil, garlic and herbs

FAGIOLINI   green string beans

FAGIOLINI IN PADELLA   green beans sautéed with onion and tomatoes

FAGIOLINI RIFATTI   string beans first boiled then sautéed in tomato sauce

FAGIOLINI VERDI CON CAROTE STUFATE E MORTADELLA   smothered green beans and carrots with ham

FAGIOLO   haricot bean (see FAGIOLI)

FAVATA   beans stewed in lard with pork sausage and spice

FAVE   broad beans

FAVE AL GUANCIALE   broad beans steamed with onions and fat bacon

FAVE FRESCHE   fresh broad beans

FAVE FRESCHE STUFATE   braised broad beans with lettuce

FAVE STUFATE   broad beans sautéed with bacon, wine, onion

FAVETA   casserole of beans with bacon, sausage and seasoning

FEDERICO   braised turnip tops, sausages and spaghetti with olive oil and garlic

FETTINE CROCCANTI DI MELANZANA   crisp-fried eggplant slices

FINOCCHIO   fennel

FINOCCHIO ALLA CASALINGA   sautéed fennel home style

FINOCCHIO ALLA PARMIGIANA   fennel with cheese

FINOCCHIO IN PINZIMONIO   raw fennel dipped in herb olive oil

FOGLIE DI RAPA STRASCINATE   turnip tops sautéed in garlic and oil

FONDI DI CARCIOFI   artichoke bottoms

FONDO DI CARCIOFO   artichoke heart

FRITTATA DI PEPERONI E PATATE   pepper and potato omelette

FRITTATA DI SPINACI AL FORNO   baked spinach omelette

FRITTEDA ALLA PALERMITANA   vegetable casserole from Palermo

FRITTO DI FIORI DI ZUCCA   fried squash flowers

FRITTO DI MELANZANE FILANTI   eggplant slices with cheese filling, battered and deep-fried

FRITTO DI VERDURA   fried vegetables

FUNGHI   mushrooms

FUNGHI AL FUNGHETTO   mushrooms with garlic and herbs

FUNGHI ALLA GRIGLIA   grilled mushrooms

FUNGHI ARROSTO   grilled mushrooms seasoned with garlic, olive oil, parsley

FUNGHI COLTIVATI   button mushrooms

FUNGHI FRESCHI   fresh mushrooms

FUNGHI FRESCHI CON PROSCIUTTO   fresh mushrooms and ham

FUNGHI FRITTI   mushrooms batter-dipped and deep-fried

FUNGHI FRITTI ALLA MODA DEI PORCINI   mushrooms dipped in egg, pepper, salt, bread crumbs and fried

FUNGHI IMBOTTITI   stuffed mushroom caps

FUNGHI PORCINI   wild mushrooms

FUNGHI PORCINI AL TEGAME   wild mushrooms sautéed in garlic and mint

FUNGHI PRATOLINI   field mushrooms

FUNGHI SECCHI   dried mushrooms

FUNGHI STUFATI   stewed mushrooms

FUNGHI TRIFOLATI ALLA FIORENTINA   sautéed thick slices of mushrooms and cucumbers

GALANTINA TARTUFATA   truffles in a meat-based gelatine

GALLINACCIO   chanterelle mushroom

GATTÒ DI PATATE   potato pudding

GIARDINIERA   diced, cooked or raw vegetable decoration

GNOCCHI AL FORNO   potato-stuffed pasta baked in sauce

GNOCCHI ALLA PARMIGIANA   potato dumplings with Parmesan cheese

GNOCCHI ALLA ROMANA   potato dumplings with Parmesan cheese

GNOCCHI DI PATATE   potato dumplings

GRANOTURCO   corn meal (polenta)
INDIVIA BELGA   Belgium endive
INDIVIA CRUDA   endive braised with garlic
INSALATA DI PATATE   potato salad
INSALATINA TENERA CON PANCETTA   smothered
   lettuce with bacon
INVOLTINI DI ASPARAGI E PROSCIUTTO   asparagus
   and cheese wrapped in ham slices
INVOLTINI DI CAVOLO VERDE   meat-filled cabbage
   leaves cooked in sauce
LEGUME (see LEGUMI)   vegetables
LEGUMI   tuber vegetables like potatoes and onions
LENTICCHIA   lentil
MACEDONIA DI LEGUMI   mixed, cooked root
   vegetables
MANFRIGUL   homemade egg barley
MARROWS   squash flowers
MELANZANE   eggplant
MELANZANE AI FERRI   eggplant slices, grilled
MELANZANE AI FUNGETIELLI   slices of eggplant
   sautéed with tomatoes, oil, olives, capers, oregano
MELANZANE AL FUNGHETTO   eggplant prepared like
   mushrooms, chopped small, seasoned with garlic, oil,
   parsley and pepper
MELANZANE ALL'AGRODOLCE   eggplant in a sweet-
   sour sauce
MELANZANE ALL'OLIO   eggplant marinated in wine
   vinegar, garlic, pepper
MELANZANE ALLA FIORENTINA   eggplant slices
   cooked in layers with cheese and tomatoes
MELANZANE ALLA LIGURE   eggplant sautéed with
   tomatoes and eggs
MELANZANE ALLA MARINARA   marinated eggplant
   with garlic and peppers
MELANZANE ALLA NAPOLETANA   eggplant slices
   layered with cheese, then baked

MELANZANE ALLA PARMIGIANA   eggplant cut into thin slices, dipped in oil, spices, buffalo cheese, tomato sauce, powdered with Parmesan cheese, browned slowly in oven

MELANZANE ALLA SARDA   eggplant baked with oil, tomatoes, garlic, basil, bread crumbs

MELANZANE E PEPERONI FRITTI   deep-fried eggplant and peppers

MELANZANE FARCITE   eggplant stuffed with tomato, anchovies, garlic, oil, parsley, baked in oven

MELANZANE GRATINATE   eggplant fried, pulp mixed with grated cheese, replaced and oven-baked

MELANZANE IMBOTTITE   eggplant stuffed with rice, cheese, parsley

MELANZANE RIPIENE   eggplant stuffed with anchovies, capers, olives and garlic

MELANZANE RIPIENE ALLA CALABRESE   eggplant stuffed with mince, onion, chopped basil, rice or bread crumbs, grated cheese, tomato sauce, baked in oven

MELANZANE RIPIENE ALLA ROMAGNA   fried eggplant alternating with slices of cheese, then oven-browned

MELANZANE RIPIENE ALLA SICILIANA   eggplant with chopped meat and tomato sauce, beaten egg and grated cheese

MELANZANINE CON MOZZARELLA   baby eggplants with mozzarella cheese

MINESTRONE ESTIVO   vegetable stew soup made without water

NAVONE   yellow turnip

ORTAGGI   garden vegetables like carrots and cabbages

ORTOLANA   peas and artichokes

PAPRICHE   sweet peppers

PAPRICHE STUFATE   sweet peppers stewed in tomato, garlic, oil

PARMIGIANA DI MELANZANE   baked eggplant and Parmesan cheese casserole

PASSATO   puree *or* creamed

PASSATO DI LEGUMI   puree of vegetables

PASSATO DI LENTICCHIE   puree of lentils

PASSATO DI MARRONI   puree of chestnuts

PASSATO DI PATATE   puree of potatoes (mashed)

PASSATO DI PISELLI   puree of split peas

PASTICCIO DI FAGIOLINI VERDI   green bean pudding

PATATE   potatoes

PATATE AL FORNO   potatoes baked with skin on

PATATE ALLA BOSCAIOLA   potatoes baked with mushrooms

PATATE ARROSTO   roasted potatoes

PATATE CON ACCIUGHE   pan-roasted potatoes with anchovies

PATATE FRITTE   deep-fried potatoes

PATATE GHIOTTE   stuffed and baked potatoes

PATATE IN PADELLA   potatoes fried in a pan

PATATE IN UMIDO   potato stew

PATATE LESSE   boiled potatoes

PATATE NOVELLE   new potatoes

PATATE NOVELLE AL FORNO   new potatoes baked with skin

PATATE NOVELLE ALLA PAESANA   new potatoes sliced, seasoned and baked

PATATE SALTATE   sliced and sautéed potatoes

PATATE ALLA TRIESTINA   pan-fried, boiled potatoes with onion, pork fat, oil

PATATINE   small, new potatoes

PEPERONATA   sautéed sweet peppers, onions and tomatoes

PEPERONCINI   pickled, small green peppers

PEPERONI   green *or* red sweet peppers

PEPERONI AL GRATIN   peppers cut down the middle, stuffed with tomato, spices, anchovies and cheese, rolled in bread crumbs, baked in oven

PEPERONI AL GUANCIALE   sweet peppers pan fried with onion, bacon, tomatoes

PEPERONI ARROSTITI   roasted sweet peppers
PEPERONI E CIPOLLE   pan-fried sweet peppers and
   onions with tomatoes, oil, basil
PEPERONI IMBOTTITI PICCANTI   stuffed sweet peppers
PEPERONI IN PADELLA   peppers pan fried with onions,
   herbs and tomatoes
PEPERONI RIPIENI   cheese-stuffed peppers
PEPERONI STUFATI   stewed bell peppers
PIATTI FREDDI DI ORTAGGI   cold mixed cooked vegetables
PIATTO DI VEGETALI AL FORNO   fresh vegetables
   roasted in oven
PISELLI   peas (also PISELLO)
PISELLI AL GUANCIALE   peas stewed with onions, ham
   or bacon
PISELLI AL PROSCIUTTO   peas with ham
PISELLI AL SUGO DI CARNE   peas and brown sauce
PISELLI ALL'UCCELLETTO   peas cooked in herb tomato
   sauce
PISELLI ALL'USO SARDO   peas baked with eggs, onion,
   cheese, bread crumbs soaked in milk
PISELLI ALLA FIORENTINA   peas cooked with ham,
   onions, herbs, tomato sauce
PISELLI ALLA TOSCANA   peas cooked with onion, ham,
   herbs and tomato sauce
PISELLI CON PEPERONI   peas and sweet peppers
PISELLI NOVELLI   young fresh peas
PIZZA DI SCAROLA   escarole pie
POLPETTINE DI MELANZANE   fried eggplant patties
POLPETTONE DI BIETOLE ALLA GENOVESE   cornmeal,
   Swiss chard and mushroom pudding
POLPETTONE DI FAGIOLINI ALLA GENOVESE   green
   beans and potato pie, in a batter of cheese, eggs and
   marjoram
POLPETTONE DI TONNO E SPINACI   tuna and spinach
   loaf
POMODORI AL GRATIN   tomatoes baked in oil, cheese,
   herbs and bread crumbs

POMODORI AL TONNO   tomatoes with tuna fish, olive oil and vinegar

POMODORI ALLA SICILIANA   tomatoes stuffed with onion, anchovy, capers, bread crumbs, oil, baked

POMODORI RIEMPITI DI MOZZARELLA   tomatoes stuffed with cheese and baked

POMODORI RIPIENI   tomatoes stuffed with bread crumbs, cheese, garlic, oil, then baked

POMODORI RIPIENI DI RISO   baked tomatoes stuffed with rice and cheese

POMODORO   tomato

POMODORO AL FORNO   stuffed baked tomato

POMODORO CON ACCIUGHE E MANDORLE   tomato with anchovies and almonds

POMODORO CON MOZZARELLA   tomato and mozzarella cheese

PORCINI   boletus kind of mushrooms

PORRI   leeks

PORRI AL BURRO E FORMAGGIO   braised leeks with Parmesan cheese

PORRI ALLA PANNA   leeks prepared in a cream sauce

PORRI DORATI   leeks batter-dipped and deep-fried

PORRI IN UMIDO   stewed leeks with tomatoes and olives

PRIMIZIE   first fruits *or* vegetables of season

PUNTE DI ASPARAGI   asparagus tips

PURÉ   pureed *or* strained (also see PASSATO)

PURÉ DI PATATE   mashed potatoes

RABARBARO   rhubarb

RADICCHIO   chicory, lettuce with bitter taste

RADICCHIO ROSSO   wild chickory *or* curly endive (red)

RAFANO   horse-radish

RAPA   turnip

RAPA ROSSA   white turnip with some red color

RAPANELLI   radishes

RAPE ROSSE AL FORNO   baked red beets *or* turnips

RAVANELLI   radishes

RICOTTA CON SPINACI E CERVELLA   cottage cheese with spinach and brains

SALMÌ   stew cooked in earthen pot

SCALOGNO   shallot

SEDANI DI TREVI IN UMIDO   white celery sticks cooked in tomato sauce

SEDANO IN UMIDO   braised celery with tomatoes and onions

SFORMATO DI CARCIOFI   baked artichoke mold with bechamel sauce

SFORMATO DI FUNGHI   baked mushroom pudding

SFORMATO DI PATATE   potato pie with Parmesan cheese, ham and mozzarella cheese

SORRENTINA   casserole of potatoes with tomato sauce and grated cheese

SOTTACETI   pickled vegetables

SOUFFLÉ DI SPINACI E RICOTTA   spinach and cheese soufflé

SPINACI   spinach

SPINACI AL BURRO E PARMIGIANO   cooked spinach with sauce of butter and grated cheese

SPINACI AL GRATIN   spinach with sauce of butter and grated cheese

SPINACI ALLA GENOVESE COI PIGNOLI   spinach with pine nuts, olive oil, anchovy paste and garlic

SPINACI ALLA PARMIGIANA   spinach with sauce of butter and grated cheese

SPINACI ALLA PIEMONTESE   spinach sautéed with anchovies, garlic

SPINACI COI FUNGHI   spinach and mushrooms

SPUGNOLA   morel mushroom

STUZZICA APPETITO   antipasti of vegetables pickled in oil and vinegar

TARTUFI   truffles

TARTUFI ALLA PIEMONTESE   truffles baked with Parmesan cheese

TARTUFI BIANCHI   white truffles

TARTUFI NERI   black truffles

TEGAME   sautéed in butter or oil in small individual pan

TIMBALLO DI FUNGHI   baked mold of mushrooms, bread crumbs, garlic, parsley, tomatoes, cheese

TIMBALLO DI MELANZANE   baked eggplant, ham and cheese pie

TIMBALLO DI SCAMORZA   baked potato and cheese pie

TIMBALLO DI ZUCCHINI   baked zucchini and egg loaf

TIMBALLO DI ZUCCHINI ALLA PIZZAIOLA   zucchini pie baked with tomato sauce, onion, cheese, anchovy

TOPINAMBUR   Jerusalem artichoke

TOPINAMBUR AL POMODORO   Jerusalem artichoke smothered with tomato and onion

TOPINAMBUR FRITTI   fried sliced Jerusalem artichoke

TORTA DI CARCIOFI   artichoke pie in a flaky crust

TORTA PASQUALINA   baked cheese and spinach pie

TORTA TARANTINA DI PATATE   baked potato pie with cheese, oil, tomato, olives

TORTINO   tart filled with cheese and vegetables

TORTINO DI CARCIOFI   tart with slices of artichoke fried together with beaten eggs

TORTINO DI FUNGHI E PATATE   baked mushroom and potato pie

TORTINO DI MELANZANE E MOZZARELLA   tart with baked eggplant, mozzarella, eggs and tomatoes

TORTINO DI PATATE   potato and cheese tart

TORTINO DI VERDURE   vegetable casserole

TORTINO DI ZUCCHINE   baked zucchini mold with bechamel sauce

VERDURE   green vegetables

VERDURE ALLA PARMIGIANA   vegetables cooked with butter, served with grated cheese

VERDURE COTTE   cooked green vegetables

VERDURE MISTE AL FORNO   mixed baked vegetables

VERZA   green cabbage

ZUCCA   large yellow squash

ZUCCHINE   Italian squash

ZUCCHINE ALL'AGRODOLCE   squash sautéed in a sweet and sour sauce

ZUCCHINE ALLA PANNA   squash in cream with rosemary

ZUCCHINE ALLA PARMIGIANA   squash sliced and sautéed in butter, garlic and lemon

ZUCCHINE ALLA SVELTA   shredded zucchini squash quick fried in butter and lemon juice

ZUCCHINE COI PEPERONI   zucchini and peppers baked with anchovies, oil, tomatoes, cheese

ZUCCHINE E PEPERONI AL FORNO   baked zucchini and peppers

ZUCCHINE FARCITE   zucchini stuffed with ham, mushrooms, herbs and cheese, baked

ZUCCHINE FRITTE   zucchini batter-dipped and deep-fried

ZUCCHINE GRATINATE   baked zucchini with tomato, herbs and cheese

ZUCCHINE IMBOTTITE DI CARNE   zucchini stuffed with meat

ZUCCHINE IN CARPIONE   marinated squash (usually cold)

ZUCCHINE IN SCAPECE   cold fried zucchini squash with vinegar sauce

ZUCCHINE RIPIENE   stuffed zucchini

ZUCCHINE SALTATE ALL'ORIGANO   sautéed zucchini with oregano

ZUCCHINE TRIFOLATE CON LE CIPOLLE   sautéed zucchini with onions

ZUPPA DI FINOCCHI SELVATICI   fennel casserole with sharp cheese, olive oil, toasted bread

Wines, Beer, Liquor

AGLIANICO   red wine with fleshy flavor and natural, lively pink foam

ALBANA   sweet white wine

ALEATICO DI GRADOLI   dessert wine made from
   muscat grapes
ALEATICO DI PORTOFERRAIO   dark red mild wine
AMABILE   slightly sweet wine
AMARONE   strong red wine from Veneto
AMERICANO   aperitif of Campari, vermouth
ANGHELU RUGU   sweet rich red dessert wine
ANSONICA   dry white wine
APERITIVO   aperitif, as vermouth
ASPRINIO   yellow, sharp wine
ASTI SPUMANTE   sparkling white dessert wine from
   Piedmont
AURUM   liqueur of tea, rum and tangerine
BALBINO ALTROMONTONE   yellow wine, licorice and
   fruity flavor
BARBAGALLO   soft red wine
BARBARANO RED   dry red wine
BARBARANO WHITE   dry white wine
BARBARESCO   red wine from Piedmont
BARBERA   dark red wine
BARDOLINO   pale red wine
BAROLO   strong red wine, best with roasts and red meat
BIANCO   white wine
BIANCO DEI COLLI FRIULANI E GORIZIANI   semi-
   sparkling dry white wine
BIANCO DEL COLLIO   dry white wine
BIANCO DELLA VAL D'ADIGE   white wine, moderately
   tart and nutty
BIANCO DI CONEGLIANO   dry white wine, slightly
   sharp taste
BIANCO DI SCANDIANO   white wine, dry or sweet
BIANCO PICENO   white wine, full-bodied
BIANCOLELLA   pale yellow wine, mellow flavor
BICCHIERE DI VINO   glass of wine
BIRRA   beer
BIRRA AL BARILE   draft beer
BIRRA ALLA SPINA   draft beer

BIRRA CHIARA   lager beer
BIRRA SCURA   dark beer
BONARDA   dark red wine
BREGANZE RED   dry red wine
BREGANZE WHITE   dry white wine
BRUNELLO DI MONTALCINO   rich red wine, good with
   game
BRUT   very dry wine
BUTTAFUCCO   rich red wine from Lombardy, good with
   beef or game
BUTTAFUOCO   red, full-bodied wine
CABERNET   dry, pleasant red wine
CABERNET DI TREVISO   dark red wine, full-bodied
CABERNET FRANC   dark red wine
CALDARO   dry red wine good with beef and veal
CALVADOS   apple brandy
CAMPARI   reddish bitter aperitif with a quinine taste
CANNONAU   dry red wine good with meat and veal
CANONAU   light red wine, full-bodied, verging on
   sweetness
CAPRI RED   dark red wine
CAPRI WHITE   pale yellow dry wine
CASTELLER   light red, slightly sweet wine
CASTELLI ROMANI   dry white wine from Rome
CENTERBE   liqueur used to aid digestion
CERASCELLA   cherry liqueur aperitif
CERASUOLO DI ABRUZZO   red wine with excellent flavor
CERTOSINO   yellow *or* green herb liqueur
CHIANTI   red wine of Tuscany
CHIARETTO   famous rosé wine
CHIARETTO DEL GARDA   pink dry wine
CINQUETERRE   delicately-flavored white wine
CIRO   robust dry red wine good with meat and game
CIRO DI CALABRIA   dark red wine, lively flavor
CLASSICO   wine from grape of controlled zone
CORONATA   dry white wine, sometimes verging on
   sweetness

CORTESE   dry white wine from Piedmont
CORTESE DI LIGURIA   dry white wine
CORVO BIANCO   dry white wine good with seafood
CORVO ROSSO   red, robust wine from Palermo, good
    with meat, rabbit, poultry
D.O.C.   Government regulated wine
DOLCEACQUA   light red wine, slightly sweet
DOLCETTO DELLE LANGHE   red wine
DORATO SORSO   gold-colored wine, nutty and robust
    with special bouquet
EPOMEO RED   dark red, mellow wine
EPOMEO WHITE   dry yellow wine, full-bodied
EST! EST! EST!   semi-sweet white wine
FALERNO   dry yellow wine
FALERNO RED   dark red wine, dry but fruity flavor
FALERNO ROSSO   red, robust wine from Campania,
    good with cheese, beef, game
FERNET-BRANCA   a bitter digestive drink
FIANO DI AVELLINO   delicate dry white wine good with
    seafood
FIASCO   a straw-covered flask
FORASTERA   dry yellow wine
FRASCATI   Roman white wine, dry
FRECCIAROSSA   white, semi-dry wine
FRECCIAROSSA RED   dark red wine
FRECCIAROSSA ROSÈ   pink dry wine
FRECCIAROSSA WHITE   dry white wine
FREISA   semi-sparkling red wine
FRIZZANTE   semi-sparkling wine
GAMBELLARA   dry white wine
GATTINARA   red, full-bodied wine from Piedmont
GHEMME   red
GHIACCIATO   iced, chilled
GIRO   sweet red wine
GRAGNANO   full red wine good with pasta and meat
GRAPPA   wine-type spirit distilled from grape mash
GRECO   yellow, slightly sweet wine

GRECO DI TUFO   dry delicate white wine great with antipasti and fish

GRECO GERACE   yellow-amber wine, delicate orange blossom bouquet

GRIGNOLINO   red wine often with high alcoholic content

INFERNO   deep red, soft-flavored wine

KIRSCH   clear cherry brandy

LACRIMA   dark red wine

LACRYMA CHRISTI DEL VESUVIO   wine from Campania

LAGO DI CALDARO   red wine, delicate and pleasing

LAGREIN   dark red, sparkling wine

LAGREIN ROSATO   rosé wine

LAMBRUSCO   sparkling red wine

LEGGERO   light

LESSONA   dry, full red wine recommended with rabbit and game

LIQUORE   liquor *or* brandy

LISCIO   straight *or* neat

LISTA DEL VINO   wine list

LOCOROTONDO   white, dry pleasant wine good with eggs and fish

LUGANA   good dry white wine

MALVASIA BOSA   brilliant yellow wine with keen bouquet, slightly dry with bitter almond aftertaste

MALVASIA CAMPIDANO   golden yellow wine, pleasantly sharp with aftertaste of bitter almonds

MARSALA   red dessert wine

MARTINI   brand of white and red vermouth

MARZEMINO   full-bodied red wine good with beef or veal

MERLOT   full dry red wine good with pasta, beef or veal

MERLOT DEL TRENTINO   dark red wine, sometimes pink

MILLEFIORI   liqueur made from herbs and flowers

MONTEPULCIANO D'ABRUZZO   dark red wine, fruity and nutty

MONTEPULCIANO DEL PICENO   dark red dry wine
MOSCATELLO, MOSCATO   dessert and table wines
MOSCATO DI CASTEGGIO   sweet, delicate, sparkling
   white wine
MOSCATO DI COSENZA   amber-yellow wine, sweet flavor
MOSCATO DI SIRACUSA   amber-yellow wine, subtle
   aroma, strong and generous, a rare wine slowly
   disappearing
MOSCATO GIALLO   white, full-flavored wine
OLIENA   vigorous dry red wine recommended with beef
   or rabbit
ORVIETO   white wine, dry or semi-dry
PELLARO   red-pink wine, slightly dry
PIENO   full-bodied
PINOT BIANCO   white wine, slightly sharp flavor
POLCEVERA   pale white, tending to sweetness
PORTO   port wine
PORTOFINO   dry white wine
PRIMITIVO   dry full-bodied red wine good with rice or
   meat
PUNT E MES   brand of vermouth
RISERVA   wines aged longer in cask at winery
ROSATELLO   rosé wine
ROSSO   red wine
ROSSO DELLA RIVIERA DEL GARDA   light red, dry wine
SACRANTINO   red, semi-dry wine
SANGIOVESE   red table wine
SANGUE DI GIUDA   dark red wine, slightly sweet and
   sparkling
SANTA GIUSTINA   red table wine
SANTA MADDALENA   light and fruity red wine
SARTICOLA   dry white wine
SASSELLA   robust, smooth red wine good with beef or
   game
SAVUTO   red, velvety wine with good bouquet
SECCO   dry wine
SILVESTRO   herb and mint liqueur

SOAVE   dry white wine

SPUMANTE   sparkling wine

STOCK   distilled wine brandy

STREGA   a strong herb liqueur

SUPERIORE   higher alcohol content than required

TAURASI   full-bodied robust red wine good with meat, game or rabbit

TERLANO   white, dry delicate wine from Venice, good with soup, fish, eggs

TEROLDEGO   red wine, full, rich, good with game

TORRE QUARTO BIANCO   light, dry, white wine, good with antipasto and seafood

TORRE QUARTO ROSSO   full, smooth red wine, good with meat or game

TRAMINER   white wine

TREBBIANO   pleasant dry white wine good with pasta, fish and antipasti

TREBBIANO D'ABRUZZO   dark yellow dry wine

VALPOLICELLA   light red wine

VECCHIA ROMAGNA   wine distilled to brandy

VERDICCHIO   dry white wine, a favorite with seafood

VERMENTINO LIGURE   dry white wine, sometimes semi-sparkling

VERNACCIA DI SAN GIMINIANO   wine from Tuscany/Florence

VIN SANTO   dessert wine

VINO   wine

VINO APERTO   open wine

VINO BIANCO   white wine

VINO DA TAVOLA   table wine

VINO DEL PAESE   local wine

VINO REGIONALE   regional *or* local wine

VINO ROSATELLO   rosé wine

VINO ROSSO   red wine

VINO TIPICO   typical wine of the area

ZUCCO   amber-yellow wine, pleasing bouquet, generous flavor

4

What It Means: A Complete Alphabetical Dictionary of Italian Food and Drink

A

A PIACERE   to your own choosing or pleasure
A PUNTINO   medium-cooked meat
A PUNTO   medium-rare cooked meat
A SCELTA   of your choosing
ABBACCHIO   milk fed grilled lamb
ABBACCHIO AI CARCIOFI   braised lamb with artichokes
ABBACCHIO AL FORNO   oven-roasted lamb chops
ABBACCHIO ALLA CACCIATORA   lamb chops with a
   dressing of olive oil, vinegar, sage, rosemary, garlic,
   anchovies
ABBACCHIO ALLA ROMANA   braised lamb Roman style
ABBACCHIO ALLO SPIEDO   lamb roasted on a spit
ABBACCHIO BRODETTATO   pieces of lamb cooked in a
   sauce of egg yolks, flavored with lemon peel
ABBASTANZA   enough
ABBESPATA   soft, mild ricotta cheese
ABRUZZESE   with red peppers and ham
ACCIUGHE   anchovies
ACCIUGHE AL LIMONE   fresh anchovies with lemon
   sauce, oil, breaded
ACCIUGHE AL POMODORO   anchovies, tomato and
   bread crumbs
ACCIUGHE E FUNGHI   anchovies and mushrooms

ACCIUGHE FRESCHE   sauce of fresh anchovies

ACCIUGHE RIPIENE   deep-fried anchovies stuffed with cheese and bread crumbs

ACCIUGHE TARTUFATE   anchovies prepared with garlic and truffles

ACCOMPAGNARE   to accompany

ACERBO   sour

ACETO   vinegar

ACETOSELLA   sorrel, succulent acid leaves, used in salads

ACQUA   water

ACQUA ALLA FIORENTINA   mushroom and tomato soup

ACQUA CON GAS   water with gas

ACQUA CON GHIACCIO   ice water

ACQUA COTTA ALLA FIORENTINA   soup of bread and vegetables, sometimes with eggs and cheese

ACQUA FREDDA   ice-cold water

ACQUA GASSATA   soda water

ACQUA MINERALE   mineral water with *or* without gas

ACQUA NATURALE   well *or* tap water

ACQUADELLA   small fish used for deep frying

ADESSO   now, at present

AFFETTATI MISTI   mixture of sliced cold meats, ham, sausages

AFFETTATO   sliced cold meat

AFFOGATO   fish poached in white wine and herbs

AFFUMICATO   smoked

AGLIANICO   red wine with fleshy flavor and natural, lively pink foam

AGLIATA   garlic sauce; garlic mashed with bread crumbs and olive oil

AGLIO   garlic

AGLIO, OLIO E ACCIUGHE   garlic, oil and anchovies

AGLIO, OLIO E POMODORO   garlic, oil and tomato

AGLIO, OLIO E SAETTINE   garlic, oil and ground hot peppers

AGNELLO   lamb

AGNELLO AI FINOCCHIETTI   lamb cooked with fennel

AGNELLO AL FORNO   oven-roasted lamb, usually leg

AGNELLO AL FORNO CON PATATE E POMODORO
baked lamb with potato and tomato

AGNELLO ALL'ARETINA   roast lamb with rosemary,
basted with oil and vinegar

AGNELLO ALL'ARRABBIATA   lamb cooked over a hot
fire, basted with oil and vinegar

AGNELLO ALLA CACCIATORA   braised lamb with
herbs, wine, garlic, vinegar and anchovy

AGNELLO ALLA PECORARA   lamb pieces and onion
casserole

AGNELLO ALLA TURCA   lamb stew

AGNELLO ARROSTO   roasted lamb, usually leg

AGNELLO CON CACIO E UOVA   lamb stew with wine,
cheese, eggs

AGNELLO DORATO IN SALSA D'UOVO   casserole of
baked baby lamb chops with ham, cheese and wine

AGNELLO IN FRICASSEA   pan-roasted lamb in white
wine, with egg and lemon sauce

AGNELLO RUSTICO   baked leg of lamb with lemon juice
and cheese

AGNELOTTI   small ravioli made with egg, stuffed with
minced meat, chopped vegetables, boiled and served
with meat sauce

AGNOLOTTI ALLA PIEMONTESE   pasta filled with
meat, spinach, cheese and eggs

AGNOLOTTI D'AGNELLO CON SALSA AL FINOCCHIO
lamb-filled ravioli with fennel sauce

AGNOLOTTI DI CARNE   pasta filled with meat

AGONI   shad-type fish

AGONI AL BURRO E SALVIA   freshwater shad cooked in
butter with sage flavoring

AGONI SECCATI ALLA GRATICOLA   grilled, dried shad fish

AGRO   dressing of lemon juice and oil

AGRODOLCE   sweet-sour dressing of sugar, vinegar and
flour

AI FERRI   on the grill, grilled

AI QUATTRO FORMAGGI sauce made with four cheeses; Parmesan, Gruyére, provolone dolce, Fontina, sometimes with anchovies

AL CONTRARIO on the contrary

AL DENTE pasta *or* noodles served firm by undercooking

AL FORNO oven-baked

AL FRESCO informal *or* outdoor dining

AL GRATIN covered with grated cheese and bread crumbs and oven-baked

AL PURGATORIO sautéed in oil with tomatoes, parsley, garlic and peppers

AL SANGUE rare

AL TONNO E ACCIUGHE with tuna and anchovies

AL, ALL', ALLA, ALLE in the style of; with

ALA wing

ALBANA sweet white wine

ALBICOCCA apricot

ALCUNI a few, some

ALEATICO DI GRADOLI dessert wine made from muscat grapes

ALEATICO DI PORTOFERRAIO dark red mild wine

ALICI salt-cured anchovies

ALICI AL LIMONE fresh anchovies baked with olive oil and lemon juice

ALL'AMATRICIANA sauce of fresh tomatoes, chopped bacon, onion and garlic

ALL'INDIANA East Indian style with curry and spices

ALL'OLIO E ACCIUGHE sauce of olive oil, anchovies, garlic

ALL'OLIO E LIMONE oil and lemon juice dressing

ALLA BOLOGNESE with tomatoes, meat or ham, cheese

ALLA BRACE on charcoal

ALLA CACCIATORA with mushrooms, herbs, shallots, wine, tomatoes, ham

ALLA CAMPAGNOLA with vegetables

ALLA CARBONARA pasta with smoked ham or bacon, cheese, eggs and olive oil

ALLA CASALINGA homemade style

ALLA CAVALLEGGERA   with eggs and walnuts

ALLA CRETA   roasted in a clay pot

ALLA DIAVOLA   grilled with pepper, chili pepper, spicy

ALLA DORIA   highly-spiced and grilled

ALLA DUCHESSA   chicken livers sautéed in butter, cheese

ALLA FIAMMA   roasted over an open fire (usually charcoal)

ALLA FIAMMINGA   braised in beer, onion, mushrooms, herbs and broth

ALLA GENOVESE   sauce with basil and other herbs, pine kernels, garlic and oil

ALLA GRATELLA   grilled

ALLA GRATICOLA   grilled

ALLA GRIGLIA   from the grill

ALLA LAZIALE   with onions

ALLA LIVORNESE   seafood braised in olive oil, garlic, onion, tomato and herbs

ALLA LUCCHESE   with ricotta and chicken livers

ALLA MARCONI   pasta stuffed with ham and cheese, breaded and fried in olive oil

ALLA MARINARA   cooked in olive oil, garlic, capers, olives

ALLA MILANESE   breaded, then fried

ALLA MONTANARA   made with different root vegetables, garlic, onion, oil, broth

ALLA NAPOLETANA   made with cheese, tomatoes, herbs and sometimes anchovies

ALLA PAESANA   made with bacon, potatoes, carrots, squash and other root vegetables

ALLA PAPALINA   with chopped ham, mushrooms, cheese and butter

ALLA PARMIGIANA   breaded and baked with Parmesan cheese

ALLA PIEMONTESE   prepared with truffles and rice

ALLA PUTTANESCA   with a sauce of tomatoes, black olives, hot peppers, garlic, oil, chopped parsley

ALLA ROMANA   sautéed in pork and bacon fat with wine, garlic and tomato paste

ALLA SICILIANA   with eggplant and provolone cheese

ALLA SIRACUSANA   with a sauce of tomatoes, eggplant, pimento, capers, olives, anchovies, garlic and oregano

ALLA VENEZIANA   with onions or shallots, white wine and mint

ALLA VIENNESE   breaded, then fried

ALLODOLA   lark

ALLORO   bay leaf

ALTRE BEVANDE   other kinds of beverages

ALZAVOLA   teal

AMABILE   slightly sweet wine

AMARELLI DI MODENA   dry biscuits of egg white, sweet and bitter almonds

AMARETTI   macaroons

AMARO   bitter

AMARONE   strong red wine from Veneto

AMBURGHESE ALLA TIROLESE   hamburger grilled and served with onions

AMBURGO AL BURRO   hamburger fried in butter with sage

AMERICANO   aperitif of Campari, vermouth

ANANAS   pineapple

ANANAS AL LIQUORE   pineapple served with a liqueur

ANATRA   duck

ANATRA ALLE OLIVE   duck sautéed in oil, herbs, olives

ANATRA ARROSTO   roast duck

ANATRA CON SALSA PICCANTE   duck stuffed with veal, sausage and cheese, baked in wine vinegar sauce

ANATRA RIPIENA   duck, stuffed with veal, sausage, cheese, baked

ANATRA SELVATICA   wild duck roasted and basted with wine and herbs

ANELLETTI GRATINATI   rings of cuttlefish, dipped in bread crumbs, oil, salt, pepper, garlic and parsley, baked in oven

ANELLI   small rings of pasta

ANGHELU RUGU   sweet rich red dessert wine

ANGUILLA   eel

ANGUILLA ALLA FLORENTINA   eel browned in oil then baked with wine and garlic

ANGUILLA ALLA VENEZIANA   eel braised with tuna and lemon

ANGUILLA CARPIONATA   eel fried and left to soak in vinegar, flavored with garlic, bay leaf and sage

ANGUILLA DEL LAGO MONTICCHIO   eels from Lake Monticchio, roasted over coals or fried, dipped into vinegar and seasoned with garlic, sage and rosemary

ANGUILLA IN UMIDO   eel braised in oil with onion and tomato paste

ANGUILLA STUFATA   baked stuffed eel

ANGUILLE DI CALDARO   eels from Lake Caldaro, grilled or marinated

ANGURIA   watermelon

ANICE   aniseed, licorice-flavored

ANICINI   aniseed cookies

ANIMELLE   sweetbreads

ANIMELLE AL MARSALA   sweetbreads cooked in wine

ANIMELLE DI VITELLO   veal sweetbreads

ANITRA   duck

ANITRA AL COGNAC   duck cooked with brandy, juniper berries and rosemary

ANITRA ALL'AGRODOLCE   duck with a sweet-sour sauce

ANITRA ALL'ARANCIA   oven-roasted duck basted with orange juice

ANITRA ALLA SALSA D'ARANCIO   roast duck with orange sauce

ANITRA ALLE OLIVE   casserole of duck and olives

ANITRA ARROSTITA ALLA SICILIANA   roasted duck stuffed with pork, peppers and black olives, with Marsala

ANITRA ARROSTO ALLA GENOVESE   duck roasted in olive oil with herbs and fresh lemon juice

ANITRA CON SALSA DI CAPPERI   duck cooked in the oven with a sauce of Marsala, capers, white truffles

ANITRA IN SALMÌ   duck marinated in red wine with onion, herbs, garlic, anchovies, fried and then cooked in the marinade

ANITRA MUTA ALLA NOVARESE   duck stuffed with
rice, meats, herbs, roasted

ANITRA SELVATICA   wild duck

ANITROCCOLO   duckling

ANNEGATI   slices of meat in white wine or Marsala wine

ANOLINI   rolls of egg paste stuffed with bread crumbs,
cooked and eaten in beef and chicken broth

ANSONICA   dry white wine

ANTIPASTI   appetizers, first course (see ANTIPASTO)

ANTIPASTI ASSORTITI   assorted appetizers of vegetables, cold cuts, olives

ANTIPASTI DI MOLLUSCHI   plate of assorted shellfish

ANTIPASTO   hors d'oeuvre, appetizer

ANTIPASTO A SCELTA   appetizer of one's own choosing

ANTIPASTO AI FUNGHI   marinated mushroom appetizer

ANTIPASTO ALLA GENOVESE   appetizer with raw
young broad beans, salami and cheese

ANTIPASTO DI BURANELLA   assorted seafood
appetizer

ANTIPASTO DI MARE   seafood appetizer

ANTIPASTO DI PESCE   appetizer of fish

ANTIPASTO MAGRO   assorted meatless appetizer

ANTIPASTO MISTO   assorted appetizer

ANTIPASTO MISTO   appetizer of assorted cured meats
and marinated vegetables

ANTIPASTO MISTO NAVE   assorted seafood appetizer

APERITIVO   aperitif, as vermouth

APRIRE   to open

ARACHIDE   peanut

ARAGOSTA   spiny lobster

ARAGOSTA ALLA MAIONESE   lobster boiled or roasted
with mayonnaise

ARANCIA   orange

ARANCIA AFFETTATA   slices of orange poached in liqueur

ARANCIA AL MARSALA   sliced orange in Marsala wine

ARANCIATA   orangeade

ARANCIATA DI NUORO   orange rind candy

ARANCINE ALLA SICILIANA   rice balls stuffed with meat, breaded and fried

ARINGA   herring

ARINGA AI CETRIOLI E BARBABIETOLE   herring in thick cream, cucumber, beets

ARINGA ALLA CALABRESE   fresh herring braised in garlic oil, mashed and spread on toast

ARISTA   loin of pork

ARISTA AL FORNO   roast loin of pork

ARISTA ALLA FIORENTINA   loin of pork seasoned with garlic, cloves, rosemary, cooked slowly in oven with water

ARISTA DI MAIALE   pork loin, rubbed with herbs and garlic, roasted in oven or on spit

ARROSTETTI DI MAIALE   small pork roast

ARROSTI MISTI FREDDI   cold sliced roast meat

ARROSTICINI ALL'ABRUZZESE   skewered marinated grilled lamb cubes

ARROSTINO ANNEGATO AI FUNGHI   small veal roast covered with mushrooms

ARROSTINO DI MAIALE ALLA SALVIA   small pork roast basted in broth with herbs

ARROSTO   roast, usually of veal, cut into large portions and prepared with potatoes, cooked in a slow oven

ARROSTO ALLA GENOVESE   pot roast cooked in gravy of onion, wine, tomato paste

ARROSTO ALLA MONTANARA   pot roast cooked in gravy of onion, olive oil, tomato, herbs

ARROSTO DI MAIALE   roast of white pork seasoned with bay leaf and spices

ARROSTO DI MAIALE AL LATTE   pork cooked in milk

ARROSTO DI MAIALE UBRIACO   roast pork braised in red wine

ARROSTO DI VITELLO   roast veal, usually slices

ARROSTO IN PASTINE   roast meat cooked in dough crust

ARROSTO MORTO AL FORNO   slowly roasted without gravy or sauce

ARSELLA   kind of mussel

ARSELLE   clams
ASIAGO   cheese made of skimmed milk
ASPARAGI   asparagus
ASPARAGI AI FUNGHI PASSATI AL BURRO   asparagus
   and mushrooms sautéed in butter
ASPARAGI ALLA BISMARK   boiled asparagus with
   butter sauce and fried egg
ASPARAGI ALLA MILANESE   asparagus baked with
   cheese, butter and eggs
ASPARAGI ALLA MILANESE CON LE UOVA   boiled
   asparagus with grated cheese, butter sauce and fried egg
ASPARAGI ALLA PARMIGIANA   boiled asparagus with
   grated cheese, butter sauce and fried egg
ASPARAGI CON SALSA TARTARA   asparagus in
   seasoned egg and oil sauce
ASPRINIO   yellow, sharp wine
ASSORTITI   assorted
ASTACO   lobster (also ASTICE)
ASTI SPUMANTE   Piedmont sparkling white dessert wine
ASTICE   lobster
ATTORTA   flaky pastry filled with fruit and almonds
AURUM   liqueur of tea, rum and tangerine
AVELLANA   hazelnut
AVENA CALDA   warm oatmeal

B

BABBALUCI   snails in olive oil with tomatoes and onions
BACCALÀ   dried codfish
BACCALÀ AGLIATA   dried salt cod with garlic sauce
BACCALÀ AL POMODORO   braised codfish cooked
   with tomatoes and herbs
BACCALÀ ALLA LIVORNESE   stewed codfish with
   tomatoes and sliced potatoes
BACCALÀ ALLA MILANESE   pan-fried dried cod fritters
BACCALÀ ALLA NAPOLETANA   pan-fried salt cod
   baked with sauce of garlic, oil, capers, tomatoes

BACCALÀ ALLA VICENTINA   dried codfish cooked in milk, flavored with onion, garlic, anchovies

BACCALÀ ALLE OLIVE VERDI   salt cod baked with oil, pickles, tomato, onion, green olives

BACCALÀ CON POLENTA   braised codfish served atop cornmeal mush (polenta)

BACCALÀ FRITTO   fried *or* deep-fried dried cod fish

BACCALÀ MANTECATO   dried codfish, boiled, then beaten in milk to make a smooth cream

BACCELLI   raw, broad beans

BACCHE DI SOTTOBOSCO   seasonal berries

BAGNA CAUDA   hot sauce for dipping raw vegetables with anchovies, wine, garlic

BAGNARE   to wet

BAICOLI   dry biscuits made of flour, sugar, salt and butter, flavored with orange

BALBINO ALTROMONTONE   yellow wine, licorice and fruity flavor

BANANE   bananas

BARBABIETOLA   beet root

BARBAGALLO   soft red wine

BARBARANO RED   dry red wine

BARBARANO WHITE   dry white wine

BARBARESCO   red wine from Piedmont

BARBERA   dark red wine

BARDELE MARAI   special green noodle with butter, pepper and cheese sauce

BARDOLINO   pale red wine

BAROLO   strong red wine best with roasts and red meat

BASILICO   basil

BASTA!   enough!

BATTUTA   ground *or* chopped beef, as hamburger

BATTUTA AL PROSCIUTTO   ground beef with ground ham

BATTUTA DI VITELLO   veal cutlet pounded thin and grilled

BATTUTO DI MANZO   ground beef either sautéed or fried

BAVETTE   small flat noodle pasta

BAVETTE AI BROCCOLI   bavette pasta with broccoli

BAVETTE ALLA TRASTEVERINA   small flat pasta with tuna and mushrooms

BECCACCIA   woodcock

BECCACCIA ALLA ROMAGNOLA   woodcock stuffed and roasted

BECCACCIA FARCITA   stuffed and roasted woodcock

BECCACCIA IN SALMÌ   woodcock sauteed in oil and butter with a sauce made of intestines

BECCACCINO   wild snipe bird

BECCAFICHI   small table birds

BECCAFICHI AL MARSALA   birds cooked in tomato, anchovies, olives, garlic, Marsala, served on fried bread with sauce

BEL PAESE   mild soft cheese

BEN COTTO   well-done

BENE   well

BENISSIMO   all right

BENONE   very well

BERE   to drink

BERGAMOT   small sweet, aromatic orange rind

BESCIAMELLA   white sauce

BESCIAMELLA CON FORMAGGIO E UOVA   white sauce, cheese and egg

BEVANDE   beverages

BIANCHETTE DI VITELLO   veal stew in herb mushroom cream sauce

BIANCHETTI   just hatched anchovies or sardines boiled, served cold

BIANCHETTI FRITTI   small fried sardines

BIANCO   white wine

BIANCO DEI COLLI FRIULANI E GORIZIANI   semi-sparkling dry white wine

BIANCO DEL COLLIO   dry white wine

BIANCO DELLA VAL D'ADIGE   white wine, moderately tart and nutty

BIANCO DI CONEGLIANO   dry white wine, slightly sharp taste

BIANCO DI SCANDIANO   white wine, dry or sweet

BIANCO PICENO   white wine, full-bodied

BIANCOLELLA   pale yellow wine, mellow flavor

BIBITE   beverages *or* drinks

BICCHIERE   glass

BICCHIERE D'ACQUA   glass of water

BICCHIERE DI LATTE   glass of milk

BICCHIERE DI VINO   glass of wine

BICCIOLANI DI VERCELLI   spiced, sweet cookies

BIETOLE   Swiss chard

BIETOLE IN PADELLA   Swiss chard pan fried in butter or oil

BIGNÉ   baked *or* fried pastry filled with custard

BIGOLI   spaghetti-like pasta

BIGOLI ALL'ANATRA   spaghetti-like pasta with duck sauce

BIGOLI CON CARNE E POMODORO ALLA VENETA
   round solid pasta with meat and tomatoes

BIGOLI CON SALSA   round solid noodles with anchovy
   or sardine sauce

BIRRA   beer

BIRRA AL BARILE   draft beer

BIRRA ALLA SPINA   draft beer

BIRRA CHIARA   lager beer

BIRRA SCURA   dark beer

BISATO   eel

BISATO IN TEGLIA   stewed eel

BISATO SULL'ARA   baked eel

BISCOTTINI AL MIELE   baked honey cookies

BISCOTTO   rusk, biscuits *or* cookies

BISCOTTO DI SAVONA   light potato flour cake with
   orange and lemon peel

BISCUIT TORTONI   dessert of whipped egg whites,
   whipped cream, macaroon crumbs and bits of almond

BISI   peas

BISTECCA   steak, usually beef

BISTECCA AL TARTUFO   grilled beef steak covered with
   grated truffle

BISTECCA ALLA BISMARK   steak pan-fried in butter
   and served with fried egg on top

BISTECCA ALLA FIORENTINA   steak salted, coated with olive oil, charcoal-broiled

BISTECCA ALLA PIZZAIOLA   beef *or* veal cutlet stewed in an open pan with tomato, olive oil, garlic and marjoram

BISTECCA ALLA SICILIANA   beefsteak pan fried in oil, garlic, tomatoes, olives, pickles and peppers

BISTECCA ARROSTO   roast loin of beef

BISTECCA DI AGNELLO   loin of lamb

BISTECCA DI MANZO   beefsteak

BISTECCA DI MANZO AI FERRI   grilled beefsteak

BISTECCA DI VITELLO   veal loin steak, grilled

BISTECCHINE ALLA GRIGLIA   hamburgers

BISTECCHINE DI CINGHIALE   thin pan-fried wild boar steaks in sweet and sour sauce

BISTECCHINE DI MANZO ALLA CACCIATORA   thin beef-steaks fried with mushrooms, olive oil, red wine and tomatoes

BOCCONCINI   diced meat with herbs

BOCCONCINI ALLA CACCIATORA   beef chunks sautéed in oil, mushroom, herbs

BOCCONCINI ALLA FIORENTINA   steak chunks sautéed in oil, garlic, onion, herbs

BOCCONCINI DI PESCE SPADA FRITTO   fried swordfish

BOCCONCINI DI VITELLO AI SAPORI E FUNGHI   herb-flavored bits of veal and mushrooms, braised

BOCCONOTTA   chocolate cookies baked with fruit, coffee and liqueur

BOCCONOTTI   pastry filled with custard

BOLLITO   boiled, as meat *or* fish stew (also LESSATI)

BOLLITO DI GALLINA   boiled chicken

BOLLITO DI MANZO   boiled beef

BOLLITO RIFATTO ALLA MODA DEI PAPI   grilled left-over boiled beef

BOMBA DI RISO   rice pudding

BOMBOLETTE DI RICOTTA   ricotta fritters

BOMBOLONI   fried cookies filled with cream

BONARDA   dark red wine

BONDIOLA DI PARMA   pork sausage from Parma

BONGO BONGA   profiteroles

BONITO   small tuna fish

BORLOTTI   red kidney beans

BOSCAIOLA   tomatoes, mushrooms, oil, garlic, basil, butter and cheese

BOSCO   wild

BOTARGUE   smoked *or* dried tuna *or* mullet roe, served with oil and lemon

BOTTARGA   hard roe of tuna fish, eaten with olive oil and lemon or lightly baked

BOTTARGA DI TONNO   tuna roe, grilled or boiled and served with oil and lemon

BOTTIGLIA   bottle

BOVE   beef fillet

BRACIOLE   rib steak

BRACIOLE AI SASSI   pan-fried steak served with pan-fried potatoes

BRACIOLE ALLA FIORENTINA   rib steak that is salted, coated with olive oil and charcoal-broiled

BRACIOLE ALLA PIZZAIOLA   grilled steak served with tomato, garlic and olive oil sauce

BRACIOLE ALLA TOSCANA   grilled steak and boiled potatoes served with sauce of wine, onion, olive oil

BRACIOLE DI ABBACCHIO ALLA SCOTTADITO   small grilled lamb chops

BRACIOLE DI CASTRATO   grilled *or* fried mutton chops or rib chops

BRACIOLE DI MAIALE   pork chops

BRACIOLE DI VITELLO AL VINO E LIMONE   veal chops braised with wine and lemon

BRACIOLETTE DI ABBACCHIO   grilled lamb chops

BRACIOLINE DI AGNELLO   baby lamb chops pan fried in wine

BRACIOLINE DI AGNELLO AI CARCIOFI   baby lamb chops and artichokes sautéed in wine

BRACIOLINE DI MAIALE AL VINO BIANCO   pork cutlets pan fried in wine

BRACIOLINE SCOTTADITO   charcoal-grilled lamb chops

BRACIOLONE DI FARSUMAGRU   beef *or* veal stuffed
with sausages, salami, cheeses, hard-boiled eggs

BRANZINO   sea bass

BRANZINO AL VINO BIANCO   marinated sea bass
baked in white wine

BRANZINO ALLA FIAMMA   sea bass braised in wine
then flamed with brandy

BRANZINO ALLA RIVIERASCA CON CARCIOFI   baked
striped bass with artichokes

BRANZINO BOLLITO   sea bass poached in wine, herbs, onion

BRASATO   braised beef

BRASATO CON LENTICCHIE   braised beef with lentils

BRASATO DI MANZO   pot roast marinated in wine

BRASATO DI MANZO CON SEDANO E CIPOLLE   beef
braised with celery and onions

BRASATO DI MANZO E CIPOLLE   beef braised with onions

BREGANZE RED   dry red wine

BREGANZE WHITE   dry white wine

BRESAOLA AL LIMONE   salted, dried beef with lemon juice

BRIGIDINI   anise seed wafers

BROCCOLETTI DI RAPA   turnip greens

BROCCOLETTI FRITTI   fried flowering broccoli

BROCCOLETTI STRASCINATI   broccoli sautéed with pork
fat and garlic

BROCCOLI AL CRUDO   broccoli sautéed in wine and garlic

BROCCOLI AL PROSCIUTTO   boiled broccoli sautéed
with ham

BROCCOLI ALL'OLIO E LIMONE   broccoli fried with oil
and lemon

BROCCOLI ALLA ROMANA   broccoli cooked in oil,
garlic and wine

BROCCOLI ALLA SICILIANA   broccoli sautéed in wine,
oil, onion, olives

BROCCOLI STUFATI AL VINO ROSSO   broccoli
smothered in red wine

BRODETTO   fish stew with onion, garlic, parsley, tomatoes

BRODETTO DI CHIETI   squid and fish broth
BRODETTO DI PESCE   single fish cooked fish-soup style
BRODETTO DI POLLO   chicken broth
BRODETTO MISTO   chicken, beef and vegetable broth
BRODETTO PASQUALE   broth of meat, vegetables, herbs, thickened with egg yolks, served with grated cheese
BRODETTO VASTESE   fish stew soup
BRODO   bouillon, broth, soup, consommé
BRODO ALLA GIARDINIERA   broth with rice and vegetables
BRODO CON ROMBETTI ALLA GIARDINIERA   clear broth served with squares of cheese and vegetable-flavored custard
BRODO DI BUE   concentrated beef broth
BRODO DI MANZO   beef broth
BRODO DI POLLO   chicken bouillon *or* stock
BRODO IN TAZZA   broth served in a cup
BRODO VEGETALE   vegetable bouillon *or* stock
BRUNELLO DI MONTALCINO   rich red wine, good with game
BRUSCHETTA   thick slice of bread, grilled with garlic and olive oil
BRUT   very dry wine
BUCATINI   pasta, like a thick spaghetti
BUCATINI AL CAVOLFIORE   pasta like a thick spaghetti with cauliflower
BUCATINI ALLA BOSCAIOLA   thick spaghetti with eggplant
BUCATINI ALLE ACCIUGHE   thick spaghetti with anchovies
BUDELLI DI MAIALE   entrails of pork
BUDINO   custard, pudding
BUDINO DI MANDORLE   almond pudding
BUDINO DI PANE   bread pudding
BUDINO DI PANETTONE   rum and wine-soaked bread pudding
BUDINO DI POLLO   chicken mousse
BUDINO DI RICOTTA   ricotta cheese pudding
BUDINO FREDDO AL GIANDUIA   pudding with chocolate custard, hazelnuts

BUE   beef
BUE AL BAROLO   beef braised in red wine
BUONO   good
BURANELLA   mixed seafood antipasto
BURRIDA   fish casserole *or* soup stew
BURRO   butter
BURRO AL LATTE E PARMIGIANO   butter with milk
   and cheese
BURRO ALLA PANNA CON LE UOVA   butter with
   cream and eggs
BURRO E ACCIUGHE   butter and anchovies
BURRO E SALVIA   butter and sage
BURRO MAGGIORDOMO   butter with lemon juice and
   parsley
BUSECCA   thick tripe and vegetable soup
BUSECCHINA   chestnuts stewed in wine and cream
BUSSOLA   baked doughnut-shaped cake made with
   lemon peel
BUTTAFUCCO   rich red wine from Lombardy, good with
   beef or game
BUTTAFUOCO   red full-bodied wine
BUTTARIGA   tuna *or* mullet roe

C

C'É   there is
CABERNET   dry, pleasant red wine
CABERNET DI TREVISO   dark red wine, full-bodied
CABERNET FRANC   dark red wine
CACCIAGIONE   game animals such as deer, also birds
CACCIUCCO ALLA LIVORNESE   spicy fish soup made
   with red wine
CACHI   persimmon
CACIO   cheese
CACIO E PEPE   pasta served with pepper and string cheese
CACIOCAVALLO   firm, slightly sweet cheese from cow's
   or sheep's milk

CACIOCAVALLO AL FUMO   sweet cheese melted by steaming

CACIOCAVALLO DI PESCOCOSTANZO   highly-spiced strong buffalo cheese

CACIOTTE   small ewe milk cheese stuffed with butter

CACIUCCO CON CECI   chick-pea soup

CAFFETTIERA   coffee pot

CAFFÉ   coffee

CAFFÉ AFFOGATO   white chocolate ice cream, espresso, whipped cream

CAFFÉ CORRETTO   espresso made with liquor *or* brandy

CAFFÉ E LATTE   coffee with half milk

CAFFÉ ESPRESSO   strong aromatic coffee

CAFFÉ ESPRESSO   strong, thick, aromatic, small coffee

CAFFÉ FREDDO   iced coffee

CAFFÉ MACCHIATO   espresso made with a few drops of warm milk

CAFFÉ NERO   black coffee

CAFFÉ RISTRETTO   small concentrated cup of coffee

CALABRESE   tomato sauce flavored with ginger

CALAMARETTI RIPIENI   broiled, stuffed squid

CALAMARETTI RIPIENI AI FUNGHI SECCHI   stuffed squid with dried wild mushrooms

CALAMARETTO   young squid (see CALAMARI, CALA-MARETTI, CALAMARO)

CALAMARI   squid

CALAMARI ALLA LUCIANA   squid stewed in olive oil, herbs and garlic

CALAMARI ALLE ERBE   squid cooked in olive oil, herbs and garlic

CALAMARI FRITTI   fried squid

CALAMARO   squid (see CALAMARI)

CALAMERETTI FRITTI   baby squid, lightly-floured

CALAMITO   grey mullet fish

CALCIONETTI   cookies with chestnut filling

CALCIONI   small ravioli made with egg, stuffed with meat and browned in oven

CALCIUNI   fried ravioli (pasta)

CALCIUNI DEL MOLISE   fried ravioli stuffed with chestnuts

CALDARO   dry red wine good with beef and veal

CALDO   hot

CALVADOS   apple brandy

CALZONCINO MEZZADRO   turnover filled with scrambled eggs, sausage, onions, potatoes, Parmesan cheese

CALZONE   pizza dough envelope baked, filled with ham, cheese and herbs

CALZONE ALLA NAPOLETANA   pizza dough envelope containing buffalo cheese, anchovies and tomato

CALZONE ALLA PUGLIESE   folded pizza dough filled with capers, olives, onions, anchovies

CAMBIO   change, exchange

CAMERIERE   waiter

CAMOSCIO   small wild deer

CAMOSCIO IN SALMÌ   deer meat cooked in sauce of wine, olive oil, garlic, herbs and anchovies

CAMPAGNA   sauce of minced beef and cottage cheese

CAMPARI   reddish bitter aperitif with a quinine taste

CANDITO   candied

CANEDERLI   large dumpling of bread with bacon in soup

CANESTRELLI DI MARE   small clams, scallops

CANESTRELLI TRIFOLATI   sautéed scallops with garlic and parsley

CANNARICULI   deep-fried honey cookies

CANNELI   tubes of pasta

CANNELLA   cinnamon

CANNELLONI   tubular pasta stuffed with meat, cheese *or* vegetables

CANNELLONI ALLA BARBAROUX   tubular pasta, chopped ham, veal, cheese and white sauce

CANNELLONI ALLA LAZIALE   tubular pasta, meat and onion filling, baked in tomato sauce

CANNELLONI ALLA NAPOLETANA   tubular pasta, cheese and anchovy filling and tomato herb sauce

CANNELLONI ALLA PARTENOPEA   tubular pasta stuffed with ricotta cheese and ham, baked in tomato sauce

CANNELLONI ALLA ROMAGNOLA   tubular pasta stuffed with meat mixture, baked in garlic and tomato sauce

CANNELLONI RIPIENI ALLA TOSCANA   pasta tubes with a stuffing of meat, chicken livers, eggs, cheese and wine

CANNOCCHIE   shrimp-type shell fish

CANNOLI   round pastry cases filled with cottage cheese, candied fruit or chocolate

CANNOLI ALLA CREMA DI CAFFÉ   fried pastry rolls filled with coffee-flavored ricotta cheese

CANNOLI ALLA SICILIANA   pastry shell filled with ricotta cream

CANNOLICCHI   pasta of small curved noodle with hole

CANNOLICCHI CON FAGIOLI FRESCHI   pasta served with white beans in tomato sauce

CANNOLO   short pasta tubes as macaroni

CANNONAU   dry red wine good with meat and veal

CANOCCHIE   prawn-type crustacean

CANONAU   light red wine, full-bodied, verging on sweetness

CAODA   hot herb oil and anchovy dip for raw vegetables

CAPARAZZOLI   like baby clams

CAPELLINI   very thin solid pasta often called Angel Hair

CAPELLINI AL POMODORO NATURALE   angel hair pasta, chopped fresh tomatoes, basil, garlic

CAPITONE   fat eel roasted in large rounds, or fried and flavored with vinegar, garlic and spices

CAPITONE MARINATO   pickled eel

CAPOCOLLO   smoked salt pork

CAPONATA   chopped eggplant, cooked in open pan with sauce of tomatoes, onion and herbs

CAPONATA ALLA MARINARA   hard biscuits covered with oil, garlic, anchovies, black olives, onions, marinated eggplant, pimentos, herbs

CAPPELLE DI FUNGHI RIPIENE   baked stuffed mushroom caps

CAPPELLETTI   small ravioli, filled with cottage cheese, minced turkey, Parmesan cheese, egg and spices

CAPPELLETTI ALLA ROMANA   ravioli pasta stuffed with cheese, pork, chicken and served with meat sauce

CAPPELLETTI CON SALSA ALLA BOLOGNESE   small ravioli pasta with meat and tomato sauce

CAPPELLETTI DI PESCE AL SUGO DI GAMBERETTI   ravioli pasta with fish stuffing and shrimp sauce

CAPPELLETTI DI ROMAGNA   ravioli stuffed with cheese

CAPPELLETTI DI ZUCCA   ravioli stuffed with pumpkin

CAPPELLO   hat

CAPPERI   capers

CAPPON MAGRO   boiled vegetable and pickled fish salad

CAPPONCELLO AL FORNO   roast capon

CAPPONE   capon

CAPPONE RIPIENO   capon stuffed with veal, ham, eggs, cheese, bread crumbs

CAPPUCCINO   black coffee with steamed milk on top

CAPRETTO   kid, baby goat

CAPRETTO AL CARCIOFI   baby goat sautéed with wine, onion, artichokes, lemon, egg yolks and ham

CAPRETTO AL FORNO   roast goat, basted with herb broth

CAPRETTO AL VINO BIANCO   goat cooked in white wine

CAPRETTO ALLA PAESANA   baby goat roasted in casserole with potatoes, oil, cheese, onions

CAPRETTO ALLA PASQUALINA   oven-roasted baby goat basted with wine, olive oil, onion and broth

CAPRETTO ALLO SPIEDO   spit-roasted baby goat

CAPRETTO RIPIENO AL FORNO   baby goat stuffed with herbs and cooked in the oven

CAPRI RED   dark red wine

CAPRI WHITE   pale yellow dry wine

CAPRINO   soft goat's cheese

CAPRINO ROMANO   hard goat's milk cheese

CAPRIOLO   female deer

CAPRIOLO ALLA CASALINGA   home style stew of wild deer

CAPRIOLO IN SALMÌ   deer with wine, herbs and vegetables

CARAFFA   decanter

CARAMELLATO   caramelized sugar coating

CARASAU   paper thin shepherds bread from Sardinia

CARATELLA   lamb pieces roasted on skewers

CARBONATA   beef stew in red wine

CARCIOFI   artichokes

CARCIOFI AI FUNGHI   artichokes stuffed with mushrooms, bread crumbs, onion and herbs

CARCIOFI AL FORNO   artichokes baked in a covered pan with olive oil, garlic and parsley

CARCIOFI AL TEGAME   young artichokes pan-fried in oil

CARCIOFI AL VINO BIANCO   artichokes stewed in oil, white wine and herbs

CARCIOFI ALLA CONTADINA   artichokes stuffed with bread crumbs, garlic, anchovies, capers, stewed in oil

CARCIOFI ALLA FIORENTINA   artichoke hearts with a cheese sauce, mushrooms and cauliflower

CARCIOFI ALLA GIUDIA   artichokes fried in olive oil and flattened out in frying pan, served crisp

CARCIOFI ALLA ROMANA   artichokes stuffed with garlic and mint, cooked with oil over slow fire

CARCIOFI ALLA VENEZIANA   artichokes stewed in oil and white wine

CARCIOFI ARROSTITI   roasted artichokes with garlic, olive oil and parsley

CARCIOFI BOLLITI   hot or cold boiled artichokes served with a dressing

CARCIOFI CON MAIONESE   artichoke hearts with mayonnaise

CARCIOFI DORATI   artichokes dipped in egg and flour and fried

CARCIOFI E PISELLI   artichokes and peas

CARCIOFI FRITTI   fried artichokes

CARCIOFI IN PINZIMONIO   artichokes eaten raw with olive oil, herb sauce

CARCIOFI RIPIENI   cheese-stuffed artichokes

CARCIOFINO   small artichoke (see CARCIOFI)

CARCIOFO   artichoke (see CARCIOFI)

CARCIOFO RIPIENO   cold artichoke stuffed with marinated artichoke hearts, tomato, bread, lemon vinaigrette

CARDI   celery-like vegetable usually blanched, stalks and leaves eaten like celery

CARDI AL GRATIN   celery-like plant, with cheese

CARDI ALLA FIORENTINA   celery-like plant boiled for a short time then sautéed

CARDI ALLA PERUGINA   chopped chards boiled and dipped into a flour batter, fried in oil

CARDOONS   thistle-like plant, leaves and stalks eaten as celery (see CARDI)

CARNE   meat

CARNE ARROSTO   roast meat

CARNE ARROSTO CON PROSCIUTTO E SPINACI   roast meat, ham and spinach

CARNE CARRARGIU   meat spit-roasted in the open air on wood with scented herbs

CARNE CON FEGATINI E TARTUFI   beef, chicken livers and truffles

CARNE CON FUNGHI SECCHI   beef and dried mushrooms

CARNE CON MELANZANE   meat and eggplant

CARNE CRUDA   steak tartar, raw, finely-ground meat and garlic, anchovy, oil

CARNE DI MANZO   roast beef

CARNE DI PICCIONE   pigeon meat

CARNE DI SUINO   pork meat

CARNE FREDDA ASSORTITA   roasted and boiled assorted cold meats

CARNE TRA DUE PIATTI   meat steamed between two plates

CARNE TRITATA   minced beef and ham

CARNIA   hard provolone type cheese

CARO   dear, expensive

CAROTA   carrot

CAROTE AL MARSALA   carrots cooked with Marsala wine

CAROTE ALLA VICHY   carrots cooked in butter and
water, sugar-coated

CAROTE CON CAPPERI   carrots with capers

CARPA   carp

CARPACCIO   thinly-sliced raw beef fillet, usually served
with a piquant sauce

CARPIONATA   carp marinated in herb oil then fried

CARPIONE   carp fish

CARPIONE AL VINO   carp, pan-fried in wine, onion, vinegar

CARPIONE FRITTO   fish fried in oil then marinated in
vinegar, served cold

CARRELLO   from the food serving cart (your choice)

CARRELLO VARIO   assorted antipasti from a rolling cart

CARRETTIERA   sauce of tuna fish and mushrooms

CARTA DI MUSICA   white bread of thin, unleavened
layers, "music paper" put one on top of another

CARTEDDATE   honey-coated fried or baked pastries
made with wine

CARTOCCIO   roasted in a sealed bag

CASEATA GELATA   dessert with custard ice cream and
whipped cream

CASONCELLI   meat-stuffed pasta-like macaroni

CASONSEI DI BERGAMO   meat, herb and cheese stuffed
ravioli

CASSATA   ice cream cake with chocolate, custard and
almonds

CASSATA ALLA SICILIANA (DOLCE)   mould of ricotta
cheese, candied fruit, chocolate, flavored with vanilla
and maraschino cherries supported with spongecakes

CASSATA ALLA SICILIANA (GELATO)   ice cream made
in several different colored layers with candied fruit and
almonds

CASSATA ALLA SICILIANA   refrigerator cake with ricotta
cheese, candied fruit, chocolate, almonds, Marsala wine

CASSATELLA   chocolate icebox cake

CASSATINE   tarts (also see TORTA)

CASSATINE DI RICOTTA   baked ricotta cheese-filled tarts

CASSERUOLA   casserole

CASSIERE   cashier

CASSOEULA   pork feet, ears, lean meat sautéed in casserole with wine

CASSOLA   highly-spiced, very tasty fish stew

CASTAGNACCIO   chestnut flour tart with nuts, raisins, candied fruits

CASTAGNACCIO ALLA TOSCANA   chestnut cake

CASTAGNE   chestnuts

CASTAGNE AL MARSALA   chestnuts with Marsala wine

CASTAGNE ALLA ROMAGNOLA IN VINO ROSSO   chestnuts boiled in red wine

CASTAGNE STUFATE   chestnuts stewed in wine

CASTAGNOLE FRITTE   sweet lemon fritters

CASTELLANA   thin veal cutlet, filled, folded then fried

CASTELLANA AL MARSALA   thin veal cutlet filled with ham, cheese, breaded and fried in wine

CASTELLANA AL PROSCIUTTO   thin veal cutlet filled with ham, breaded, fried in brown sauce

CASTELLANA TARTUFATA   veal cutlet filled with ham, cheese, breaded, fried in white wine

CASTELLER   light red, slightly sweet wine

CASTELLI ROMANI   dry white wine from Rome

CASTRADINA   roast mutton

CASTRATO   castrated sheep *or* mutton

CATALOGNA   green salad leaf

CATTIVO   bad

CAVEDANO   chub

CAVIALE   caviar

CAVOLATA   pork and cauliflower soup

CAVOLFIORE   cauliflower

CAVOLFIORE AL POMODORO   cauliflower with tomato

CAVOLFIORE ALLA BESCIAMELLA   boiled cauliflower covered with white sauce, cheese and baked

CAVOLFIORE ALLA MILANESE   cauliflower breaded with cheese, fried

CAVOLFIORE DORATO   cauliflower, batter-coated and fried

CAVOLFIORE FRITTO IN PASTELLA AL PARMIGIANO
fried cauliflower with Parmesan cheese batter
CAVOLINO   brussel sprouts
CAVOLO   cabbage
CAVOLO ROSSO   red cabbage
CAVOLO STUFATO ALLA VENEZIANA   stuffed green
cabbage
CAVOLO VERDE   green cabbage
CAZZOEULA   casserole of pork, cabbage and spices
CECHINE   eels
CECI   chick-peas
CEFALO   gray mullet fish
CELESTINA   clear soup with little stars of pasta
CENA   dinner, supper
CENARE   to have supper
CENCI   fried cookies
CENETTA   a little supper
CENTERBE   liqueur used to aid digestion
CERASCELLA   cherry liqueur aperitif
CERASUOLO DI ABRUZZO   red wine with excellent flavor
CERFOGIO   parsley
CERNIA   grouper-type fish
CERTO   sure
CERTOSINO   yellow *or* green herb liqueur
CERTOSINO PANETTONE   Christmas fruit bread
CERVELLA   brains, usually veal
CERVELLA AI PISTACCHI   brains and pistachio nuts
CERVELLA AL BURRO   brains poached, floured, pan
fried in butter
CERVELLA AL TEGAMINO   diced brains dipped in flour
and egg batter, fried in butter
CERVELLA ALLA FINANZIERA   brains sliced, poached,
served with brown mushroom sauce
CERVELLA ALLA SALVIA   brains sautéed with butter
and sage
CERVELLA E ZUCCHINI   brains and zucchini breaded
and pan-fried

CERVELLA FRITTA CON CARCIOFI   brains and artichokes breaded and fried

CERVELLA FRITTA CON CARCIOFI E MOZZARELLA   brains with artichokes and mozzarella cheese, breaded and fried

CERVO   large wild-horned deer

CESSARE   to cease, stop

CESTINI   small cases of puff *or* flaky pastry with tasty fillings

CESTINO DI FRUTTA   large basket of fruit

CETRIOLI   cucumbers

CETRIOLI ALL'ACETO   pickled cucumbers

CETRIOLINI   small pickles

CHIANTI   red wine of Tuscany

CHIARETTO   famous rosé wine

CHIARETTO DEL GARDA   pink dry wine

CHIOCCIOLE   snails

CHIODO DI GAROFANO   cloves

CHIUSO   closed

CHIZZE   squares of pastry filled with anchovy or cheese

CI SONO   there are

CIALDE   wafers *or* cookies

CIALZON DI FRUTTA   turnover filled with assorted fruits, sprinkled with crystallized sugar and cinnamon

CIAMBELLA   ring-shaped bun

CIAMBELLA ALLA BOLOGNESE   fruit and nut cake made with wine

CIAMBELLA DI PASQUA   sweet Easter bread

CIAMBOTTA   vegetable stew

CIARAMICOLA   cake with liqueur, lemon rind, covered with meringue

CIBO   food

CICALA AL SALMORIGLIO   broiled lobster tail with olive oil, lemon juice and oregano

CICCIA   meat

CICCIOLI   fried pork sausage

CICERCHIATA   deep-fried honey cake balls

CICORIA   endive, chicory

CILIEGE AL BAROLO   cherries, sautéed in wine, sugar and cream

CILIEGIA   cherry

CIMA   cold, stuffed veal breast

CIMA ALLA GENOVESE   beef *or* veal stuffed with sweetbreads, pork, peas

CIMA DI MANZO   beef breast stuffed, cooked, sliced, served cold

CIMALINO DI MANZO   boiled stuffed beef breast and beans

CINGHIALE   wild boar

CINGHIALE ALLA CACCIATORA   boar with wine and vegetables

CINGHIALE ARROSTO   roast wild boar

CINGHIALE IN AGRODOLCE ALLA ROMANA   wild boar marinated with wine and spices, cooked in sweet-sour sauce

CINQUETERRE   delicately-flavored white wine

CIOCCOLATA   chocolate

CIOCIARA   sauce of fat bacon, ham and sausage

CIPOLLATA DI TONNO   tuna fish fried with sliced onions

CIPOLLE   onions

CIPOLLE AL POMODORO   onions stewed with tomatoes

CIPOLLE AL PROSCIUTTO E ROSMARINO   onions with ham and rosemary

CIPOLLE ALL'AGRODOLCE   onions cooked in sweet and sour tomato sauce

CIPOLLE CON PISELLI   button onions and peas

CIPOLLE DI NAPOLI   onions baked with oil and Marsala wine

CIPOLLE GLASSATE   onions sugar-coated and cooked in herb broth

CIPOLLINA   pearl onion

CIPOLLINE D'IVREA   pearl onions sautéed in herb wine

CIPOLLINE NOVELLE   green onions (scallions)

CIPOLLINE STUFATE E TOPINAMBUR   braised scallions and Jerusalem artichokes

CIRIOLE   little eels

CIRO   robust dry red wine good with meat and game

CIRO DI CALABRIA   dark red wine, lively flavor
CIUPPIN   thick fish stew *or* sauce
CLASSICO   wine from grape of controlled zone
COCKTAIL DI PESCE   fish cocktail
COCOMERO   watermelon
CODA ALLA VACCINARA   pieces of oxtail stewed in tomato sauce, seasoned with celery
CODA DI BUE   oxtail
CODA DI BUE ALLA CAVOUR   oxtail stew
CODA DI VITELLO AL FORNO   veal tail braised then oven roasted
COLAZIONE   a main meal (usually lunch)
COLTELLO   knife
COMPOSTA   stewed fruit
COMPOSTA DI FRUTTA   fruit compote
COMPRARE   to buy
CON   with
CONCHIGLIE   shells of pasta
CONCHIGLIE CON BACON, PISELLI E RICOTTA   pasta shells with bacon, peas and ricotta cheese
CONDIGLIONE   mixed salad
CONIGLIO   rabbit
CONIGLIO AI CAPPERI   braised marinated rabbit with wine, anchovy, onion, vinegar
CONIGLIO AL FORNO   rabbit baked in oven, with wine, onion, broth
CONIGLIO AL MARSALA   rabbit cooked in Marsala with onions, pimentos, tomatoes, eggplant
CONIGLIO ALL'AGRO   rabbit stewed in red wine and lemon juice
CONIGLIO ALL'AGRODOLCE   sweet-sour rabbit
CONIGLIO ALLA BORGHESE   rabbit sautéed in white wine, herbs, onions and mushrooms
CONIGLIO ALLA BUONGUSTAIO   rabbit with vegetables and Marsala wine
CONIGLIO ALLA CACCIATORA   rabbit braised in wine, mushrooms, tomato and garlic

CONIGLIO ALLA CAMPAGNOLA   rabbit with garlic, rosemary and wine

CONIGLIO ALLA FRIULANA   rabbit with egg and lemon sauce

CONIGLIO ALLA LIVORNESE   rabbit casserole with tomatoes and anchovies

CONIGLIO ALLA MOLISANA   grilled rabbit and sausage chunks

CONIGLIO ALLA ROMAGNOLA   pieces of rabbit breaded, batter-dipped then fried in butter

CONIGLIO CON POLENTA   rabbit braised in sauce and served on cornmeal mush

CONIGLIO FARCITO AL FORNO   rabbit stuffed and roasted

CONIGLIO FRITTO   rabbit fried in bacon fat and oil, with sage and garlic

CONIGLIO FRITTO ALLA LOMBARDA   rabbit dipped in egg and chopped herbs, then coated with bread crumbs and fried

CONIGLIO IN PADELLA   rabbit sautéed in oil with bacon, tomatoes, garlic, wine and parsley

CONIGLIO IN SALMÌ   rabbit marinated in wine, cooked with chopped vegetables, oil, wine and herbs

CONIGLIO IN SALSA CON UOVA   rabbit poached in sauce thickened with eggs and lemon juice

CONIGLIO IN SALSA PICCANTE   rabbit in spicy sauce with vegetables, wine, capers and anchovies

CONIGLIO IN UMIDO   rabbit stew

CONIGLIO IN UMIDO DI BERGAMO   rabbit stewed with basil, parsley, onion and vermouth

CONIGLIO RIPIENO AL FORNO   stuffed and roasted rabbit

CONIGLIO SELVATICO   wild rabbit

CONSOMMÉ   broth *or* clear soup (also see CREMA MINESTRA, MINESTRONE, ZUPPA)

CONSOMMÉ ALLA MADRILENA   jellied beef broth flavored with tomato juice

CONSOMMÉ ALLE MILLE FANTI   consommé with egg shreds

CONSOMMÉ BENSO   chicken broth gelatine with white truffles

CONSOMMÉ CALDO O FREDDO IN TAZZA   hot *or* cold consommé served in a cup

CONSOMMÉ CON PASSATELLI   consommé with pasta pieces

CONSOMMÉ CON PASTINA   consommé with very small pasta pieces added

CONSOMMÉ DI TARTARUGA   clear turtle soup

CONSOMMÉ DOPPIO   double strength consommé soup

CONSOMMÉ GELLÉ   jellied beef broth

CONSOMMÉ JULIENNE   consommé with small pieces of vegetables

CONSOMMÉ REALE   consommé with pastry garnish

CONSOMMÉ RISTRETTO   consommé cooked down for added strength

CONSUM   dough dumplings filled with sautéed greens

CONTENTO   content, happy

CONTO   count *or* restaurant check

CONTORNI   vegetables, side dishes

CONTORNO   garnish

CONTORNO DI CIPOLLE E FUNGHI   garnish of onions and mushrooms

CONTROFILETTO DI VITELLO AI FERRI   veal loin steak grilled

CONTRONOCE DI VITELLO AL FORNO   oven roast veal bottom round

CONTRONOCE DI VITELLO ALLA GENOVESE   veal bottom round braised in wine, mushroom, vegetable broth

COPATA   small wafer of honey and nuts

COPERTO   place setting

COPPA   kind of raw ham, usually smoked, sliced and served cold

COPPA DI FRUTTA   cup of fruit cocktail

COPPA DI GAMBERETTI   shrimp cocktail

COPPIETTE   small meatballs with ham, cheese, garlic, cheese, deep-fried

CORATELLA   lamb's heart, lung, liver and spleen cooked in olive oil, seasoned with pepper and onion

CORATELLA DI CAPRETTO   lung and intestines of kid

CORDA   long strips of tripe, either roasted or stewed in tomato sauce, with peas

CORNETTI   crescent rolls

CORONATA   dry white wine, sometimes verging on sweetness

CORTESE   dry white wine from Piedmont

CORTESE DI LIGURIA   dry white wine

CORVO BIANCO   dry white wine good with seafood

CORVO ROSSO   red, robust wine from Palermo, good with meat, rabbit, poultry

COSCE DI RANA   frogs' legs

COSCIA   leg, thigh

COSCIA DI VITELLO AL FORNO   oven-roasted leg of veal

COSCIOTTO   leg

COSCIOTTO DI AGNELLO   leg of lamb, usually roasted

COSCIOTTO DI CONIGLIO   rabbit leg braised in gravy

COSCIOTTO DI DAINO   leg of venison, usually roasted

COSCIOTTO DI PORCELLO AL FORNO   roast leg of young pig

COSTA   meat with bone in (see COSTOLETTA)

COSTA DI BUE ALLA FIORENTINA   bone-in steak, salted, coated with olive oil and charcoal-broiled

COSTA DI BUE ALLA MAITRE D'   bone-in steak grilled with seasoned butter and lemon juice sauce

COSTA DI BUE ALLA TIROLESE   bone-in steak, served with fried onions

COSTA DI CAPRETTO ALLA BRACE   broiled baby goat chops

COSTA DI CAPRETTO ALLA MILANESE   pan-fried breaded baby goat chops

COSTA DI MAIALE   pork chop

COSTAGELLA   meat with bone in (see COSTOLETTA)

COSTALLATA   meat with bone in (see COSTOLETTA)

COSTARELLE PANUNTELLA   pork chops grilled and
served over bread slices

COSTATA   meat with bone in (see COSTOLETTA)

COSTATA AL FINOCCHIO   pork chops pan-fried with
wine and herbs

COSTATA ALLA FIORENTINA   thick cut of beef grilled
over coal

COSTATA DI MANZO   beef rib steak

COSTATA DI MANZO AL BAROLO   marinated boned rib
of beef in red wine

COSTATA DI MANZO DISOSSATO   boned rib steak

COSTATA DI VITELLO   veal chop, bone in

COSTE   meat with bone in

COSTE DI BIETE SALTATE   sautéed Swiss chard stalks

COSTE DI MAIALE CON CARCIOFI   pork chops with
artichokes

COSTICINE DI MAIALE AI FERRI   grilled marinated
spareribs

COSTICINE DI MAIALE ALLA TREVIGIANA   pan-
roasted spareribs with garlic, sage and red wine

COSTOLA DI VITELLO   veal ribs with bone

COSTOLE DI AGNELLO ALLA MILANESE   lamb chops
breaded and pan-fried

COSTOLETTA   veal *or* pork cutlet with bone or chop

COSTOLETTA AL PROSCIUTTO   steak and ham slice
breaded, fried, then topped with melted cheese

COSTOLETTA AL SOAVE   steak braised in white wine

COSTOLETTA ALLA BOLOGNESE   breaded veal cutlet,
ham, cheese and tomato sauce

COSTOLETTA ALLA FIORENTINA   grilled steak in oil,
garlic, onion, herb sauce

COSTOLETTA ALLA MAITRE D'   steak grilled and
served with herb butter

COSTOLETTA ALLA MILANESE   veal cutlet, batter
dipped in bread crumbs and cheese, pan-fried in butter

COSTOLETTA ALLA PALERMITANA   grilled, breaded veal cutlets

COSTOLETTA ALLA PARMIGIANA   steak fried and covered with melted cheese

COSTOLETTA ALLA PETRONIANA   marinated veal chop, breaded and fried with onion, cream sauce and oven-browned

COSTOLETTA ALLA PIZZAIOLA   steak partially fried then sautéed in tomato sauce with garlic, herbs and oregano

COSTOLETTA ALLA SALVIA   steak braised in wine served with grated cheese and sage

COSTOLETTA ALLA TIROLESE   steak grilled in and served with onions

COSTOLETTA ALLA VALDOSTANA   veal chop stuffed with cheese

COSTOLETTA ALLA ZINGARA   steak pan fried in wine, mushrooms, butter, basil and pieces of pickled tongue

COSTOLETTA CARPIONATA   veal chop floured, fried, served cold in herbal vinegar

COSTOLETTA DI AGNELLO CON PEPERONI   baby lamb chop baked with sweet peppers

COSTOLETTA DI MAIALE AL VINO   pork chop braised with Marsala and red wine

COSTOLETTA DI MAIALE ALLA MODENESE   pork chop, braised with sage and tomatoes

COSTOLETTA DI MAIALE CON FUNGHI   braised pork chop with mushrooms

COSTOLETTA DI VITELLO ALLA MILANESE   veal cutlet breaded and fried

COSTOLETTA DI VITELLO PROFUMATA ALL'AGLIO E ROSMARINO   veal chop sautéed with garlic and rosemary

COSTOLETTA FRITTA COI FUNGHI   fried steak with mushrooms

COSTOLETTA RIPIENA   veal steak stuffed with seasoned chopped meat, floured and pan-fried

COSTOLETTA TRIFOLATA   pan-fried steak served with truffles

COSTOLETTE DI ABBACCHIO ALLA GRIGLIA   grilled lamb chops

COSTOLETTE DI MAIALE   pork chops

COSTOLETTE DI MAIALE ALLA MARCONI   pork chops stuffed with cheese and ham breaded and fried in oil

COSTOLETTINE   breast of chicken (also see POLLO)

COSTOLETTINE DI POLLO CON POMODORI E FUNGHI chicken breasts braised in tomato and mushroom sauce

COTECHINO   boiled spiced pork sausage

COTICHE   pork skin preserved in lard

COTOLETTA   meat without bone (as cutlet see COSTOLETTA)

COTOLETTA AL PROSCIUTTO   veal cutlet pan fried with slice of ham or bacon

COTOLETTA ALLA BOLOGNESE   veal cutlet with slices of ham and cheese, baked in oven and sprinkled with white wine

COTOLETTA ALLA MILANESE   veal cutlet, dipped in egg and bread crumbs, fried in olive oil

COTOLETTA ALLA VIENNESE   veal cutlet, dipped in egg and bread crumbs, baked in olive oil

COTOLETTA DI VITELLO   veal steak without bone

COTOLETTE ALLA CALABRESE   thin slices of meat, sautéed with olive oil, red peppers, garlic, tomato paste

COTTO   cooked

COTTO A PUNTINO   cooked medium

COURGETTES   zucchini

COZZE   mussels

COZZE ALLA MARINARA   mussel stew with garlic, pepper or ginger and gravy, in which there is some of the sea water taken up with the mussels themselves

COZZE CON RISO   mussels pan fried with tomatoes, rice, garlic, oil

COZZE E VONGOLE   baby clams and mussels

COZZE FRITTE   mussels breaded and deep-fried

COZZE GRATINATE   mussels with half of their shell removed, covered in oil, parsley, garlic and bread crumbs, then browned in oven

COZZE IMPEPATE   mussels highly flavored with pepper

COZZE PELOSE   mussels with hairy shells

CRAUTI   sauerkraut

CRAUTI CON SALUMI   pickled sauerkraut with sausage

CREMA   cream, cream soup *or* custard

CREMA CARAMELLA   custard topped with caramel sauce

CREMA CON CECI   pasta served with chick-peas

CREMA DI ASPARAGI   cream of asparagus soup

CREMA DI FAGIOLI   cream of haricot bean soup

CREMA DI FUNGHI   cream of mushroom soup

CREMA DI GALLINA   cream of chicken soup

CREMA DI MASCARPONE   soft cream cheese with rum and sugar added

CREMA DI ORZO   cream of barley soup

CREMA DI PISELLI   cream of green pea soup

CREMA DI POLLO   cream of chicken soup

CREMA DI POMODORO   cream of tomato soup

CREMA DI PORRI   cream of leek soup

CREMA DI RISO E ASPARAGI   cream of rice and asparagus soup

CREMA DI SEDANI   cream of celery soup

CREMA DI SPINACI   cream of spinach soup

CREMA DI VERDURE   cream of vegetable soup

CREMA FREDDA DI UVA NERA   chilled grape pudding

CREMA FRITTA   fried cream

CREMA PASTICCERA   custard cream sauce

CREMINO   soft cheese *or* type of ice cream bar

CREPES ALLA PIEMONTESE   pancakes with anchovy and truffle butter, glazed in brandy

CRESCENTE   savory bread, baked with ham or bacon bits

CRESCENTINE   eggless pie dough snack, eaten by itself or with salami or ham

CRESCIONE   watercress

CRESPOLINA   pancake filled with veal, grated cheese, baked in tomato sauce

CRESPOLINO   spinach-filled pancake baked in cheese sauce

CRISPELLE   pastry deep-fried then honey-coated

CROCCANTE DI MANDORLE   almond brittle

CROCCHETTA   potato *or* rice croquette

CROCCHETTA DI CARNE ARROSTITA   meatballs roasted in skewer with pork fat and toast

CROCCHETTA DI CERVELLA E ZUCCHINI FRITTI   croquettes of brains and zucchini, breaded and fried

CROCCHETTA DI PATATE   potato croquette with salami and cheese

CROCCHETTA DI POLLO   fried chicken croquette

CROCCHETTA DI RISO   rice croquette with cheese center, deep-fried

CROCCHETTE DI PATATE   potato croquettes

CROCCHETTE DI PATATE ALLA ROMAGNOLA   potato and ham croquettes

CROCHETTE DI POLLO   chicken croquettes, usually fried

CROCHETTE DI RISO   rice croquettes

CROSTACEO   shellfish

CROSTATA   pie *or* tart

CROSTATA DI CREMA   custard tart

CROSTATA DI VISCIOLE   sour cherry tart

CROSTINI   small pieces of toast, croutons

CROSTINI ALLA NAPOLETANA   small toast with anchovies and melted cheese

CROSTINI ALLA PROVATURA   slices of bread dipped in egg and put in oven with a slice of cheese melted on top

CROSTINI CON FEGATINI DI POLLO E PROSCIUTTO   toasts with chicken liver and ham

CROSTINI CON TARTUFI BIANCHI   rarebit with white truffle

CROSTINI DI MOZZARELLA   cheese toast

CROSTINI MARCHESE   toast with chicken liver

CROSTOLI   fried ribbon cookies

CRUDO   raw
CUCCHIAINO   teaspoon
CUCCHIAIO   tablespoon
CULATELLI   spicy ham, specialty of Parma
CULATELLO   type of raw ham cured in white wine
CULATELLO DI ZIBELLO   loin of pork dried in warm air
   and eaten raw
CULINGIONES   pasta stuffed with spinach and cheese
CUORE   heart
CUORE DI BUE   bull's heart
CUORE DI SEDANO   celery heart
CUORI DI CARCIOFI   artichoke hearts
CUSCINETTI   pasta dumplings stuffed with jam
CUSCINETTI PANDORATI   egg-fried bread stuffed with
   ham, anchovy, cheese, deep-fried
CUSCUSU   fish soup with macaroni
CUSCUSU DI TRAPANI   fish stew soup with semolina flakes
CUTTURIDDI   lamb stew flavored with rosemary

D

D.O.C.   Government regulated wine
DAINO   large wild horned deer
DATTERI DI MARE   mussels *or* small clams
DATTERI MARINATI   little shellfish in sauce of olive oil,
   vinegar, sage and garlic
DATTERO   date
DEL GIORNO   of the day
DELIZIOSO   delicious
DELLA CASA   chef's specialty
DENTICE   a flat Mediterranean fish
DI BUON'ORA   early
DIAVOLO   spicy tomato sauce
DIETA   diet
DINDO   turkey
DIVERSO   varied

DOLCE   sweet, soft, mild
DOLCE DI CASTAGNE   chestnut chocolate soufflé
DOLCE DI CASTAGNE E RISO   sweet chestnut and rice
    pudding
DOLCEACQUA   light red wine, slightly sweet
DOLCETTO DELLE LANGHE   red wine
DOLCI   pastries, cakes, sweets, desserts
DOLCI DI MELE   apple cakes
DOLCI DI TORINO   rich chocolate dessert
DOMANDA   question, request
DONNE   women
DOPPIO FORMAGGIO   sauce with more than the usual
    amount of cheese
DORATINI DI RICOTTA   cheese fritters served without
    sugar at beginning of meal, with sugar at end of meal
DURO   tough, hard

E

ECCELLENTE   excellent
ECCO   here is, there are
ENTRATA   entrance
ENTRECÔTE   boneless beef *or* veal steak
ENTRECÔTE ALLA BISMARK   boneless steak fried in
    butter and served with fried egg on top
ENTRECÔTE ALLA PIZZAIOLA   boneless steak fried in
    oil with garlic and tomato sauce
ENTRECÔTE ALLA TIROLESE   boneless steak fried and
    served with onions
ENTRECÔTE DI BUE   boneless beef steak
EPOMEO RED   dark red, mellow wine
EPOMEO WHITE   dry yellow wine, full-bodied
ERBAZZONE   spinach pie with onions, ham, cheese,
    garlic
ERBETTE   boiled Swiss chard
ERBETTE SALTATE   sautéed greens
EST! EST! EST!   semi-sweet white wine

F

FAGIANO   pheasant

FAGIANO ALLA CREMA   pheasant cooked in butter and cream with lemon juice

FAGIANO ALLA MILANESE   pheasant sautéed with liver, pork, beef, onions, wine

FAGIANO ARROSTO TARTUFATO   pheasant stuffed with truffles and roasted

FAGIANO CON FUNGHI   pheasant sautéed with mushrooms

FAGIANO DI CASSERUOLA   pheasant cooked in butter and cognac

FAGIANO TARTUFATO   pheasant stuffed with truffles and roasted

FAGIOLI   beans

FAGIOLI AL FORNO   baked white beans with tomatoes

FAGIOLI AL FORNO CON FUNGHI   baked white beans with tomatoes and mushrooms

FAGIOLI AL TONNO   French beans with tuna fish

FAGIOLI ALL'UCCELLETTO   white beans boiled with tomato sauce, garlic and herbs

FAGIOLI ALLA FIORENTINA   boiled white beans with olive oil

FAGIOLI CON COTICHE   beans cooked in tomato sauce with pork

FAGIOLI E CAVOLI ALLA GALLORESE   beans and cabbage

FAGIOLI FRESCHI   fresh kidney beans

FAGIOLI FRESCHI AL POMODORO   fresh beans cooked with tomato, onion and ham

FAGIOLI DI FIASCO   beans cooked in wine bottle over open fire

FAGIOLI LESSATI AL FORNO   beans first boiled then baked

FAGIOLI ROSSI   red kidney beans

FAGIOLI SGRANATI FRESCHI   fresh shelled and boiled beans

FAGIOLI TOSCANI   white beans boiled with olive oil, garlic and herbs

FAGIOLINI   green string beans

FAGIOLINI DI PADELLA   green beans sautéed with onion and tomatoes

FAGIOLINI RIFATTI   string beans first boiled then sautéed in tomato sauce

FAGIOLINI VERDI CON CAROTE STUFATI E MORTA-DELLA   smothered green beans and carrots with ham

FAGIOLO   haricot bean (see FAGIOLI)

FAGOTTINI DI POLLO E FUNGHI   chicken livers with mushrooms

FAGOTTINI DI RICOTTA E MOZZARELLA   chicken livers with ricotta and mozzarella cheese

FALERNO   dry yellow wine

FALERNO RED   dark red wine, dry but fruity flavor

FALERNO ROSSO   red, robust wine from Campania, good with cheese, beef, game

FARAONA   guinea hen

FARAONA AL CARTOCCIO   guinea hen sautéed then baked with herbs and liver, in a sealed bag

FARAONA AL COCCIO   guinea hen baked in a clay case

FARAONA ALL'ARANCIA   oven roasted guinea hen basted with orange juice

FARAONA ALL'OLIVA   guinea hen braised in oil, herbs and olive

FARAONA ALLA CAMPAGNOLA   guinea fowl sautéed with wine and vegetables

FARAONA ALLA CRETA   guinea hen baked in a layer of clay

FARAONA ALLA FIAMMA   guinea hen roasted over open fire

FARAONA ALLA PANNA   guinea hen baked in the oven in a paper case with sage, juniper and rosemary and served with hot cream

FARAONA ALLA PIEMONTESE   guinea hen stuffed with herbs, juniper berries, bread crumbs, liver, wine and baked

FARAONA ALLA TEGLIA   guinea hen cooked in an open earthenware pan

FARAONA ALLO SPIEDO   guinea hen roasted on a spit

FARAONA ARROSTO   roasted guinea fowl

FARAONA CON SALSA AI CAPPERI   guinea fowl cooked with a caper sauce

FARAONA IN SALMÌ   guinea hen cooked in wine and vegetable sauce

FARAONA INCROSTATA   guinea fowl pie

FARAONA O FAGIANO ARROSTO   roast marinated guinea hen or pheasant

FARAONA RIPIENA   stuffed guinea fowl

FARCITO   stuffed

FARFALLETTE   pasta shaped like butterflies

FARINATE   soup made with flour

FARMACIA   pharmacy

FARSUMAGRU   breast of veal or beef, stuffed with spices and hard-boiled eggs

FATTO IN CASA   homemade

FAVATA   beans stewed in lard with pork sausage and spice

FAVE   broad beans

FAVE AL GUANCIALE   broad beans steamed with onions and fat bacon

FAVE DEI MORTI   All Soul's Day cookies with almonds and pine nuts

FAVE DOLCI   "bean" size and shape almond cinnamon cookies

FAVE FRESCHE   fresh broad beans

FAVE FRESCHE STUFATE   braised broad beans with lettuce

FAVE STUFATE   broad beans sautéed with bacon, wine, onion

FAVETA   casserole of beans with bacon, sausage and seasoning

FAVETTE   rum cookies

FAVORE   favor

FEDERICO   braised turnip tops, sausages and spaghetti with olive oil and garlic

FEGATELLI ALLA FIORENTINA   pork liver breaded with garlic, fennel, sage and oven roasted in olive oil

FEGATELLI DI MAIALE   pork liver

FEGATINI DI MAIALE   pigs' livers, seasoned and roasted on a spit between two slices of bread

FEGATELLI DI POLLO AL MARSALA   chicken livers
  with Marsala wine
FEGATINI   chicken livers
FEGATINI DI MAIALE   pork liver braised in wine and
  onions with or without tomatoes
FEGATINI DI POLLO   sautéed chicken livers
FEGATINI DI POLLO AL CARCIOFI   chicken livers, arti-
  chokes, chopped ham, cooked in butter with chopped
  parsley and lemon juice
FEGATINI DI POLLO AL POMODORO   chicken livers
  and tomatoes
FEGATINI DI POLLO ALLA SALVIA   chicken livers with sage
FEGATINI DI POLLO CON FUNGHI FRESCHI   chicken
  livers with fresh mushrooms
FEGATINI DI POLLO CON SALSA ALLA BOLOGNESE
  chicken livers and Bolognese sauce
FEGATO   liver
FEGATO AL BURRO   liver, floured and pan fried in butter
FEGATO ALL'AGRODOLCE   liver, battered and fried,
  sweet and sour
FEGATO ALLA FIORENTINA   liver, floured and cooked
  in oil, garlic and tomatoes
FEGATO ALLA SALVIA   liver breaded and fried in butter
  and sage
FEGATO ALLA TOSCANA   broiled pork liver and bread
  chunks
FEGATO ALLA VENETA   liver sautéed in oil and onions
FEGATO ALLA VENEZIANA   calf's liver fried with onions
FEGATO DI LAME   liver slices
FEGATO DI LAMELLE   very thin slices of liver sautéed in
  butter
FEGATO DI OCA   goose liver
FEGATO DI VITELLO   calf's, veal liver
FEGATO DI VITELLO AL POMODORO   pan-fried calf's
  liver in tomato sauce
FEGATO DI VITELLO ALLA GRIGLIA   calf's liver steak,
  charcoal-grilled

FEGATO DI VOLATILI   various fowl livers

FEGATO PICCANTE   calf's liver with vinegar

FERMATA   stop

FERNET-BRANCA   a bitter digestive drink

FESA   round steak cut from leg fillet of veal

FESA AL FORNO   veal leg fillet baked in oven

FESA AL VINO BIANCO   roast veal slices served in wine sauce

FESA ARROSTO   veal leg fillet roasted in oven

FESA CON FUNGHI   veal leg fillet pot roast with mushrooms, peas, stock, herbs

FESA IN GELATINA   veal round steak in gelatin

FESA PRIMAVERILE   leg of veal larded with ham, carrot, celery and bacon

FETTINA   small slice

FETTINE CROCCANTI DI MELANZANA   crisp-fried eggplant slices

FETTINE DI MANZO ALLA PIZZAIOLA   beef slices pan fried with tomato, wine, garlic, oil

FETTINE DI MANZO FARCITE   pan-fried, stuffed thin beefsteaks with cheese and ham

FETTUCCINE   long, thin, narrow noodles

FETTUCCINE AL DOPPIO BURRO   fettuccine noodles with double butter

FETTUCCINE ALLA GOLOSA   fettuccine with creamy ham and mushroom sauce

FETTUCCINE ALLA PAPALINA   fettuccine with butter, ham, mushrooms and Parmesan cheese

FETTUCCINE ALLA RICOTTA   thin noodles with cheese

FETTUCCINE CON SALSA   fettuccine in tomato cheese sauce

FETTUCCINE CON ZUCCHINE FRITTE   noodles with fried zucchini

FETTUCCINE VERDI   green noodles made with spinach

FETTUCCINE VERDI ALLA BORAGGINE   green noodles with black butter

FETTUCCINE VERDI CON FUNGHI FRESCHI   green noodles with fresh mushrooms

FIADONE   baked cheese pie

FIAMMA   flamed usually with brandy

FIAMMIFERO   match

FIANO DI AVELLINO   delicate dry white wine good with seafood

FIASCO   a straw-covered flask

FICHI   figs

FICHI AL CIOCCOLATO   chocolate-covered, nut-stuffed figs

FICHI ALLO SCIROPPO   cooked, rum-soaked fresh figs

FICHI CON PROSCIUTTO   figs with prosciutto ham

FICO   fig (see FICHI)

FILETTI DI BACCALÀ   thin strips of codfish dipped in batter of flour and water, fried in boiling oil

FILETTI DI SOGLIOLA   sauce made with fillets of sole

FILETTI DI TACCHINO   slices of turkey breast with ham and cheese, baked in oven and sprinkled with white wine

FILETTO   fillet (see COSTOLETTA)

FILETTO DI BACCALÀ FRITTO   fried fillets of salt codfish

FILETTO DI BUE AL BAROLO   beef fillet with red wine

FILETTO DI BUE ALLA BISMARK   boneless steak grilled, served with fried egg

FILETTO DI BUE ALLA TARTARA   raw ground steak served with egg, onion, anchovy

FILETTO DI PESCE ALLA MILANESE   fish breaded with egg batter and fried

FILETTO DI TACCHINO   turkey breast meat

FILETTO DI TACCHINO AL MARSALA   turkey breast sautéed in wine

FILETTO DI VITELLO ALLA ROSSINI   butter-fried veal steak topped with liver and red wine

FINANCIERE SAUCE   bechamel sauce with Marsala wine and cheese

FINE   end

FINOCCHIO   fennel

FINOCCHIO ALLA CASALINGA   sautéed fennel home style

FINOCCHIO ALLA PARMIGIANA   fennel with cheese

FINOCCHIO IN PINZIMONIO   raw fennel dipped in herb olive oil

FINOCCHIONA ALLA TOSCANA   pork salami flavored with fennel

FINTA ZUPPA DI PESCE   fish soup sauce with olive oil, garlic, tomatoes, anchovies

FIORENTINA   herbs, oil and often spinach

FITASCETTA   baked onion bread ring

FLAMBÉ   flamed usually with brandy

FLUMMERI AL CIOCCOLATO   whipped chocolate pudding

FOCACCETTE FRITTE   cheese-filled pasta fritters

FOCACCIA   flat bread, with olive oil, onions or cheese

FOCACCIA ALLA MORTADELLA E PEPERONI   pizza bread, pork sausage, roasted peppers

FOCACCIA ALLA SALVIA   bread baked with sage

FOCACCIA COI CICCIOLI   flat bacon bread

FOCACCIA DOLCE   sweet ring-shaped cake

FOGLIE DI RAPA STRASCINATE   turnip tops sautéed in garlic and oil

FOIE GRAS DI POLLO   chicken liver pâté

FOIOLO   tripe (stomach lining of cow or calf)

FOIOLO AL SUGO   tripe braised in onion, tomato and herbs

FOIOLO ALLA BOLOGNESE   tripe braised in tomato sauce with wine, garlic, cheese

FOIOLO ALLA GENOVESE   tripe braised in tomato sauce with wine, garlic, cheese

FOIOLO ALLA MILANESE   tripe braised in onion, herbs, with wine, garlic, cheese

FONDI DI CARCIOFI   artichoke bottoms

FONDO DI CARCIOFO   artichoke heart

FONDUA ALLA PIEMONTESE   melted Fontina cheese with white truffles

FONDUTA - FONDUA   fondue melted with Fontina cheese, white truffle

FONDUTA   sauce of melted Fontina cheese, egg yolks, butter and milk flavored with white truffles

FONTINA   soft, creamy cheese used in cooking

FORASTERA   dry yellow wine
FORCHETTA   fork
FORMAGGI ASSORTITI   assorted cheeses
FORMAGGIO   cheese
FORMAGGIO ALL'ARGENTIERA   sweet cheese melted
   by pan frying
FORTE   hot, spicy, strong
FRACOSTA ALLA GRIGLIA   grilled rib steak
FRACOSTA DI BUE   bone-in rib steak
FRAGOLE   strawberries
FRAGOLE AL VINO   strawberries with wine
FRAGOLINE   wild strawberries
FRAGOLINE DI BOSCO   small wild strawberries
FRAGOLINE DI MARE   tiny squids "little sea strawberries"
FRAGOLONE   very large strawberries
FRAPPÉ   milk shake
FRASCATI   Roman white wine, dry
FRATTAGLIE   chicken giblets
FRECCIAROSSA   white, semi dry wine
FRECCIAROSSA RED   dark red wine
FRECCIAROSSA ROSÈ   pink dry wine
FRECCIAROSSA WHITE   dry white wine
FREDDO   cold
FREGOLATA   almond cookies
FREGULA   soup with semolina and saffron dumplings
FREISA   semi-sparkling red
FRESCO   cool, fresh, uncooked
FRETTA   hurry
FRICASSEA   a white veal stew with mushrooms, sauce
   thickened with egg yolks
FRICASSEA DI CONIGLIO   stew in wine sauce thickened
   with egg yolks, flavored with lemon
FRICASSEA DI POLLO   pieces of chicken poached in a
   cream sauce with onions and rosemary
FRICASSEA DI POLLO ALLA MARCHIGIANA   sautéed
   chicken with egg and lemon sauce
FRICO DI FRIULI   pan-fried eggs with pork and cheese

FRITOLE   spiced rum fritters

FRITTATA   egg pancake *or* omelette (also see OMELETTES)

FRITTATA AI CARCIOFI   omelette with artichoke hearts

FRITTATA AI FUNGHI   mushroom omelette

FRITTATA AI TARTUFI   omelette made with truffles

FRITTATA AL BASILICO   omelette flavored with basil

FRITTATA AL FORMAGGIO   cheese omelette

FRITTATA ALLA GENOVESE   spinach omelette

FRITTATA ALLA MOZZARELLA E CROSTINI   omelette
   with cheese and bread cubes

FRITTATA ALLA TRENTINA   fluffy omelette filled with
   either a sweet or savory mixture

FRITTATA ALLE CIPOLLE   open-faced omelette with
   onions

FRITTATA CON ARSELLE   omelette with mussels

FRITTATA CON ZOCCOLI   omelette with bacon chunks

FRITTATA DI MELE   apple omelette

FRITTATA DI PASTA   spaghetti omelette

FRITTATA DI PATATE   potato omelette

FRITTATA DI PATATINE FRITTE   open-faced omelette
   with pan-fried potatoes

FRITTATA DI PEPERONI E PATATE   pepper and potato
   omelette

FRITTATA DI PISELLI   omelette with onion, ham, peas, fennel

FRITTATA DI RICOTTA   omelette made with ricotta cheese

FRITTATA DI SPINACI AL FORNO   baked spinach omelette

FRITTATA DI ZUCCHINI   omelette with zucchini,
   chopped tomato, potato, rosemary

FRITTATA SEMPLICE   plain omelette

FRITTE ALLA PIEMONTESE   fried eggs on a bed of rice
   with grated cheese, tomatoes and sliced truffles

FRITTEDA ALLA PALERMITANA   vegetable casserole
   from Palermo

FRITTELLE   fritters *or* croquettes (also see CROCCHETTA)

FRITTELLE ALLA VALTELLINA   cheese fritters deep-fried

FRITTELLE CON SCIROPPO D'ACERO   pancakes with
   butter and maple syrup

FRITTELLE DI CARCIOFI   fritters of artichokes, fava
  beans and peas, fennel
FRITTELLE DI FRUTTA   fried fruit fritters
FRITTELLE DI MITILI   mussel fritters in batter
FRITTELLE DI PROSCIUTTO   fritters made from ham,
  cheese and cooked vegetables
FRITTELLE DI RICOTTA   deep-fried ricotta cheese balls
FRITTELLE DI RICOTTA DOLCE   pan-fried ricotta cheese
  sweet fritters
FRITTELLE DI SEGALA   little rolls of dark rye flour and
  egg, spiced and fried in olive oil
FRITTO   fried
FRITTO ALLA NAPOLETANA   fried fish, vegetables and
  cheese
FRITTO ALLA ROMANA   fried sweetbreads, artichokes
  and cauliflower
FRITTO DI FIORI DI ZUCCA   fried squash flowers
FRITTO DI MELANZANE FILANTI   eggplant slices with
  cheese filling, battered and deep-fried
FRITTO DI PESCE SPADA   swordfish pan fried in oil and
  lemon juice
FRITTO DI VERDURA   fried vegetables
FRITTO MISTO   fry of fish, cottage cheese, cauliflower,
  potatoes and sweetbreads
FRITTO MISTO DI PESCE   fried fish such as sole, octo-
  pus, shrimp, mullet and cod
FRITTO STECCO   veal, sweetbreads, brains and
  mushrooms dipped in egg yolk and bread crumbs
  and fried
FRITTURA   fritter
FRITTURA DI RICOTTA   fried fritters of ricotta cheese
  with almond macaroon flour
FRITTURA DI VITELLO PICCATA   veal cutlets breaded
  battered and fried
FRIZZANTE   semi-sparkling wine
FRUSTENGA   cornmeal fruit cake with figs
FRUTTA   fruit

FRUTTA CANDITA   crystallized oranges, tangerines, figs, or other fruits

FRUTTA COTTA   stewed fruit

FRUTTA FRESCA   fresh fruit

FRUTTA MARTURANA   almond paste baked in fruit shapes and colored

FRUTTA SCIROPPATA   fruit in syrup, usually canned

FRUTTI DI MARE   small shellfish

FUMARE   to smoke

FUNGHETTI ALLA GIUDIA   mushrooms in oil with garlic and parsley

FUNGHI   mushrooms

FUNGHI AL FUNGHETTO   mushrooms with garlic and herbs

FUNGHI ALLA GRIGLIA   grilled mushrooms

FUNGHI ARROSTO   grilled mushrooms seasoned with garlic, olive oil, parsley

FUNGHI COLTIVATI   button mushrooms

FUNGHI CON PISELLI   sauce of mushrooms, bacon and green peas

FUNGHI FRESCHI   fresh mushrooms

FUNGHI FRESCHI E PROSCIUTTO   fresh mushrooms and ham

FUNGHI FRITTI   mushrooms batter-dipped and deep-fried

FUNGHI FRITTI ALLA MODA DEI PORCINI   mushrooms dipped in egg, pepper, salt, bread crumbs and fried

FUNGHI IMBOTTITI   stuffed mushroom caps

FUNGHI PORCINI   wild mushrooms

FUNGHI PORCINI AL TEGAME   wild mushrooms sautéed in garlic and mint

FUNGHI PRATOLINI   field mushrooms

FUNGHI SECCHI   dried mushrooms

FUNGHI STUFATI   stewed mushrooms

FUNGHI TRIFOLATI ALLA FIORENTINA   sautéed thick slices of mushrooms and cucumbers

FUSILLI   pasta made as solid spiral coils

FUSILLI AI VEGETALI   corkscrew pasta, fresh vegetables, herbs

FUSILLI AL RAGÙ   macaroni in the form of long thin tubes, boiled and served with meat sauce and grated cheese

G

GABINETTO PER DONNE   ladies' room

GABINETTO PER UOMINI   men's room

GALANTINA DI CAPPONE   fine chopped capon loaf in meat gelatine

GALANTINA DI POLLO   fine chopped chicken loaf in meat gelatine

GALANTINA DI PROSCIUTTO   fine chopped ham loaf in meat gelatine

GALANTINA IN GELATINA   fine chopped meat loaf in meat gelatine

GALANTINA TARTUFATA   truffles in a meat-based gelatine

GALLINA   hen

GALLINA AL MIRTO   hen with myrtle leaves

GALLINACCIO   chanterelle mushroom

GALLINACCIO BRODETTATO   turkey cock stewed with wine, vegetables, herbs and served with a cream sauce thickened with egg yolks

GALLINELLA   water hen

GALLO CEDRONE   grouse

GAMBA   leg

GAMBELLARA   dry white wine

GAMBERETTI   very small shrimps

GAMBERETTI ALLA GRIGLIA   shrimps broiled in lemon juice

GAMBERI   shrimp (also SCAMPI)

GAMBERI AI FERRI E CANNOCCHIE   grilled shrimp, marinated in olive oil, salt and black pepper

GAMBERI ALLA PANNA   shrimps sautéed in cream

GAMBERI DI FIUME   freshwater crayfish

GAMBERI DORATI   shrimp fried in batter containing yeast

GAMBERO   crayfish, crawfish *or* prawns (see GAMBERI)
GAMBERONI   large prawns
GAROFOLATO   beef stew
GAROFOLATO AL SUGO IN UMIDO   potted beef with
   wine, herbs, onions
GATTINARA   red, full-bodied wine from Piedmont
GATTÒ DI PATATE   potato pudding
GELATERIA   place that makes and serves ice cream,
   pastries and coffee
GELATI MISTI   assortment of Italian ice creams and sorbets
GELATINA   a meat jelly
GELATINI DI CREMA   biscuit tortoni
GELATO   ice cream, iced dessert often with fresh fruit
GELATO AL COCOMERO   watermelon ice
GELATO AL TARTUFO   ice cream with chocolate sauce
GELATO ALL'UVA NERA   black grape ice cream
GELATO ALLA BANANA COL RUM   banana ice cream
   with rum
GELATO ALLA CREMA   custard cream ice cream
GELATO ALLA FRAGOLA   strawberry ice cream
GELATO ALLA NOCCIOLA   hazelnut ice cream
GELATO ALLA PRUGNA   prune ice cream
GENERALMENTE   ordinarily
GERMANO   mallard
GERMINUS   baked almond macaroons
GHEMME   red
GHIACCIATO   iced, chilled
GHIACCIO   ice cubes
GIACCA   jacket
GIALLETTI   fruited cornmeal cookies
GIAMBONETTE   boned chicken leg, stuffed with chicken,
   ham, cheese and fried
GIANCHETTI   tiny white boneless fish for antipasti
GIARDINIERA   diced, cooked or raw vegetable decoration
GINEPRO   juniper berry
GIRARROSTO   roasted on a spit
GIRELLO   round steak from the leg (also see FESA)

GIRELLO AL FORNO   roast of veal round steak

GIRELLO AL MADERA   roast of veal fried or braised in red wine

GIRELLO AL SOAVE   roast of veal fried or braised in white wine

GIRELLO ALLA GENOVESE   roast of veal served in cold olive oil, capers and anchovy

GIRELLO DI VITELLO   veal fillet steak roasted

GIRO   sweet red wine

GIÙ   down

GNOCCHI   potato dumplings boiled and served with meat sauce and grated cheese

GNOCCHI AL FORNO   potato-stuffed pasta baked in sauce

GNOCCHI AL PESTO   dumplings of dough boiled and served with pesto

GNOCCHI ALLA BAVA   potato dumplings with cheese

GNOCCHI ALLA FONTINA   dumplings of semolina, boiled in spiced milk with melted Fontina cheese, rolled in bread crumbs and fried

GNOCCHI ALLA GENOVESE   potato-stuffed pasta served in basil, garlic, pine nut, Pecorino cheese sauce

GNOCCHI ALLA PARMIGIANA   potato dumplings with Parmesan cheese

GNOCCHI ALLA PIEMONTESE   dumplings with Parmesan cheese, Emmenthal cheese and white truffle

GNOCCHI ALLA ROMANA   potato dumplings with Parmesan cheese

GNOCCHI DI LATTE   milk dumplings

GNOCCHI DI MAIS   dumplings of cornflour, served with tomato sauce and Parmesan cheese

GNOCCHI DI PATATE   potato dumplings

GNOCCHI DI POLENTA   baked pie of cornmeal, mushrooms, meat

GNOCCHI TENERI AL LATTE   pasta stuffed with cheese and baked

GNOCCHI VERDI   spinach and cheese-filled potato dumplings

GNUMMARIELLI   entrails of baby lamb, roasted on a spit

GORGONZOLA   creamy blue-veined salad cheese, tangy flavored

GOULASCH ALL'UNGHERESE   chunks of veal or beef braised in paprika sauce

GRAGNANO   full-red wine good with pasta and meat

GRANA   hard, tasty cheese

GRANA LODIGIANO   goat milk strong-flavored cheese

GRANATINA   fruit syrup on crushed ice

GRANCEOLA   sea crab

GRANCEOLA ALLA VENEZIANA   sea crab boiled in lemon juice, oil

GRANCHIO   crab (see GRANCEOLA)

GRANERESI   sauce of pounded walnuts, cream cheese and garlic

GRANITA   water ice crystals made with flavorings

GRANITA DI CAFFÉ   cold coffee poured over crushed ice

GRANITA DI CAFFÉ CON PANNA   coffee ice crystals served with whipped cream

GRANITA DI FRAGOLE E LAMPONI   strawberry *or* raspberry ice crystals

GRANITE   general term to describe sweets

GRANOTURCO   cornmeal (polenta)

GRAPPA   wine-type spirit distilled from grape mash

GRASSO   rich with fat or oil

GRATINATA   sprinkled with bread crumbs and cheese and oven-browned

GRATTUGIATO   grated

GRAZIE   thank you

GRECO   yellow, slightly sweet wine

GRECO DI TUFO   dry delicate white wine great with antipasti and fish

GRECO GERACE   yellow-amber wine, delicate orange blossom bouquet

GREMOLADA   sauce of lemon, oil, garlic, sage, parsley, served over cooked meat

GRIGNOLINO   red wine often with high alcoholic content

GRISSINI   dry bread sticks
GRIVE   little thrushes stewed with myrtle leaves
GROVIERA SVIZZERA   Swiss cheese
GRUVIERA   mild cheese with holes, like Swiss Gruyère
GUANCIALE   streaky bacon meat
GUASTO   out of order
GUAZZETTO   meat stew with garlic, rosemary, tomatoes
   and pimentos
GUSTO   taste

I

IMBROGLIATA D'UOVO AL POMODORO   scrambled
   eggs fried with bacon and tomato
IN BIANCO   poached in white wine, herbs and onions
   (usually fish)
IN UMIDO   stewed in broth with onions, carrots, toma-
   toes and herbs
INCANESTRATO   hard, salty cheese, usually grated
INCASCIATA   lasagna-type pasta with meat sauce, eggs
   and cheese
INCAVOLATA   bean and red cabbage soup
INDIVIA   chicory, endive
INDIVIA BELGA   Belgium endive
INDIVIA CRUDA   endive braised with garlic
INFERNO   deep red, soft-flavored wine
INSALATA   salad
INSALATA AI TARTUFI   green salad with truffles
INSALATA ALL'AMERICANA   shrimp, salad greens with
   mayonnaise
INSALATA ALLA SICILIANA   salad of tomato, bean,
   mushroom, peas with mayonnaise dressing
INSALATA CARICCIOSA   mixed vegetables with ham in
   mayonnaise sauce
INSALATA CONDIGLIONE   mixed salad
INSALATA CRUDITA   salad of mixed raw vegetables
   with sauce or mayonnaise

INSALATA DI ARANCIA   orange and cucumber salad

INSALATA DI ARINGHE   herring salad

INSALATA DI BORLOTTI E RADICCHIO   cranberry beans and endive salad

INSALATA DI CAMPO   lettuce salad

INSALATA DI CARNI   chopped-up meat salad with cold cooked vegetables and hard boiled eggs

INSALATA DI CAVOLFIORE   cauliflower salad

INSALATA DI CECI   chick-pea salad

INSALATA DI CIME DI RAPE ROSSE   red beet tops salad

INSALATA DI COMPOSTA COTTA   salad of cold cooked vegetables with sauce or mayonnaise

INSALATA DI FINNOCHIO   salad of fennel

INSALATA DI FONTINA   salad of cooked peppers, olives and cheese with cream sauce

INSALATA DI FRUTTI DI MARE   seafood salad, dressing of oil, lemon juice, mustard, garlic

INSALATA DI GAMBERETTI   shrimp salad in mayonnaise

INSALATA DI LATTUGA E GORGONZOLA   romaine lettuce with gorgonzola cheese and walnuts

INSALATA DI LENTICCHIE   lentil salad

INSALATA DI PATATE   potato salad

INSALATA DI PESCE   seafood salad with oil and lemon sauce

INSALATA DI POLLO   chicken salad with mayonnaise sauce

INSALATA DI POLLO ARROSTO   salad of roast chicken, mixed greens, chopped bacon, croutons, Parmesan cheese, vinaigrette

INSALATA DI RISO   salad of cold rice with vegetables and seafood, mayonnaise sauce

INSALATA DI SEDANI   cold salad of celery and truffles with mayonnaise

INSALATA DI SPAGHETTI   salad of cold spaghetti with anchovies, olives, olive oil

INSALATA DI SPINACI E TACCHINO   salad with spinach, tomato, bacon, roasted turkey, vinaigrette

INSALATA DI TONNO   tuna fish salad

INSALATA DI VERDURA   salad of green vegetables

INSALATA DI VERDURA COTTA salad of cooked green
vegetables

INSALATA DI VERZA CRUDA raw savoy cabbage salad

INSALATA MASCHERATA mixed salad with mayonnaise

INSALATA MISTA salad of mixed raw vegetables with
sauce or mayonnaise

INSALATA NOSTRANA local *or* home grown salad

INSALATA PANZELLA salad of fresh tomatoes, cucumbers, onions, bread, vinaigrette

INSALATA RUSSA salad with diced cooked vegetables,
hard eggs in mayonnaise dressing

INSALATA VIENNESE salad of tuna, eggs, onions,
cooked beans

INSALATINA TENERA CON PANCETTA salad of
smothered lettuce with bacon

INVECE instead

INVOLTINI stewed rolls of veal, stuffed with mince and
spices

INVOLTINI AL COGNAC stuffed veal rolls cooked in
butter then flamed in brandy

INVOLTINI AL GROVIERA veal rolls stuffed with
Gruyère cheese sautéed in butter

INVOLTINI ALLA MILANESE meat roll stuffed with
chicken livers, cheese, wine

INVOLTINI DI ASPARAGI E PROSCIUTTO asparagus
and cheese wrapped in ham slices

INVOLTINI DI BUE ALLA SICILIANA beef rolls filled
with parsley, ham, onion, nutmeg

INVOLTINI DI CAVOLO VERDE meat-filled cabbage
leaves cooked in sauce

INVOLTINI DI FAGIOLONI veal slices stuffed with ham
and cheese, sautéed with beans

INVOLTINI DI MAIALE AL FORNO stuffed, baked pork
rolls

INVOLTINI DI POLLO E PROSCIUTTO chicken and
ham slices, floured and pan fried in wine

IO BEVO I drink

IO DEVO   I must, I have to
IO POSSO   I can, I may, I am able to

K

KIRSCH   clear cherry brandy

L

L'INSALATA DI ARINGHE   herring salad
L'UFFICIO DI CAMBIO   exchange office
LACCETTI ALL'AGRODOLCE   sweetbreads in a sweet-
   sour sauce
LACIADITT   deep-fried apple fritters
LACRIMA   dark red wine
LACRYMA CHRISTI DEL VESUVIO   wine from Campania
LAGANELLE   pasta of small stuffed lasagne
LAGO DI CALDARO   red wine, delicate and pleasing
LAGREIN   dark red, sparkling wine
LAGREIN ROSATO   rosé wine
LAMBRUSCO   sparkling red wine
LAMPONE   raspberry
LAMPREDA   sea eel
LAPIS   pencil
LARDO   bacon
LARDO E FUNGHI   bacon and mushrooms
LASAGNE   pasta of broad noodles with tomato, meat
   sauce baked in oven
LASAGNE AI CARCIOFI   broad ribbon noodles with
   artichokes
LASAGNE AI FUNGHI E PROSCIUTTO   broad ribbon
   noodles with mushrooms and ham
LASAGNE AL FORNO   thin layers of macaroni dough
   alternating with others of ragout, butter, cheese and
   baked in oven
LASAGNE ALL'ANATRA   pasta sheets layered with duck
   ragout, bechamel sauce, baked in oven

LASAGNE ALLA BOLOGNESE   baked pasta with meat
sauce, mushrooms, cheese, bechamel sauce

LASAGNE ALLE OLIVE NERE, MALANZANE E
PEPERONI   lasagne with black olives, eggplant and
peppers

LASAGNE CON RICOTTA   baked pasta with tomato
paste, olive oil, wine, cheese, pork sausage

LASAGNE DI CARNEVALE   baked pasta with sausage
and meat sauce

LASAGNE IMBOTTITE   timbale of macaroni dough with
egg, in alternate layers with ragout, cheese, meatballs, baked

LASAGNE VERDI CON SALSA ALLA BOLOGNESE
green lasagne pasta with tomato, meat

LATTE   milk

LATTE AL CACAO   chocolate milk drink

LATTE ALLA PORTOGHESE   baked custard with liquid
caramel

LATTERIA   milk bar with sandwiches, coffee and pastries

LATTERINI   sand smelts fish

LATTUGA   lettuce

LATTUGA ROMANA   romaine lettuce

LAURO   bay leaf

LAVARE   to wash

LAVATOIO   lavatory

LEGGERO   light

LEGUME (see LEGUMI)   vegetable

LEGUMI   tuber vegetables like potatoes and onions

LEI   you (formal)

LENTICCHIA   lentil

LEPRE   hare

LEPRE AL BAROLO   hare stewed with red wine and
vegetables

LEPRE AL DOLCE-FORTE   hare marinated in wine,
onions, spices, with sauce of chocolate, candied fruits,
raisins and nuts added after cooking

LEPRE ALL'AGRODOLCE   marinated hare, pan fried in
wine, chocolate, herbs, onions

LEPRE ALLA CACCIATORA   hare with wine, sage, rosemary, garlic, olive oil and tomatoes

LEPRE ALLA CAMPAGNOLA   hare marinated in wine and herbs, cooked in casserole with wine

LEPRE ALLA TRENTINA   hare stewed in olive oil, garlic, onion and white wine, highly-seasoned

LEPRE IN SALMÌ   stew made with marinated hare

LEPRE IN UMIDO   hare casserole with mushrooms, vegetables, tomato, garlic and Marsala

LEPROTTO   young hare

LESSATI (also see BOLLITI)   boiled

LESSO   boiled meat

LESSONA   dry, full red wine good with rabbit and game

LIBRETTI   pizza folded double enclosing toppings, baked

LIMONATA   lemonade

LIMONE   lemon

LINGUA   tongue

LINGUA AL POMODORO   boiled tongue slices served in tomato sauce

LINGUA AL PROSCIUTTO E MADERA   boiled tongue slices with ham served in wine sauce

LINGUA ALL'AGRODOLCE   tongue in a sweet-sour sauce

LINGUA ALL'ESCARLATE   boiled tongue sliced, served cold

LINGUA ALLA FIAMMINGA   tongue braised in beer with onion, mushrooms, herbs and broth

LINGUA ALLA PARMIGIANA   boiled tongue slices with Parmesan cheese melted atop

LINGUA DI VITELLO   veal *or* calf's tongue boiled or corned

LINGUA DI VITELLO SALMISTRATA   marinated veal tongue

LINGUA IN SALSA VERDE   boiled tongue served cold in sauce of capers, anchovy, oil

LINGUA PICCANTE   spiced *or* pickled tongue

LINGUA SALMISTRATA   pickled beef tongue served cold

LINGUINE   flat noodles

LINGUINE GHIOTTE   pasta with zucchini and sausage

LIQUORE   liquor *or* brandy

LISCIO   straight *or* neat
LISTA DEL VINO   wine list
LO STRACOTTO   overcooked meat sauce
LOCOROTONDO   white, dry pleasant wine good with eggs and fish
LODIGIANO   kind of Parmesan cheese
LOMBATA   loin
LOMBATA DI MAIALE   pork loin, can be roasted or fried
LOMBATA DI VITELLO   veal loin
LOMBATA DI VITELLO AL CARBONE   large grilled veal chop
LOMBATINE   flattened veal cutlets
LOMBATINE ALLA PARMIGIANA   flattened veal cutlets pan fried with ham, cheese
LONZA   loin (usually pork)
LUCCIO   pike-type fish
LUCCIO ALLA MARINARA   pike sautéed in onion, carrot, herb and wine
LUCIANA   fish braised with oil, garlic, peppers, tomato and wine
LUGANA   good dry white wine
LUGANEGA   pork sausage made with Parmesan cheese
LUGANEGA E UOVA SODE   eggs and sausages
LUGANICA   long thin sausage
LUMACHE   boiled snails cooked in sauce of tomatoes and ginger
LUMACHE ALLA BORGOGNONA   snails stuffed with garlic and parsley butter
LUMACHE ALLA BOURGUIGNONNE   snails cooked in garlic butter
LUMACHE ALLA FRANCESE   snails filled with onion, carrot, celery, parsley, butter, garlic, bread crumbs and leeks, served in their shells
LUMACHE ALLA MILANESE   snails sautéed in garlic, oil, butter, anchovies, onions
LUMACHE ALLA PARIGINA   snails cooked in garlic butter

LUMACHE ALLA ROMANA   snails cooked in tomato, anchovy and garlic

LUMACHE ALLA VALDOSTANA   snails braised in oil, garlic, mushrooms, tomato and herbs

LUME   light

LUPO DI MARE   sea perch

M

MACCARELLO   mackerel-type fish

MACCHERONI   macaroni

MACCHERONI AI CARCIOFI   macaroni with artichokes

MACCHERONI AI GAMBERI   shelled prawns mixed in with macaroni

MACCHERONI AL FORNO   pie made of macaroni, filled with buffalo cheese and meatballs, then put in oven

MACCHERONI ALLA BOSCAIOLA   macaroni with mushrooms

MACCHERONI ALLA CALABRESE   macaroni served with garlic, hot pepper, cheese, tomatoes, ham, chili pepper

MACCHERONI ALLA CARRETTIERA   macaroni with sauce containing capers, olives, garlic, spices, olive oil and ginger

MACCHERONI ALLA CHITARRA   macaroni spread over an object resembling a "guitar" and cut into square strips

MACCHERONI ALLA CIOCIARA   macaroni with a sauce of bacon, ham and sausage

MACCHERONI ALLA TRAINIERA   macaroni with sauce containing capers, olives, garlic, spices, olive oil and ginger

MACCHERONI CON ALICI FRESCHE   macaroni with fresh anchovies

MACCHERONI CON PISELLI E PEPERONI   macaroni with peas and peppers

MACCHERONI CON RICOTTA   macaroni in a sauce or cream made of cottage cheese

MACCHERONI CON SAFFI   macaroni with asparagus, cream and ham

MACCHERONI CON SARDE   macaroni with sauce containing pine seeds, fennel, olive oil, chopped sardines

MACCHERONI GRATINATI AL PROSCIUTTO   macaroni with ham, bread crumbs and cheese

MACCHERONI NERI   macaroni with a sauce of garlic, oil and hot red peppers

MACEDONIA D'UVA BIANCA E NERA   bowl of white and black grapes

MACEDONIA DI FRUTTA   fruit salad

MACEDONIA DI LEGUMI   mixed cooked root vegetables

MAGGIORANA   marjoram, a mint-flavored herb

MAGRO   lean meat *or* vegetarian antipasti

MAIALE   pork

MAIALE AL LATTE   pork cooked in milk

MAIALE ALLA PIZZAIOLA   pork slices braised in tomato, garlic, oil, capers

MAIALE ALLO SPIEDO   spit-roast pig

MAIALE CON SPINACI   pork and spinach

MAIALE PICCANTE   spicy pork

MAIALE UBRIACO   pork cooked in red wine

MAIONESE   mayonnaise

MALATTIA   sickness

MALE   bad

MALFATTINI   very small egg pasta pieces boiled and served with cheese

MALLOREDDUS   dumplings of cornflour and saffron, with spiced sauce and sprinkled with grated goat cheese

MALTAGLIATI   small pasta tubes

MALVASIA BOSA   brilliant yellow wine with keen bouquet, slightly dry with bitter almond aftertaste

MALVASIA CAMPIDANO   golden yellow wine, pleasantly sharp with after taste of bitter almonds

MANCIA   tip

MANDARINO   mandarin orange *or* tangerine

MANDARINO FARCITO   frozen tangerine dessert with rum

MANDORLA   almond

MANDORLATO   made with almonds

MANFRIGUL   homemade egg barley

MANGO E FRAGOLE AL VINO BIANCO   mangoes and
strawberries steeped in white wine

MANICOTTI   wide pasta ribbons filled with ricotta
cheese, meat, herbs, tomato sauce, baked

MANTECATO   very fluffy air-filled ice cream

MANZO   beef

MANZO AL LIMONE   beef cooked in lemon juice

MANZO ALL'ACETO   beef pot roasted with vinegar and
capers

MANZO ALLA CERTOSINA   spicy pot roast

MANZO ALLA GENOVESE   beef braised with vegetables, wine, tomatoes

MANZO ALLA PIZZAIOLA   grilled steak served with
sauce of garlic, oil, tomato and herbs

MANZO ARROSTO   roast beef

MANZO BOLLITO   boiled beef

MANZO BRASATO   beef pot roasted with wine

MANZO CON CIPOLLE   beef braised with onions, oil,
butter and stock

MANZO LESSO   boiled beef

MANZO RIPIENO   stuffed beef

MANZO SALATO   corned beef

MANZO SALMISTRATO CON UOVA AFFOGATE
Italian corned beef hash with herbs, poached eggs,
polenta, cheese

MANZO STUFATO AL BAROLO   marinated beef in red
wine

MARINATO   marinated

MARITOZZO   soft roll

MARITOZZO FORNAIO ALLA ROMANA   buns baked
with raisins, pine nuts, orange peel

MARMELLATA   jam

MARMELLATA DI ARANCE   orange marmalade

MARRONE   chestnut

MARROWS   squash flowers

MARSALA   red dessert wine

MARSIONI small Adriatic fish
MARTINI brand of white and red vermouth
MARZEMINO full-bodied red good with beef or veal
MASCARPONE delicate cream cheese
MAZZACUOGNI very large prawns
MAZZAFEGATI sausages of pigs' liver, seasoned with
garlic, pepper, coriander, fried in olive oil
MAZZANCOLLE large prawns
MEDAGLIONE round fillet of beef *or* veal
MEDAGLIONE AL BAROLO beef pieces braised in wine
MEDAGLIONE AL MADERA beef steaks fried in red wine
MEDAGLIONE ALLA PROVINCIALE beef pieces fried
and served with brains, sweetbreads, broth and peas
MEDAGLIONE ALLA ZINGARA beef steaks fried in
sauce of onion, tomato and mushrooms
MEDAGLIONE PRIMAVERA beef steaks fried with
mushrooms, onions and tomato sauce
MELAGRANA pomegranate
MELANZANE eggplant
MELANZANE AI FERRI eggplant slices, grilled
MELANZANE AI FUNGETIELLI slices of eggplant
sautéed with tomatoes, oil, olives, capers, oregano
MELANZANE AL FUNGHETTO eggplant prepared like
mushrooms, chopped small, seasoned with garlic, oil,
parsley and pepper
MELANZANE ALL'AGRODOLCE eggplant in a sweet-
sour sauce
MELANZANE ALL'OLIO eggplant marinated in wine
vinegar, garlic, pepper
MELANZANE ALLA FIORENTINA eggplant slices
cooked in layers with cheese and tomatoes
MELANZANE ALLA LIGURE eggplant sautéed with
tomatoes and eggs
MELANZANE ALLA MARINARA marinated eggplant
with garlic and peppers
MELANZANE ALLA NAPOLETANA eggplant slices
layered with cheese, then baked

MELANZANE ALLA PARMIGIANA   eggplant cut into thin slices, dipped in oil, spices, buffalo cheese, tomato sauce, powdered with Parmesan cheese, browned slowly in oven

MELANZANE ALLA SARDA   eggplant baked with oil, tomatoes, garlic, basil, bread crumbs

MELANZANE E PEPERONI FRITTI   deep-fried eggplant and peppers

MELANZANE FARCITE   eggplant stuffed with tomato, anchovies, garlic, oil, parsley, baked in oven

MELANZANE GRATINATE   eggplant fried, pulp mixed with grated cheese, replaced and oven-baked

MELANZANE IMBOTTITE   eggplant stuffed with rice, cheese, parsley

MELANZANE RIPIENE   eggplant stuffed with anchovies, capers, olives and garlic

MELANZANE RIPIENE ALLA CALABRESE   eggplant stuffed with mince, onion, chopped basil, rice or bread crumbs, grated cheese, tomato sauce, baked in oven

MELANZANE RIPIENE ALLA ROMAGNA   fried eggplant alternating with slices of cheese, then oven-browned

MELANZANE RIPIENE ALLA SICILIANA   eggplant with chopped meat and tomato sauce, beaten egg and grated cheese

MELANZANINE CON MOZZARELLA   baby eggplants with mozzarella cheese

MELE   apples

MELE COTOGNE   sour quince apples

MELE RENETTE AL FORNO CON AMARETTI   baked apples with macaroons

MELONE   melon

MELONE COL PROSCIUTTO   melon with prosciutto ham

MENTA   mint

MENÙ TURISTICO   fixed price set for meal

MERINGA   meringue

MERINGA AL CHANTILLY   meringue shells filled with whipped cream

MERINGA AL GELATO   meringue shells filled with ice cream
MERLANO   whiting-type fish
MERLI   blackbirds
MERLOT   full dry red wine good with pasta, beef or veal
MERLOT DEL TRENTINO   dark red wine, sometimes pink
MERLUZZO   codfish
MESSICANI   stuffed veal scallops
MESSICANI ALLA MILANESE   veal rolls stuffed with
    meat, cheese, braised in wine sauce
MESSICANI ALLA VILLERECCIA   veal ribs stuffed with
    meat, cheese, braised in vegetable sauce
MESSICANI DI VITELLO   veal rolls stuffed with pork
    and cheese
MEZZA PORZIONE   half-portion
MEZZELUNE ALLE ERBE AMARE   half-moon ravioli,
    ricotta, bitter herbs, brown butter, sage
MI DISPIACE   I am sorry
MI PIACE   I like
MIASCIA TRAMEZZO   bread and grape cake
MICHETTE   sweet cakes, bread rolls
MIDOLLO   bone marrow
MIELE   honey
MIGLIACCIO ALLA NAPOLETANA   baked casserole of
    cornmeal, sausage, cheeses
MIGNESTRIS DE RIS VERT   rice cooked with spinach and
    other vegetables
MILLEFIORI   liqueur made from herbs and flowers
MILLEFOGLIE   custard slice
MINESTRA   soup (also see MINESTRINA AND MINE-
    STRONE, ZUPPA, CONSOMMÉ)
MINESTRA CON PASSATELLI   consommé with meat
    dumplings
MINESTRA DI CASTAGNE   chestnut soup
MINESTRA DI CECI   soup made with chick-peas
MINESTRA DI ERBE MARITATA   soup with chopped
    meat and greens
MINESTRA DI FAGIOLI   thick bean soup

MINESTRA DI FUNGHI   cream of mushroom soup
MINESTRA DI LENTICCHIE E BIETE   lentil soup with chard
MINESTRA DI PASTA E CECI   soup with pasta and chick-peas
MINESTRA DI PASTA GRATTATA   soup with grated
   pasta and cheese
MINESTRA DI PISELLI FRESCHI E CARCIOFI   soup of
   fresh peas and artichokes
MINESTRA DI POMODORO   tomato soup
MINESTRA DI RISO E FAGIOLI   rice and bean soup
MINESTRA DI RISO E SCAROLA   rice and escarole soup
MINESTRA DI SEDANI   thick celery rice soup
MINESTRA DI TRIPPA   tripe soup
MINESTRA IN BRODO   pasta *or* rice cooked in broth
MINESTRA PARADISO   soup of meat stock, eggs, bread
   crumbs and cheese
MINESTRINA DI BROCCOLI E MANFRIGUL   broccoli
   and barley soup
MINESTRINA DI MANZO   thin clear beef broth
MINESTRINA DI POLLO   thin clear chicken broth
MINESTRINA DOPPIA   double strength clear broth
MINESTRONE   thick vegetable broth with pieces of
   macaroni, seasoned with herbs and spices
MINESTRONE AL PESTO   vegetable soup with mush-
   rooms, garlic, cheese and pesto
MINESTRONE ALL'ABBRUZZESE   very thick soup of
   beans, vegetables, meat, lentil and cheese
MINESTRONE ALL'ITALIANA   vegetable soup with
   chopped ham
MINESTRONE ALLA FIORENTINA   vegetable soup with
   white beans
MINESTRONE ALLA GENOVESE   vegetable soup with
   spinach, basil, macaroni
MINESTRONE ALLA MILANESE   vegetable soup with
   rice, bacon, garlic and herbs
MINESTRONE ALLA NOVARESE   hearty vegetable soup
MINESTRONE ALLA TOSCANA   vegetable soup with
   white beans, chopped ham, rosemary

MINESTRONE DI ASTI vegetable soup with beans, pork, cheese

MINESTRONE DI FAGIOLI bean soup with tomatoes and celery

MINESTRONE DI PASTA vegetable soup with pasta included

MINESTRONE DI RISO vegetable soup with rice included

MINESTRONE ESTIVO vegetable stew soup made without water

MINESTRONE SEMIFREDDO vegetable soup with rice served cold

MINESTRONE VERDE vegetable soup with green beans

MINUICCHI pasta of small stuffed pockets

MIO my

MIRABELLA yellow plum

MIRTILLO blueberry *or* huckleberry

MISSOLTITT shad fish which are dried with bay leaves

MISTO mixed

MISTO NAVE mixed seafood antipasto

MITILI mussels

MODINO small, round fillet slices, usually veal or beef

MODINO AI SASSI small round fillet slices fried in wine and herbs

MODINO AL BURRO small round fillet slices fried in butter

MODINO AL SOAVE small round fillet slices fried in wine and herbs

MODINO ALLA PANNA small round fillet slices fried in cream sauce with onions

MODINO ALLA PIZZAIOLA small round fillet slices fried with tomatoes, garlic, oil

MOKA flavor of coffee

MOLECHE soft-shell crabs

MOLLE soft

MOLLETTE CON FUNGHI E FORMAGGIO soft-boiled eggs with grated cheese and mushrooms cooked in butter

MOLLICA sauce with bread crumbs and anchovies fried in oil

MOLTO much

MONTE BIANCO   chestnuts cooked and grated covered with chilled whipped cream

MONTEPULCIANO D'ABRUZZO   dark red wine, fruity and nutty

MONTEPULCIANO DEL PICENO   dark red dry wine

MONTONE   mutton

MONZETTE   snails (see LUMACHE)

MORA   blackberry *or* mulberry

MORMORA   flounder type fish

MORTADELLA   pork sausage made of pork fat, peppercorns and pistachio nuts

MORTADELLA CAMPOTOSTO   dry and spicy sausage, strong garlic flavor

MOSCARDINI   small squid

MOSCARDINO   small squid

MOSCATELLO, MOSCATO   dessert and table wine

MOSCATO DI CASTEGGIO   sweet, delicate, sparkling white wine

MOSCATO DI COSENZA   amber-yellow wine, sweet flavor

MOSCATO DI SIRACUSA   amber-yellow wine, subtle aroma, strong and generous, a rare wine slowly disappearing

MOSCATO GIALLO   white, full-flavored wine

MOSTACCIOLI   hard sweets made of flour and honey

MOSTARDA   sweet-sour pickle

MOZZARELLA   cheese made from whey

MOZZARELLA ALLA MILANESE   cheese slices battered with bread crumbs, deep-fried

MOZZARELLA ALLA ROMANA   cheese slices breaded and pan-fried

MOZZARELLA CON CROSTINI   bread and cheese pieces baked and served with butter and anchovies

MOZZARELLA CON POMODORI E ACCIUGHE   mozzarella cheese with tomatoes and anchovies

MOZZARELLA CON RICOTTA E PROSCIUTTO   mozzarella with ricotta and ham

MOZZARELLA CON UOVA E ACCIUGHE   mozzarella with egg, cheese and anchovies

MOZZARELLA DI BUFALA   pear-shaped mild buffalo
milk cheese
MOZZARELLA FRITTA   fried mozzarella cheese
MOZZARELLA IN CARROZZA   mozzarella cheese like
Welsh rarebit, made of buffalo cheese
MUSCOLETTI DI VITELLO CON FUNGHI   veal shank
stewed in wine, tomato, mushroom sauce
MUSCOLI   mussel type shellfish
MUSCOLI ARROSTO   mussels in half shell, breaded with
ham and cheese and baked
MUSCOLI GRATINATI   mussels in half shell braised in
wine and white sauce
MUSCOLO ALLA FIORENTINA   casserole of shin of
beef, wine, vegetables and herbs
MUSTACCIOLI DI ERICE   baked almond cookies
MUSTACCIOLI DI NATALE   Christmas spice cookies

N

NASELLO   whiting-type fish
NASELLO BIANCO   codfish *or* whiting poached in wine
and herbs
NASELLO BOLLITO   codfish *or* whiting stewed in herbs,
onion, olive oil
NATURALE   plain, without sauce or filling
NAVE   fish *or* seafood
NAVONE   yellow turnip
NEPITELLE   sweet Christmas pies
NESPOLA   a tart wild fruit
NIENTE   nothing
NOCCIOLA   hazelnut *or* filbert
NOCCIOLINI DI VITELLO IN BRODO   broth with veal
meatballs
NOCE   walnut
NOCE DI COCCO   coconut
NOCE DI SOTTOFILETTO   veal top round *or* roast veal
cutlet

NOCE DI VITELLO   best end of veal roast, roast or grilled
   sirloin of veal
NOCE MOSCATA   nutmeg
NODINI DI VITELLO AL SUGHETTO CON ACCIUGHE
   veal chops sautéed with anchovy sauce
NODINO DI MAIALE ALLA GRIGLIA   small grilled
   pork steaks
NON FUMARE   no smoking
NOSTRANO   local *or* home grown
NOVELLI   tomato sauce with anchovies and herbs
NOVELLO   first, new *or* young

O

OCA   goose
OCA ARROSTITA RIPIENA ALLA SALVIA E CIPOLLA
   goose roasted and stuffed with sage and onion
OCA ARROSTO AL FORNO   goose stuffed with sausage,
   herbs, chestnuts and bread crumbs and oven-roasted
OCA ARROSTO RIPIENA   stuffed roast goose
OCA IN SALMÌ   goose cooked with wine, herbs, vege-
   tables, mushrooms and truffles
OCCHIATE   flat sea bream-type fish
OGGI   today
OLIENA   vigorous dry red wine recommended with beef
   or rabbit
OLIO   oil
OLIO D'ARACHIDE   peanut oil
OLIO D'OLIVA   olive oil
OLIO DI SEMI   seed oil
OLIVE AGRODOLCI   olives in vinegar and sugar
OLIVE AL FORNO   olives wrapped in bacon and baked
OLIVE ALL'AGLIO   garlic black olives
OLIVE CONDITE CON CAPPERI   olives with capers
OLIVE NERE   black olives
OLIVE RIPIENE   olives stuffed with meat, cheese *or*
   pimento

OLIVE VERDI   green olives

OLIVETTE   small chunks of veal with olive-like appearance, cooked in white wine

OMBRELLO   umbrella

OMBRINA   fish

OMELETTE   fried whipped eggs (see FRITTATA)

OMELETTE ALLA CONTADINA   omelette with red onion, bacon, potatoes

OMELETTE ALLA FIAMMA   a fluffy, sweet omelette with jam, flambeed with brandy at the table

OMELETTE ALLA PIEMONTESE   omelette made with truffles

OMELETTE CON VERDURE   omelette with fresh seasonal vegetables

OMELETTE DI GAMBERETTI   shrimp omelette

OMELETTE DI PATATE E MAIALE   omelette filled with diced potato and lean pork

OMELETTE DI RISO   omelette with rice, Gruyère cheese and salami

ORATA   fish (like pompano)

ORATA AL CARTOCCIO   bream-type fish baked in bag with mussels, shrimp, mushrooms

ORATE AL LIMONE E MAGGIORANA   pan-roasted porgies with marjoram and lemon

ORECCHIETTE   pasta of semolina made into small shells

ORECCHIETTE AL POMODORO   pasta shells with sauce of tomato, garlic, oil, onion, basil, cheese, meat

ORIGANO   oregano

ORTAGGI   garden vegetables like carrots and cabbages

ORTOLANA   peas and artichokes

ORVIETO   white wine, dry or semi-dry

OSS DA MORD   anise-flavored buns

OSSIBUCHI ALLA MILANESE   veal shank braised with tomatoes and wine

OSSO   bone

OSSO DI PROSCIUTTO CON FAGIOLI   ham bone with white beans

OSSOBUCO   veal shank

OSSOBUCO AI FUNGHI   veal shank braised in
   mushroom gravy
OSSOBUCO AL VINO BIANCO   veal shank braised in
   white wine, garlic and herbs
OSSOBUCO ALLA GREMOLADA   veal shank breaded
   and fried with garlic, lemon, herb sauce
OSSOBUCO ALLA LOMBARDA   veal shank braised then
   floured and butter-fried, served with lemon juice
OSSOBUCO ALLA MILANESE   veal shank braised in
   wine, tomato sauce with lemon juice
OSSOBUCO CON PUREA   veal shank braised and served
   over pureed potatoes
OSTERIA   neighborhood restaurant bar
OSTREGHE   (Venetian) oysters
OSTRICA   mushroom sauce
OSTRICHE   oysters
OSTRICHE ALLA TARANTINA   baked fresh oysters
OTTIMO   very good
OVALINA   small mozzarella cheese from buffalo's milk

P

PAETA   young turkey
PAETA ARROSTO CON MELAGRANE   roast turkey with
   pomegranates
PAGARE   to pay
PAGARO   pompano-type fish
PAGLIA E FIENO CON GAMBERETTI   spinach and egg
   linguine, marinated grilled shrimp, garlic
PAGLIA E FIENO   called straw and hay, egg pasta and
   spinach pasta
PAGLIARINO   medium-soft cheese
PAGNOTTA   loaf of bread
PAGNOTTA CACCIATORE   game birds baked inside
   bread loaf
PAGNOTTINE BRUSCHE   bread baked with fine diced
   salami and cheese

PAIATA   hen turkey

PAIATA MALGARAGNO   turkey roasted and basted with drippings

PAILLARD   beef rib steak

PALLOTTOLINE   meatballs (see POLPETTA)

PALOMBA   wood pigeon

PALOMBACCE ALLO SPIEDO   wood pigeons roasted on a spit with various seasonings

PALOMBACCIO   wild pigeon

PALOMBO CON PISELLI   halibut with peas

PAN DEI SANTI   bread with lemon, raisins, almonds (Saint's Bread)

PAN DEMEI   anise-flavored buns

PAN DI GENOVA   almond cake

PAN DI RAMERINO   baked buns with raisins and rosemary

PAN DI SPAGNA   spongecake

PAN PEPATO   spicy nut bread cookies

PAN TOSTATO   toasted Italian bread

PANATA   bread soup with grated cheese and egg

PANCETTA   bacon salted and spiced then rolled, eaten raw

PANCETTA AFFUMICATA   bacon and egg

PANCOTTO   bread slices soaked in "soup" of tomatoes, bay leaves, garlic, oil, chili

PANDOLCE   heavy cake with dried fruit and pine kernels

PANDOLCE ALLA GENOVESE   baked sweet bread

PANDORATO   bread dipped in whipped egg and fried (French Toast)

PANDORO   golden bread

PANDORO DI VERONA   very light fluffy cake usually star-shaped

PANE   bread

PANE ALLA TIROLESE   confection of flour, eggs, butter, almonds, cinnamon and lemon peel

PANE CASARECCIO   homemade-style bread

PANE DI SEGALE   rye flour bread

PANE E COPERTO   a charge on the bill for bread and table setting

PANE GIALLO DI GRANO DURO   hard wheat bread
PANE INTEGRALE   whole wheat bread
PANE SCURO   dark bread
PANETTONE   tall light cake with raisins and crystallized fruit
PANFORTE   a hard cake of nuts, cocoa, spices, candied
   orange and lemon peel, melon and honey
PANFORTE DI SIENA   dry, nougat-like sweet made of
   almonds, candied fruits, spices, flour, butter and eggs
PANGRATTATO   bread crumbs
PANINI   various bread and rolls
PANINO   like a French hard roll
PANINO IMBOTTITO   sandwich made with hard roll
PANISCIA ALLA NOVARESE   rice cooked with
   vegetables and red wine added to vegetable soup
PANISSA   rice and bean dish with bacon, onion and tomato
PANNA   cream
PANNA ACIDA ALLE ERBE AROMATICHE   sour cream
   and herbs
PANNA MONTATA   whipped cream
PANNA MONTATA CON I CIALDONI   whipped cream
   served with wafers
PANZANELLA   tomatoes, cucumbers, green onions,
   bread, vinaigrette
PANZAROTTI   fried *or* baked meat filled dough envelopes
PANZENELLA   special bread dish made with olive oil,
   tomato, onion and French dressing
PANZEROTTI   ravioli filled with buffalo cheese, anchovies,
   eggs and butter, first fried and then browned in oven
PANZONI   pasta pillows stuffed with cheese, walnuts,
   basil, garlic
PAPAROT   spinach soup
PAPPA AL POMODORO   tomato soup with bread, herbs,
   olive oil
PAPPARDELLE   long, broad noodles
PAPPARDELLE AI CANTUNZEIN   yellow and green
   broad noodles with sweet peppers and sausage
PAPPARDELLE ALL'ANATRA   long broad noodles with duck

PAPPARDELLE ALL'ARETINA   duck cooked with red wine, tomatoes, herbs, served with wide ribbon pasta

PAPPARDELLE ALLA LEPRE   noodles with stew of hare giblets, well-seasoned

PAPRICHE   sweet peppers

PAPRICHE STUFATE   sweet peppers stewed in tomato, garlic, oil

PARMIGIANA DI MELANZANE   baked eggplant and Parmesan cheese casserole

PARMIGIANO   Parmesan cheese

PARMIGIANO REGGIANO   a hard strong-flavored cheese, generally grated

PARROZZO   baked almond and chocolate cake

PASSATELLI   pasta mixed with egg, cheese, bread crumbs, cooked in broth

PASSATELLI ALLA BOLOGNESE   pasta made with eggs, cheese, bread crumbs in cooked broth

PASSATELLI DI CARNE IN BRODO   meat dumpling soup

PASSATEMPI   small portions of seafood, pizza, vegetables, from pushcarts

PASSATO   puree *or* creamed

PASSATO DI LEGUMI   puree of vegetables

PASSATO DI LENTICCHIE   puree of lentils

PASSATO DI MARRONI   puree of chestnuts

PASSATO DI PATATE   puree of potatoes (mashed)

PASSATO DI PISELLI   puree of split peas

PASSATO DI VERDURA   mashed vegetable soup, with croutons

PASTA   dough made in various shapes

PASTA 'NCACIATA   pasta with cheese, eggplant, tomato, salami, hard eggs, garlic, oil

PASTA - AGNOLOTTI   pasta square filled with a savory meat stuffing

PASTA - ALL'UOVO   egg noodles

PASTA - BAVETTE   pasta one size larger than linguine

PASTA - BAVETTINE   next smallest of ribbon-like pasta

PASTA - BOMBOLOTTI   short smooth cylinders of pasta

PASTA - BUCATINI   smallest tubular pasta

PASTA - CANNELLONI   tubes of pasta filled with a savory meat stuffing

PASTA - CAPELLINI   very small cylindrical pasta

PASTA - CAPPELLETTI   discs of stuffed pasta, twisted into a small tricorn hat shape

PASTA - CONCHIGLIE   pasta shaped like seashells

PASTA - DENTI DI ELEFANTE   short and tubular pasta with a ribbed exterior

PASTA - FARFALLE   pasta like butterflies

PASTA - FEDELI, FEDELINI   cylindrical pasta, smaller than spaghetti

PASTA - FETTUCCINE   flat ribbon-like form of egg pasta

PASTA - FIOCCHETTI   small bows of pasta

PASTA - FISCHIETTI   smallest tubular pasta

PASTA - FUSILLI   twisted ribbon-like pasta

PASTA - LASAGNE SECCHE   largest of the flat ribbon-like pasta

PASTA - LINGUE DI PASSERO   smallest of flat ribbon-like pasta

PASTA - LINGUINE   pasta one size larger than bavettine

PASTA - LUMACHE   pasta shaped like snail shells

PASTA - MACCHERONCINI   small tubular pasta

PASTA - MACCHERONI   macaroni

PASTA - MACCHERONI CHITTARA   flat ribbon-like forms of egg pasta

PASTA - MALTAGLIATI   short and tubular pasta with a smooth exterior

PASTA - MEZZI RIGATONI   short and tubular pasta with a ribbed exterior

PASTA - MEZZI ZITI   large macaroni

PASTA - MILLE RIGHE   curved, elbow-like, and ribbed pasta

PASTA - MILLE RIGHE GRANDI   same as MILLE RIGHE, but larger

PASTA - PAPPARDELLE   flat ribbon-like forms of pasta uovo (with egg)

PASTA - PENNE   short and tubular pasta with a smooth exterior

PASTA - PERCIATELLI   small tubular pasta

PASTA - RAVIOLI   pasta squares stuffed with spinach and ricotta

PASTA - RIGATONI   biggest of the short tubular pasta

PASTA - ROTOLI   giant stuffed pasta tubes

PASTA - SECCA   hard pasta

PASTA - SPAGHETTI   cylindrical pasta, usually hard wheat

PASTA - SPAGHETTINI   cylindrical pasta, smaller than spaghetti

PASTA - TAGLIATELLE   flat ribbon-like form of egg pasta

PASTA - TAGLIERINI   flat ribbon-like form of egg pasta

PASTA - TAGLIOLINI   pasta one size larger than BAVETTE

PASTA - TORTELLINI   round stuffed pasta

PASTA - TORTIGLIONI   twisted ribbon-like pasta

PASTA - TRENETTE, LASAGNETTE   pasta larger than TAGLIOLINI

PASTA - VERDE   spinach and egg pasta

PASTA - VERMICELLI   pasta like spaghetti but bigger

PASTA - ZITI   very large macaroni

PASTA - ZITONI   largest of all macaroni

PASTA AL FORNO   partially cooked pasta, mixed with other ingredients and baked

PASTA ALLA FINOCCHIELLA   pasta boiled in fennel water served with cheese

PASTA AMMUDDICATA   pasta served with bread crumbs, anchovies, oil, chili

PASTA ASCIUTTA   any pasta not eaten in a broth or soup

PASTA ASCIUTTA ALLA CALABRESE   spaghetti or macaroni served with thick tomato sauce with ginger

PASTA CON SARDE   pasta with fennel, sardines, anchovy, onions, oil, pepper, raisins

PASTA CON SARDE ALLA PALERMITANA   pasta with sardines, anchovies, raisins, saffron, fennel

PASTA DEL GIORNO   pasta of the day

PASTA DELLA NONNA   pasta with spinach and ham

PASTA E FAGIOLI   pasta in a broth of beans, with onions, bacon and tomatoes, sprinkled with grated cheese

PASTA E FASOI   soup of beans and pork rind with pieces of pasta

PASTA E FASOI COL PISTELO DI PARSUTO   pasta with beans, cheese and ham bone

PASTA FREDDA   cold pasta salad

PASTA FROLLA   sweet pastry dough

PASTA GENOVESE CLASSICA   baked dessert from eggs, sugar, flour

PASTA GIALLA   pasta made with egg

PASTA IN BRODO   pasta in a soup

PASTA RIPIENA   pasta stuffed, then cooked

PASTICCERIA   cake and pastry shop

PASTICCINO   tart, cake, small pastry

PASTICCIO   pie *or* baked type of pasta like lasagne

PASTICCIO ALLA FERRARESE   pasta tubes with meat, mushroom sauce and bechamel sauce, oven-baked

PASTICCIO DI FAGIOLINI VERDI   green bean pudding

PASTICCIO DI FEGATO   chopped liver with pistachio nuts

PASTICCIO DI LASAGNE   lasagne with mozzarella, Bolognese sauce and mushrooms

PASTICCIO DI MACCHERONI   macaroni and chicken liver

PASTICCIO DI MACCHERONI E PICCIONI   macaroni and pigeon pie

PASTICCIO DI PATATE E SALSICCE   baked sausage and potato pie

PASTICCIO DI TACCHINO   turkey with a cream sauce in pastry

PASTIERA   short pastry containing filling of cottage cheese and candied fruit

PASTINA   small pasta in various shapes

PASTINA IN BRODO   pasta cooked and served in soup

PASTINE RUSTICHE   pie filled with ricotta cheese, eggs, citron, raisins, pine nuts, chocolate

PASTISSA DI MANZO AI FUNGHI   beef baked in pastry shell with gravy and mushrooms

PASTIZADA   beef pot roast
PASTIZADA ALLA VENETA   beef pot roast made with
   wine, onion, herbs
PASTO   meal
PATATE   potatoes
PATATE AL FORNO   potatoes baked with skin
PATATE ALLA BOSCAIOLA   potatoes baked with
   mushrooms
PATATE ALLA TRIESTINA   pan-fried, boiled potatoes
   with onion, pork fat, oil
PATATE ARROSTO   roasted potatoes
PATATE CON ACCIUGHE   pan-roasted potatoes with
   anchovies
PATATE FRITTE   deep-fried potatoes
PATATE GHIOTTE   stuffed and baked potatoes
PATATE IN PADELLA   potatoes fried in a pan
PATATE IN UMIDO   potato stew
PATATE LESSE   boiled potatoes
PATATE NOVELLE   new potatoes
PATATE NOVELLE AL FORNO   new potatoes baked with skin
PATATE NOVELLE ALLA PAESANA   new potatoes
   sliced, seasoned and baked
PATATE SALTATE   sliced and sautéed potatoes
PATATINE   small, new potatoes
PATÉ   finely ground meat *or* liver paste served cold
PATÉ D'OCA   fine ground goose liver loaf sliced and
   served cold
PATÉ DI FEGATO   fine liver paste usually served cold
PATÉ DI POLLO TARTUFATO   fine chicken liver with truffles
PEARA   peppery sauce for boiled meats
PECORA   sheep
PECORINO   hard strong-flavored cheese
PELLARO   red-pink wine, slightly dry
PENNA   feather, *also* feather pen
PENNE   short pasta tubes
PENNE AL SUGO DI CAVOLFIORE   pasta tubes with
   cauliflower, garlic and oil

PENNE ALL'ARRABBIATA   short, thick pasta with red hot sauce

PENNE ALLA RUSTICA   pasta tubes, fresh tomato sauce, pancetta, oregano

PENNE CON SPINACI E RICOTTA   pasta tubes with ricotta cheese and spinach sauce

PENNE CONTADINE ALLA GROSSETANA   pasta tubes with mushrooms and tomatoes

PEOCI   mussels

PEPATO   peppered

PEPE   pepper

PEPERONATA   sautéed sweet peppers, onions and tomatoes

PEPERONCINI   pickled small green peppers

PEPERONI   green *or* red sweet peppers

PEPERONI AL FORNO   sweet peppers baked in the oven with olive oil

PEPERONI AL GRATIN   peppers cut down the middle, stuffed with tomato, spices, anchovies and cheese, rolled in bread crumbs, baked in oven

PEPERONI AL GUANCIALE   sweet peppers pan-fried with onion, bacon, tomatoes

PEPERONI ARROSTITI   roasted sweet pepper

PEPERONI E CIPOLLE   pan-fried sweet peppers and onions with tomatoes, oil, basil

PEPERONI IMBOTTITI PICCANTI   stuffed sweet peppers

PEPERONI IN PADELLA   peppers pan fried with onions, herbs and tomatoes

PEPERONI RIPIENI   cheese stuffed peppers

PEPERONI STUFATI   stewed bell peppers

PER FAVORE   if you please

PERE   pears

PERE AL FORNO   baked pears

PERE CARAMELLATE   pears dipped in boiling sugar

PERE COTTE ALLA CREMA E CIOCCOLATO   cooked pears with custard cream sauce and chocolate

PERE COTTE BIANCHE/ROSSE   pears baked in white or red wine

PERE HELÈNE   pears poached in vanilla syrup served
with ice cream and chocolate sauce
PERICOLO   danger
PERLA DI VITELLO   braised veal with diced ham,
flavored with spices, herbs and onions
PERNICE   partridge
PERNICE AL FORNO   roast partridge
PERNICE ALLA SARDA   partridge served cold with
dressing of oil, vinegar, capers, parsley
PERNICE ARROSTO   partridge stuffed with bacon, juniper
berries, mushrooms, roasted and served on fried bread
PERNICE IN SALMÌ   partridge cooked in vegetable and
brandy sauce
PERNICI   partridges
PERNICI ALLE OLIVE   partridges pan-fried with wine,
ham, olives, oil, tomatoes, herbs
PERNICI IN SALSA D'ACETO   partridges pan-fried in
wine vinegar sauce
PERSICO   lake perch
PESCA   peach (also PESCHE)
PESCA AL BAROLO   peach baked in wine
PESCA ALLA PIEMONTESE   peach stuffed with maca-
roons and baked
PESCA MELBA   peach poached in syrup, vanilla ice-
cream, raspberry sauce
PESCANOCE   nectarine
PESCATRICE   angler fish
PESCE   fish
PESCE AI DUE PIATTI   fish steamed between two plates
PESCE AI FINOCCHI   fish with fennel
PESCE AI FINOCCHI FRESCHI   sea bass with fresh
fennel
PESCE AL CARTOCCIO   marinated fish baked in a bag
with seafood or anchovy sauce
PESCE AL FORNO   fish baked with potatoes and cheese
PESCE AL FORNO PICCANTE   baked marinated spiced
swordfish *or* tuna steak

PESCE AL TAGLIO IN SALSA   turbot fish with white wine and anchovy sauce

PESCE ALLA GRATELLA   grilled fish

PESCE AMMOLLICATO   small fish browned with bread crumbs

PESCE FRESCO   fresh fish

PESCE IN CARPIONE   fried fish marinated with onions in vinegar

PESCE MARINATO   marinated fish stew

PESCE PASSERA   flounder

PESCE PERSICO ALLA SALVIA   perch filets pan fried in oil and herbs

PESCE RIPIENO AL FORNO   fish stuffed with mushrooms, egg, anchovy, crumbs and baked

PESCE SPADA   swordfish

PESCE SPADA AL FORNO   swordfish baked in tomato sauce

PESCE SPADA AL LIMONE   swordfish steaks made with lemon and capers

PESCE SPADA AL SALMORIGLIO   swordfish with sauce of olive oil, lemon, oregano

PESCE TURCHINO AL FORNO CON PATATE   baked bluefish with potatoes, garlic, oil, parsley

PESCHE   peaches (see PESCA)

PESCHE RIPIENE   peaches stuffed with pumpkin, fruit and wine

PESCI   fish

PESTO   sauce of basil leaves, garlic, cheese, pine kernels and marjoram

PESTO ALLA GENOVESE   sauce with basil, garlic, pine nuts, cheese and olive oil

PESTRINGOLO   baked fruit cake with figs

PETITS PATÉS   little filled pastry cases

PETTICINI   breast of chicken (see PETTO DI POLLO)

PETTO   breast

PETTO D'ANITRA   breast of duck

PETTO DI POLLO   chicken breast

PETTO DI POLLO AI FUNGHI   chicken breast braised in
butter with mushrooms

PETTO DI POLLO AL BURRO   chicken breast floured,
fried in butter, then oven-braised

PETTO DI POLLO AL MARSALA   breast of chicken fried
in butter, flavored with Marsala and grated Parmesan

PETTO DI POLLO AL PROSCIUTTO   chicken breast pan
fried with ham and cheese covered and broiled

PETTO DI POLLO AL VINO BIANCO   chicken breast
floured, pan fried in wine and butter sauce

PETTO DI POLLO ALL'ARANCIA   chicken breast
sautéed in brown sauce with orange juice

PETTO DI POLLO ALLA BOLOGNESE   chicken breast
floured, pan fried with ham, cheese, butter

PETTO DI POLLO ALLA FIORENTINA   breast of chicken
fried in butter

PETTO DI POLLO ALLA GRIGLIA   grilled breast of chicken

PETTO DI POLLO ALLA MILANESE   chicken breast
floured, egg-battered, breaded and pan-fried

PETTO DI POLLO ALLA PANNA   chicken breast braised
in cream sauce with wine and herbs

PETTO DI POLLO ALLA PANNA E FUNGHI   chicken
breast braised in wine, cream sauce with mushrooms
and lemon juice

PETTO DI POLLO ALLA PARIGINA   chicken breast
braised in cream sauce with mushrooms

PETTO DI POLLO ALLA PRINCESSA   chicken breast pan
fried and served with fried egg

PETTO DI POLLO ALLA SOVRANA   breast of chicken
with artichokes and a cream sauce

PETTO DI POLLO ALLA VALDOSTANA   breast of
chicken cooked with slices of cheese, white truffles,
white wine and brandy

PETTO DI POLLO DORATO   chicken breast braised in oil

PETTO DI POLLO TONNATO   chicken breast, tuna sauce
with lemon and capers

PETTO DI TACCHINO   turkey breast

PETTO DI TACCHINO ALLA NAPOLETANA   turkey
breast baked with cheese and tomatoes

PEVERADA DI TREVISO   sauce of pork sausage, chicken
livers, onion, white wine, pickles, pepper

PEZZENTE   sausage of liver, lung and meat scraps, garlic,
pepper, smoked

PEZZO   piece

PIACENTINO   hard, peppery cheese, usually grated

PIADINA ALLA ROMAGNOLA   griddle-baked thin flat
bread

PIASTRA   grilled on steel sheet

PIATTI   dishes

PIATTI DA FARSI   plates prepared to order

PIATTI DEL GIORNO   dish of the day *or* main dish

PIATTI FREDDI   main meals served cold

PIATTI FREDDI DI ORTAGGI   cold mixed cooked vegetable dishes

PIATTI PRONTI   meals served quickly, precooked

PIATTO   plate

PIATTO DEL GIORNO   the day's specialty

PIATTO PRINCIPALE   main course

PICCAGGE AL PESTO E RICOTTA   broad ribbon noodles
with ricotta cheese pesto

PICCANTE   highly-seasoned

PICCATA   thin veal scallop

PICCATA AL MADERA   veal scallops pan-fried then
braised in red wine

PICCATA AL MARSALA   thin veal scallop braised in
Marsala sauce

PICCATA ALLA LOMBARDA   veal scallops pan-fried in
butter and lemon juice

PICCATA ALLEGRA   veal scallops pan-fried in butter
and lemon sauce

PICCATA CON CAPPERI   veal scallops pan-fried in
butter with capers and herbs

PICCATA DI FEGATO DI VITELLO AL LIMONE   sautéed
calf's liver, thin sliced with lemon juice

PICCATA DI VITELLO   pounded veal scallops floured and sautéed in lemon and wine

PICCATA DORATA   veal scallops egg-dipped, pan-fried in butter

PICCIONE   pigeon, squab

PICCIONE ALLA DIAVOLA   grilled deviled squabs

PICCIONE ALLA FIORENTINA   pigeon stuffed and braised in a wine, mushroom casserole

PICCIONE IN CASSERUOLA   pigeon braised in a wine, mushroom casserole

PICCIONE IN SALMÌ   pigeon stewed in wine vinegar sauce with oil, garlic, anchovy

PICCIONI SELVATICI   wood pigeons

PICCOLO   small, little

PICONI   baked turnovers filled with ricotta cheese

PIEDE   foot

PIENO   full-bodied

PIGNOLI   pine kernels

PINCIGRASSI   dish made of layers of macaroni dough, separated by layers of ragout, cheese, bechamel and tiny meatballs, browned in oven

PINOCCHIATE   pine kernel and almond cake

PINOCCHIO   pine nuts

PINOT BIANCO   white wine, slightly sharp flavor

PINZIMONIO   raw vegetable dressing of oil, salt and pepper

PISCI OVO   egg fritters with cheese, garlic, bread crumbs

PISELLI   peas (also PISELLO)

PISELLI AL GUANCIALE   peas stewed with onions, ham or bacon

PISELLI AL PROSCIUTTO   peas with ham

PISELLI AL SUGO DI CARNE   peas and brown sauce

PISELLI ALL'UCCELLETTO   peas cooked in herb tomato sauce

PISELLI ALL'USO SARDO   peas baked with eggs, onion, cheese, bread crumbs soaked in milk

PISELLI ALLA FIORENTINA   peas cooked with ham, onions, herbs, tomato sauce

PISELLI ALLA TOSCANA   peas cooked with onion, ham, herbs and tomato sauce

PISELLI CON PASTA   pasta with peas

PISELLI CON PEPERONI   peas and sweet peppers

PISELLI NOVELLI   young fresh peas

PISTACCHI   pistachio nuts

PIVIERE   plover bird

PIZZA   flat, baked open pie, bread dough bottom, variety of toppings

PIZZA AI CECINIELLE   baked pizza with small fish

PIZZA AI FUNGHI   baked pizza with mushrooms

PIZZA AL FORMAGGIO   cheese pizza

PIZZA ALL'AGLIO E OLIO   baked pizza with garlic and olive oil

PIZZA ALL'AGLIO, OLIO E POMODORO   baked pizza with garlic, olive oil and tomatoes

PIZZA ALLA CALABRESE   pizza dough sandwich enclosing tuna, anchovies, olives, capers, then baked

PIZZA ALLA MARINARA   pizza with tomato, garlic, olive oil

PIZZA ALLA NAPOLETANA   light, leavened dough onto which is spread olive oil, buffalo cheese, anchovies, marjoram and tomato sauce, baked in oven, served very hot

PIZZA ALLA ROMANA   baked pizza with cheese, basil, oil

PIZZA ALLA SICILIANA   baked pizza with tomatoes, anchovy, capers, olives

PIZZA ALLE COZZE   baked pizza with mussels

PIZZA ALLE QUATTRO STAGIONI   baked pizza in 4 sections with shrimp, anchovy, squid, tomatoes, cheese

PIZZA ALLE VONGOLE   baked pizza with clams

PIZZA BIANCA ALLA ROMANA   pizza with mozzarella, olive oil, anchovies and Parmesan

PIZZA CON LUGANEGA   pizza with tomato sauce, mozzarella, sausage, roasted peppers, oregano

PIZZA D'UOVA E CIPOLLE   baked pizza with onions, hard eggs

PIZZA DI PASQUA   bread dough without yeast (Easter Cake)

PIZZA DI SAN VITO   baked pizza with tomato, onion, sardines, caciocavallo cheese, oil

PIZZA DI SCAROLA   escarole pie

PIZZA DOLCE   ricotta pie

PIZZA FINOCCHIONA   pizza topped with tomato sauce, mozzarella, fennel, salami, roasted peppers, oregano

PIZZA INCHIUSA   pizza dough sandwich enclosing pork renderings then baked

PIZZA LIEVITATA CON LE VERDURE   baked vegetable pizza with garlic, capers, olive oil

PIZZA MARGHERITA   pizza with tomato, mozzarella, olive oil and Parmesan

PIZZA RUSTICA   pie made of macaroni dough filled with green vegetables, cottage cheese, sausage, baked in oven

PIZZAIOLA   tomato sauce with garlic, hot peppers, olive oil and parsley

PIZZERIA   eating place that makes and serves pizza, sandwiches and drinks

PIZZETTA   small pizza

PIZZETTA AL GORGONZOLA   baked cheese biscuits

PIZZETTA ALLA PAPALINA   pizza topped with eggs, bacon, asparagus

PIZZOCCHERI   buckwheat noodles with Swiss chard and potatoes

PIÙ   more

POLASTRO IN TEGLIA   chicken casserole with onion, wine, tomato, mushrooms

POLCEVERA   pale white, tending to sweetness

POLENTA   baked, thick, cornmeal porridge

POLENTA ALLA LODIGIANA   cooked cornmeal slices with Gruyère cheese, battered, pan-fried

POLENTA ALLA SARDA   cornmeal mixed with parsley, basil, tomatoes, sausages, pecorino cheese

POLENTA CON SALSICCE   cornmeal porridge and sausages

POLENTA CON STUFATINO   cornmeal baked with sausage, cheese, chili

POLENTA E OSEI   small roast birds served on polenta

POLENTA E UCCELLETTI   spit-roasted birds served on cornmeal

POLENTA E UCCELLI   small birds spit-roasted with dumplings

POLENTA OROPA   cornmeal porridge with cheeses

POLENTA PASTICCIATA   dumpling with meat sauce, mushrooms, butter and cheese

POLENTA PASTICCIATA AI FUNGHI   baked cornmeal porridge with mushrooms

POLENTA STUFATA   cornmeal baked with sausage, cheese, tomato, chili

POLENTA TARAGNA   cooked cornmeal with cheese

POLLAME   fowl

POLLASTRA   hen

POLLASTRO   chicken (also see POLLO)

POLLO   chicken (also see PETTO DI POLLO)

POLLO AI FUNGHI   pieces of chicken sautéed in butter with mushrooms and tomato sauce

POLLO AI PEPERONI   chicken cooked with pimentos, tomatoes, white wine, herbs and onions

POLLO AI TARTUFI   chicken and truffles

POLLO AL CHIANTI   chicken braised in red wine, onion and herbs

POLLO AL COCCIO   chicken baked in a clay case

POLLO AL DIAVOLO   grilled chicken

POLLO AL FORNO   baked *or* roast chicken

POLLO AL GIAMBONETTE   boned chicken stuffed with ham, bacon, garlic, cheese, herbs, then fried

POLLO AL GIRARROSTO   chicken roasted on a spit

POLLO AL LATTE   chicken cooked in milk

POLLO AL LIMONE   chicken cooked in lemon juice

POLLO AL MARCUGO   chicken fried in oil and butter with tomato sauce and mushrooms

POLLO AL POMODORO   chicken and tomato

POLLO AL POTACCHIO   chicken sautéed in wine, onion, garlic, tomato sauce, with chili powder

POLLO AL PROSCIUTTO   chicken and ham

POLLO AL ROSMARINO   chicken roasted with rosemary and other spices

POLLO AL TARTUFO E COGNAC   chicken with brandy, truffle and cream

POLLO AL TEGAME CON LIMONE   pan-roasted chicken with lemon juice

POLLO AL VINO BIANCO   chicken in white wine

POLLO AL VINO ROSSO   chicken in red wine

POLLO ALL'ABRUZZESE   chicken sautéed with onion, tomato, peppers

POLLO ALL'ARANCIO   chicken roasted or braised in orange juice

POLLO ALL'ARRABBIATA   chicken sautéed in wine, tomatoes, chili powder

POLLO ALL'INDIANA   chicken curry with spices and curry powder

POLLO ALLA CACCIATORA   chicken with tomatoes and hot peppers

POLLO ALLA DIAVOLA   chicken roasted and sprinkled with lemon juice

POLLO ALLA FINANZIERA   stew made of chicken giblets, with sweetbreads, mushrooms and truffles, cooked in a thick meat or tomato sauce

POLLO ALLA FIORENTINA   chicken with mushrooms, olive oil, bacon, onion, white wine, tomatoes

POLLO ALLA GHIOTTONA   pieces of chicken sautéed in butter with white wine, milk and tomatoes

POLLO ALLA LIVORNESE   chicken poached in a casserole with broth, butter, parsley and lemon juice

POLLO ALLA MACERATESE   chicken sautéed in broth with lemon, egg yolks

POLLO ALLA MARENGO   chicken sautéed in brown mushroom sauce with truffles

POLLO ALLA MARESCIALLA   boneless fried chicken, pan fried in butter

POLLO ALLA MONTANARA   chicken braised in olive oil with garlic, onion, brandy and broth

POLLO ALLA NAPOLETANA   chicken jointed and cooked slowly with mushrooms, onions, garlic, tomato and wine

POLLO ALLA PADOVANA   chicken roasted on the spit and highly spiced

POLLO ALLA PORCHETTA   chicken stuffed with ham, garlic and fennel

POLLO ALLA ROMANA   chicken sautéed in pork and bacon fat with garlic, wine and tomato paste

POLLO ALLA SICILIANA   chicken sautéed in onion, butter with vegetables and Marsala wine

POLLO ALLA ZINGARA   chicken baked in a clay case

POLLO ALLO SPIEDO   chicken broiled on a spit

POLLO ARROSTITO ALLA GENOVESE   chicken stuffed with its giblets, onion, celery, herbs, bread crumbs, butter and roasted

POLLO ARROSTO   roasted chicken

POLLO BOLLITO   boiled chicken

POLLO FARCITO TARTUFATO   roasted chicken stuffed with spinach, ham, cheese, truffles

POLLO FRITTO ALLA FIORENTINA   chicken fried in olive oil with lemon pieces added

POLLO FRITTO ALLA TOSCANA   fried egg batter-dipped chicken with lemon juice added

POLLO IMBOTTITO   stuffed and roasted chicken

POLLO IN BELLAVISTA   roasted chicken served on fried bread with cooked vegetables

POLLO IN BIANCO   pieces of chicken sautéed with onions, celery, herbs

POLLO IN CASSERUOLA   chicken cooked in a casserole

POLLO IN PADELLA ALLE ERBETTE   chicken fried with herbs

POLLO IN SALSA PICCANTE   pieces of chicken cooked with oil, garlic, white wine, vinegar, black olives and chopped anchovy

POLLO IN SUPREMA GELATINA   chicken breast in aspic jelly

POLLO IN TEGLIA   chicken baked in a shallow earthenware pan

POLLO IN UMIDO   chicken stewed in broth with onion, tomato, carrot and herbs

POLLO IN UMIDO COL CAVOLO NERO   chicken fricassee with red cabbage

POLLO LESSO   chicken boiled in vegetable broth

POLLO NOVELLO   spring chicken

POLLO PICCANTE   spicy chicken

POLLO RIPIENO   stuffed boned chicken

POLLO RUSPANTE   chicken farm-grown *or* free-ranging

POLLO SCHIACCIATO   chicken grilled with bacon

POLLO AI SOTT'ACETI   roasted chicken served with vinegar, pickles and onion

POLLO SPEZZATO CON LE MELANZANE   chicken braised in wine, tomatoes, herbs, eggplants

POLMONE DI VITELLO   calves' lung

POLPETTA   meatball

POLPETTE AI CAPPERI   meatballs with capers

POLPETTE AL SUGO   meatballs stuffed with cheese, deep-fried and served with tomato sauce

POLPETTE CASSARECCE   meatballs cooked and served in tomato sauce

POLPETTE COI FAGIOLI   meatballs served with boiled white beans

POLPETTE DI CARNE   meatballs in sauce with tomato, onion, cheese

POLPETTE DI GNOCCHI   dumplings stuffed with chopped meat or vegetables

POLPETTE DI MAIALE AL PITAGGIO   pan-fried pork meatballs with vegetables

POLPETTE DI MANZO   beef meatballs cooked in gravy

POLPETTE IN BRODO   meatball and pasta soup

POLPETTE INVERNALI CON LA VERZA   meatballs with savoy cabbage

POLPETTINE   meat patties (see POLPETTA)

POLPETTINE DI MELANZANE   fried eggplant patties

POLPETTINE DI POLENTA   cornmeal croquettes

POLPETTONE   loaf of beef, veal, or vegetables.

POLPETTONE DI BIETOLE ALLA GENOVESE   cornmeal, Swiss chard and mushroom pudding

POLPETTONE DI FAGIOLINI ALLA GENOVESE   green beans and potato pie, in a batter of cheese, eggs and marjoram

POLPETTONE DI POLLO E VITELLO   chopped chicken and veal roll

POLPETTONE DI TACCHINO   turkey meatballs with cheese, breaded and fried

POLPETTONE DI TONNO E SPINACI   tuna and spinach loaf

POLPETTONE IN BRODO   meat loaf in chicken broth

POLPETTONE SORPRESA   veal loaf with cheese, onion, garlic, oil and tomato paste

POLPO   octopus, small squid

POLPO AL PURGATORIO   octopus cooked in oil, tomato, parsley, garlic and pepper

POLPO ALLA LUCANA   cuttlefish slowly cooked in sauce of olive oil, parsley and ginger

POMAROLA   mild tomato sauce with onions, carrots, basil and olive oil

POMODORI AL GRATIN   tomatoes baked in oil, cheese, herbs and bread crumbs

POMODORI AL TONNO   tomatoes with tuna fish, olive oil and vinegar

POMODORI ALLA SICILIANA   tomatoes stuffed with onion, anchovy, capers, bread crumbs, oil, baked

POMODORI RIEMPITI DI MOZZARELLA   tomatoes stuffed with cheese and baked

POMODORI RIPIENI   tomatoes stuffed with bread crumbs, cheese, garlic, oil, then baked

POMODORI RIPIENI DI RISO   baked tomatoes stuffed with rice and cheese

POMODORO   tomato

POMODORO AL FORNO   stuffed baked tomato

POMODORO CON ACCIUGHE E MANDORLE   tomato with anchovies and almonds

POMODORO CON MOZZARELLA   tomato and mozzarella cheese

POMODORO CON RICOTTA   tomato and ricotta

POMPELMO   grapefruit

PONCE GELATO ALLA ROMANA   frozen fruit juices with rum and wine

POPONE   melon

PORCEDDU   suckling pig flavored with myrtle and roasted between hot stones in a hole in the ground, covered with earth

PORCELLO   very young pig

PORCHETTA   roast suckling pig

PORCHETTA AL FORNO   baked suckling pig

PORCHETTA DI MAIALE ARROSTO   roast suckling pig

PORCINI   boletus kind of mushrooms

PORRI   leeks

PORRI AL BURRO E FORMAGGIO   braised leeks with Parmesan cheese

PORRI ALLA PANNA   leeks prepared in a cream sauce

PORRI DORATI   leeks batter-dipped and deep-fried

PORRI IN UMIDO   stewed leeks with tomatoes and olives

PORTAFOGLIO   veal cutlet stuffed with chopped meat, ham, cheese, fried or sautéed

PORTAFOGLIO AL VITELLO   stuffed veal cutlet braised in sauce

PORTAMONETE   purse

PORTO   port wine

PORTOFINO   dry white wine

PORZIONE   charge depends on portion size

POSILLIPO   seafood served in a tomato herb sauce

PREBOGGION AL PESTO   greens and rice soup with basil sauce

PREGARE   to ask

PREGO   if you please

PRESNITZ   Easter fruitcake

PRESTO   quickly

PREZZEMOLO   parsley

PREZZO   price

PREZZO FISSO   fixed-price meal

PREZZO MODERATO   reasonably priced

PRIMA COLAZIONE   breakfast

PRIMITIVO   dry full-bodied red wine good with rice or meat

PRIMIZIE   first fruits *or* vegetables of season

PRIMO PIATTO   first course

PROFITEROLE   cream puff pastry covered with hot chocolate sauce

PROFITEROLE AL CIOCCOLATO   cream puff pastry with chocolate frosting

PROIBITO   forbidden

PROIBITO ENTRARE   do not enter

PRONTO   ready

PROSCIUTTO   salted air-cured ham

PROSCIUTTO AFFUMICATO   cured, smoked ham

PROSCIUTTO AI TARTUFI E FUNGHI   ham with white sauce, truffles and mushrooms

PROSCIUTTO AL MADERA   cooked ham served in wine sauce

PROSCIUTTO COI FICHI   ham with ripe figs

PROSCIUTTO COI FUNGHI   ham, with cheese and mushrooms

PROSCIUTTO COI FUNGHI COLTIVATI   ham with button mushrooms

PROSCIUTTO CON LINGUA E TARTUFI   ham with tongue and truffles

PROSCIUTTO COTTO   cured smoked ham which is cooked

PROSCIUTTO CRUDO   salted cured ham which is air-dried

PROSCIUTTO DI CINGHIALE   smoked wild boar

PROSCIUTTO DI LANGHIRANO   ham from the province of Parma

PROSCIUTTO DI MONTAGNA   ham from a mountain district

PROSCIUTTO DI PARMA   cured ham from Parma

PROSCIUTTO DI TACCHINO   turkey breast fried, topped with ham and Parmesan and broiled

PROSCIUTTO E MELONE   ham with melon
PROSCIUTTO E POMODORO   ham and tomatoes
PROVATURA   soft, mild cheese made from buffalo's milk
PROVATURA ALLO SPIEDO   diced bread and provatura
   cheese toasted on a spit
PROVOLE DI BUFALA   hard cheese of buffalo milk
PROVOLONE   white, medium-hard cheese
PRUGNE   plums
PRUGNE FARCITE   prunes stuffed with walnuts and
   chocolate
PRUGNE SECCHE   prunes
PUNT E MES   brand of vermouth
PUNTA DI VITELLO ARROSTO   roast breast of veal
PUNTA DI VITELLO RIPIENA   stuffed veal breast
   usually roasted
PUNTE DI ASPARAGI   asparagus tips
PURÉ   pureed *or* strained (also see PASSATO)
PURÉ DI PATATE   mashed potatoes

Q

QUÀ   here
QUAGLIE   quails
QUAGLIE AI TARTUFI   quails sautéed with truffles
QUAGLIE AL MATTONE   quails roasted in a brick oven
QUAGLIE AL VINO BIANCO   quails stuffed with pine
   nuts and raisins, cooked in wine, cream, garlic and onion
QUAGLIE ALLA MONTANARA   quails braised in red
   wine
QUAGLIE ALLA PIEMONTESE   quails roasted, served
   with rice and truffles and Marsala and truffle-flavored
   cream sauce
QUAGLIE ALLO SPIEDO   quails roasted on a spit
QUAGLIE ARROSTO CON LA POLENTA   roasted quails
   with fried polenta
QUAGLIE COI PISELLI   quails roasted and served with
   peas and onions

QUAGLIE COL PURÉ DI PISELLI   quails in a casserole with pureed peas, ham and bacon

QUAGLIE COL RISO   quails with rice, ham, onion, bacon, grated cheese, cooked in a pan

QUAGLIE CON RISOTTO   quails with herbs, vegetables, wine

QUAGLIE DI CROSTONE   quails roasted and served over cornmeal mush

QUAGLIE IN CASSERUOLA   quails braised with herbs, mushrooms in sauce

QUARESIMALI   dry biscuits of flour, egg and toasted almond

R

RABARBARO   rhubarb

RADICCHIO   chicory, lettuce with bitter taste

RADICCHIO ROSSO   wild chickory *or* curly endive (red)

RADICI   radishes

RAFANO   horseradish

RAGNO   sea bass *or* sea perch

RAGUSANO   hard sweet cheese

RAGÙ   meat sauce for pasta (also called BOLOGNESE)

RAGÙ AL TONNO   pan-fried tuna fish with wine, tomato, onion, garlic

RAGÙ ALLA NAPOLETANA   thick meat and tomato sauce

RAGÙ DI AGNELLO   braised lamb with tomatoes, basil and black olives

RAGÙ DI AGNELLO COI PEPERONI   thick lamb meat sauce with peppers

RALLENTARE   to slow down

RANE   frog *or* frogs' legs

RANE AL GUAZZETTO   stewed frogs' legs made with wine

RANE DORATE   skinned frogs' legs dipped in egg and fried in olive oil

RANE FRITTE   fried frogs' legs

RANOCCHI   frogs (also see RANE)

RAPA   turnip

RAPA ROSSA   white turnip with some red color
RAPANELLI   radishes
RAPE ROSSE AL FORNO   baked red beets *or* turnips
RAVANELLI   radishes
RAVIGGIOLO   sharp cheese from sheep or goat milk
RAVIOLI   pillow-shaped pasta stuffed with meat, cheese, vegetables, boiled, served with sauce
RAVIOLI ALLA BOLOGNESE   pillow-shaped pasta served in a tomato meat sauce
RAVIOLI ALLA GENOVESE   pillow-shaped pasta served in a tomato meat sauce
RAVIOLI ALLA PIEMONTESE   pasta with beef and brown sauce
RAVIOLI ALLA ROMANA   pasta pillows stuffed with ricotta cheese served in an herbal meat sauce
RAVIOLI DI RICOTTA   pockets of macaroni dough filled with cottage cheese, boiled and served with tomato sauce and grated cheese
RAVIOLI DI RICOTTA E SPINACI   pasta with ricotta cheese and spinach
RAVIOLI DI SAN GIUSEPPE   baked pasta stuffed with jam
RAVIOLI DOLCI   sweet pasta made with jam and brandy
RAZZA   ray fish
RECCHIATELLE   macaroni in the form of little ears, served with a chopped green vegetable sauté and garnished with cottage cheese
REGINA   large carp
RIBES   currants
RIBES NERO   black currants
RIBES ROSSO   red currants
RIBOLLITA   bean soup with leeks, onion, garlic, cheese, oil, herbs, on bread, baked
RICCI   sea urchins
RICCI DI MARE   sea urchins, served raw with lemon
RICCIARELLI DI SIENA   marzipan cookies from Siena
RICOTTA   cottage cheese made from whey
RICOTTA CON SALSICCE   cottage cheese with sausages

RICOTTA CON SPINACI E CERVELLA   cottage cheese
with spinach and brains

RICOTTA FRITTA   ricotta cheese fritters

RIFREDDO MISTO   assorted cold roast meat

RIGAGLIE   giblets

RIGAGLIE DI POLLO   chicken giblets and livers sautéed
with herbs

RIGATONI   pasta of large tube shape, in short pieces

RIGATONI AI PEPERONI   pasta tubes with sweet
peppers and tomato sauce

RIGATONI AL PROSCIUTTO   pasta tubes with ham

RIGATONI ALLA CARBONARA   pasta tubes with bacon,
cheese, garlic, eggs, oil

RIGATONI ALLA NAPOLETANA CON PEPERONI
FRESCHI   rigatoni with roasted sweet peppers

RIGHINI   sweet water sunfish

RIPIENE   stuffed

RIPIENI FRITTI   fried stuffed dumplings

RISERVA   wines aged longer in cask at winery

RISI   rice (also see RISO and RISOTTO)

RISI E BISI   rice and peas cooked in broth with onions

RISO   boiled rice with various ingredients

RISO AI QUATTRO FORMAGGI   rice with four different
cheeses

RISO AL BURRO   rice with butter, onions and broth

RISO AL CAVROMAN   rice with mutton, onion, tomato,
cheese

RISO AL LIMONE   rice with eggs and lemon

RISO AL SALTO   rice pan-fried with grated cheese

RISO AL SUGO   rice with meat sauce, tomatoes, herbs

RISO AL VERDE   rice with sage and chopped spinach

RISO ALL'ANITRA   rice cooked in sauce of chopped duck
meat and giblets

RISO ALL'UOVO E LIMONE   egg and lemon juice beaten
up and mixed into the rice

RISO ALLA BOLOGNESE   rice with meat sauce, tomatoes, garlic, broth

RISO ALLA CAMPAGNOLA   rice with tomatoes, onion, bacon, mushrooms

RISO ALLA CAPPUCCINA   rice with anchovies, onion, butter and oil

RISO ALLA CERTOSINA   rice with fish stock and served with shrimp and fish

RISO ALLA FINANZIERA   rice with meat sauce, brandy, bacon, chicken livers and broth

RISO ALLA GENOVESE   rice with onion, mushroom, tomatoes

RISO ALLA MARINARA   rice with onion, clams, tomatoes, butter, garlic

RISO ALLA MILANESE   rice with wine and saffron

RISO ALLA PARMIGIANA   rice with onion, mushrooms, livers, sausage, meat sauce

RISO ALLA PESCATORA   rice cooked in fish broth with pieces of fish

RISO ALLA PIEMONTESE   rice boiled in meat broth with cheese and butter

RISO ALLA SARACENA   rice with finely-chopped shellfish

RISO ALLA SBIRRAGLIA   rice with chicken broth, chopped chicken, wine, cheese

RISO ALLA TOSCANA   rice sautéed with liver, vegetables, wine, cheese, tomato paste

RISO ALLA VALENCIANA   rice with pork, sausage, clams, tomato, pepper, onion, garlic

RISO ALLA VALTELLINESE   rice with cabbage, beans, cheese

RISO ALLA VENETA   rice sautéed with mussels, garlic, onion, fish broth

RISO ARANCINO ALLA SICILIANA   large rice ball stuffed with meat and fried

RISO ARROSTO ALLA GENOVESE   casserole of rice, sausage, peas, artichokes, mushrooms, cheese and onion, browned in oven

RISO BISATI   rice cooked with eel and herb olive oil

RISO COI CECI   broth of rice and chick-peas, flavored with tomatoes and spice

RISO COI FINOCCHI   rice with fennel, onion, cheese

RISO COI FUNGHI   rice with butter and mushrooms

RISO COI GAMBERI   rice with sauce of shrimp, garlic, olive oil, pepper and tomato

RISO COI PISELLI   rice with peas, onion, meat, butter

RISO COI ROGNONCINI TRIFOLATI   rice cooked in broth with butter and oil, chopped vegetables, kidneys and cheese

RISO COI TARTUFI   rice with ham, cheese and truffles

RISO COL POMODORO   with tomatoes

RISO CON ASPARAGI   rice cooked with asparagus, onion and butter

RISO CON CAPAROZZOLI   rice with shellfish, garlic, wine

RISO CON RIGAGLIE   rice with giblets, veal, white wine, tomato

RISO CON SALSICCE   rice with sausage

RISO CON SCAMPI   shrimp pan fried with rice and wine

RISO CON SEDANI   rice with celery

RISO CON SEPPIE   rice with cuttlefish, olive oil, wine, tomato, garlic

RISO CON VERZA   rice with savoy cabbage

RISO CON VONGOLE   rice with clams, onion, olive oil, broth

RISO CON ZUCCA   rice with pumpkin, onion, oil, grated cheese

RISO CON ZUCCHINE   rice with zucchini, onion, cheese

RISO DI MARE   rice with oil, onion, seafood, wine, broth

RISO E FAGIOLI   rice with butter and beans

RISO E LATTE   rice and milk soup flavored with cheese

RISO E LUGANEGA   rice and sausage

RISO GRECO   rice cooked in broth with vegetables, sausage, lemon juice

RISO IN BIANCO   white rice with butter

RISO IN BIANCO COI FEGATINI   rice cooked with white wine, chicken livers

RISO IN BIANCO COI TARTUFI BIANCHI   boiled rice
   and white truffles, served with grated Parmesan cheese
   and butter
RISO IN CAGNONE   rice with butter, cheese, garlic
RISO IN TAZZA   rice served in a cup
RISO MANTECATO   rice cooked in butter and milk
RISO COI PEOCI ALLA VENETA   rice with butter, olive
   oil, mussels and broth
RISO PRIMAVERA   rice with spring vegetables
RISOTTO   cooked rice (see RISO)
RISOTTO ALLA CERTOSINA   rice with a sauce of peas,
   crayfish tails or prawns and mushrooms
RISOTTO ALLA CHIOGGIOTTA   fish rice
RISOTTO ALLA GENOVESE   rice with a meat sauce
   containing wine, herbs and vegetables
RISOTTO ALLA MARINARA   rice with seafood
RISOTTO ALLA MILANESE   rice cooked in consommé,
   mixed with butter, saffron, chicken giblets, beef marrow,
   mushrooms and Parmesan cheese
RISOTTO ALLA MONZESE   rice with sausage meat,
   tomato and Marsala wine
RISOTTO ALLA PAESANA   thick soup of rice with beans,
   cabbage, salami, bacon
RISOTTO ALLA PARMIGIANA   rice in beef broth with
   chicken livers, sausage, mushrooms, herbs, bacon and
   vegetables
RISOTTO ALLA PESCATORA   rice with fish
RISOTTO ALLA SBIRRAGLIA   chicken and rice dish,
   with herbs, vegetables, sausage and wine
RISOTTO COI CARCIOFI   hearts of baby artichokes cut
   up and cooked with rice
RISOTTO COI FEGATINI   rice with chicken livers
RISOTTO COI FRUTTI DI MARE   rice with shellfish
RISOTTO COI FUNGHI   rice with mushrooms and
   chopped onions
RISOTTO COI GAMBERI   rice with prawns
RISOTTO COI TARTUFI   rice with truffles

RISOTTO CON LUMACHE   rice with snails in a highly flavored sauce

RISOTTO CON SCAMPI   rice with prawns, butter and cheese

RISOTTO CON SECOLE   rice with small pieces of beef or veal

RISOTTO CON TELLINE   rice with clams and a tomato sauce with peppers

RISOTTO CON VONGOLE   rice cooked in sauce of oil, parsley, tomato, garlic and clams

RISOTTO DI MAGRO   rice with anything but meat

RISOTTO DI ZUCCA   rice with small pieces of pumpkin

RISOTTO IN BIANCO   rice cooked with water and white wine instead of broth

RISOTTO IN CAGNONE   rice flavored with sage and garlic, butter and cheese

RISTORANTE   restaurant offering full food and beverage service

RISTRETTO   consommé

RITIRATA   lavatory

ROBIOLA   soft, sweet sheep milk cheese

ROCCIATA DI ASSISI   fruit roll with raisins, walnuts, dry figs, almonds, citrus

ROGNONCINI D'AGNELLO SALTATI CON CIPOLLA sautéed lamb kidneys with onion

ROGNONE   kidney

ROGNONI AI FUNGHI TRIFOLATI   kidneys braised with broth, garlic, mushroom and truffles

ROGNONI AL MADERA   kidneys braised in red wine

ROGNONI DI SALSA   sauce of chopped kidneys, herbs and spices in a tomato sauce

ROGNONI DI VITELLO ALLA GRIGLIA   pan-fried veal kidneys

ROLLATINE DI VITELLO   rolled and stuffed breast of veal

ROLLE DI FILETTO   rolled fillet of beef pot roasted with wine

ROMBO   turbot, fish

ROQUEFORT   strong-flavored cheese used mainly in
   salads and dressings
ROSATELLO   rosé
ROSBIF   roast beef
ROSMARINO   rosemary
ROSSO   red wine
ROSSO DELLA RIVIERA DEL GARDA   light red, dry wine
ROSTICCERIA   snack bar serving sandwiches and drinks
ROTOLO   stuffed meat roll
ROTOLO DI TACCHINO   turkey meat boned and rolled
ROTOLO DI VITELLO E SPINACI   veal and spinach roll,
   stuffed with ham
ROTTAMI DI POLLO IN PADELLA   chicken cut up and
   sautéed

S

SA CASSOLA   fish soup of Sardinia
SACRANTINO   red, semi-dry wine
SAINT HONORÉ   custard-filled pastry with cream puffs
SALAME   salami
SALAME ALL'UNGHERESE   Hungarian salami of pork
   and beef
SALAME ALLA CACCIATORA   hard-dried salami
SALAME ALLA FINOCCHIONA   salami from Tuscany,
   flavored with fennel seed
SALAME ALLA GENOVESE   salami of pork, veal and
   pork fat
SALAME DI FABRIANO   salami with a mixture of pork
   and veal, from Marches
SALAME DI FELINO   pure pork salami from village of
   Felino near Parma
SALAMINI   sauce of tomatoes and fresh sausage
SALARE   to marinate, usually in herb vinegar or wine
SALATO   salty, salted
SALE   salt
SALITA RAPIDA   steep grade

SALMISTRATA   rabbit stew pickled in herb vinegar or wine and served cold

SALMONE   salmon fish

SALMONE AFFUMICATO   smoked salmon

SALMONE RIPIENO ALL'ANETO   salmon filled with onions and fresh dill, baked, served cold

SALMONE SCOZZESE   Scotch salmon

SALMORIGLIO   sauce of olive oil, lemon juice, parsley, oregano, salt

SALMÌ   stew cooked in earthen pot

SALSA   sauce

SALSA ABRUZZESE   sauce with oil, garlic and bell peppers

SALSA AI CAPPERI   tomato-based caper sauce

SALSA AI FRUTTI DI MARE   sauce with olive oil, tomatoes and seafood

SALSA AI FUNGHI   mushroom sauce

SALSA AL BURRO   melted butter and herb sauce

SALSA AL BURRO E AL PARMIGIANO   sauce with melted butter and grated Parmesan cheese

SALSA AL COGNAC   brandy sauce

SALSA AL FORMAGGIO   cheese sauce

SALSA AL PROSCIUTTO   tomato, herb and ham sauce

SALSA AL RAGÙ   sauce with ground meat, bacon, garlic, tomato, olive oil

SALSA AL SARMORIGLIO   sauce served hot for meat or cooked vegetables with oil, lemon, oregano, tabasco

SALSA AL SUGO   sauce of ground meat, bacon, garlic, tomato, olive oil, like Bolognese

SALSA AL TONNO   sauce with tuna, garlic, olive oil, capers, anchovies

SALSA ALL'AGLIO E OLIO   sauce of olive oil in which garlic was cooked

SALSA ALL'AMATRICIANA   sauce of oil, garlic, tomato, onion, peppers

SALSA ALL'ARRABBIATA   sauce with tomato, pepper, bacon, sausage

SALSA ALL'OLIO DI MANDORLE E LIMONE   sauce for
boiled fish with almonds, garlic, lemon, olive oil

SALSA ALL'UOVO   sauce with eggs, mozzarella and
anchovies

SALSA ALLA BOLOGNESE   sauce with ground meat,
bacon, garlic, tomatoes, olive oil

SALSA ALLA BOSCAIOLA   sauce with tuna, anchovy,
tomato, olive oil, mushroom, garlic

SALSA ALLA BUCANIERA   sauce with clams, octopus,
tomato, olive oil, mushroom, garlic

SALSA ALLA CACCIATORA   sauce of tomato, meat,
white wine, mushrooms

SALSA ALLA CAMPAGNOLA   sauce with mushrooms,
olive oil, garlic, seasoning

SALSA ALLA CARBONARA   sauce with olive oil, butter,
garlic, diced bacon

SALSA ALLA CARRETTIERA   sauce with tuna, garlic,
mushrooms, olive oil, meat sauce

SALSA ALLA CIOCIARA   sauce with meat, butter,
Parmesan cheese

SALSA ALLA CONTADINA   sauce with butter, tomato
paste, mushrooms, parmesan cheese

SALSA ALLA CREMA   sauce with butter, milk, flour, egg
yolks, cheese

SALSA ALLA DIAVOLA   sauce of tomato, meat, peppers

SALSA ALLA FINANZIERA   sauce with giblets, bacon,
onion and broth

SALSA ALLA FIORENTINA   sauce of tomato, meat,
herbs, peas

SALSA ALLA GENOVESE   sauce of basil leaves, garlic,
olive oil, pine nuts, pecorino cheese

SALSA ALLA GHIOTTONA   sauce with meat, onion,
chicken livers, wine, mushrooms

SALSA ALLA LEPRE   tomato hare sauce with garlic,
herbs, olive oil

SALSA ALLA MARINARA   sauce of capers, olive oil,
garlic, olives

SALSA ALLA NAPOLETANA   sauce of tomatoes, cheese, herbs, garlic

SALSA ALLA NORCINA   sauce with melted mozzarella cheese, butter, sausage, peas

SALSA ALLA PANNA   sauce with cream and grated cheese

SALSA ALLA PIEMONTESE   mild brown meat sauce

SALSA ALLA PIRATA   sauce with tomatoes, anchovies, capers, olives

SALSA ALLA PIZZAIOLA   meat sauce with garlic, tomato, olive oil, oregano

SALSA ALLA POSILLIPO   tomato, herb sauce, usually with seafood

SALSA ALLA PROVENZALE   sauce with onion, oil, tomato, mushrooms, olives

SALSA ALLA RICOTTA ROMANA   sauce with tomato, garlic and ricotta cheese

SALSA ALLA ROMANA   meat sauce with butter, cheese, seasonings

SALSA ALLA TARTARA   sauce with hard egg yolks, oil, mustard, herbs

SALSA ALLE ACCIUGHE   sauce of anchovies, garlic, olive oil

SALSA ALLE ALICI   anchovy sauce

SALSA ALLE MELANZANE   eggplant sauce with olive oil, meat, spices

SALSA ALLE NOCI   sauce with walnuts, cream, basil, garlic, Parmesan cheese

SALSA BESCIAMELLA   sauce with butter, flour and milk

SALSA BIANCA   white sauce

SALSA COI FEGATINI DI POLLO   chicken liver sauce

SALSA CON COZZE   sauce with olive oil, mussels, garlic

SALSA CON SALSICCIA   sauce with sausage meat

SALSA CON SARDE   sauce with olive oil, onion, sardines, anchovy, fennel, pine nuts

SALSA CON ZUCCHINE ALLA FRIULANA   sauce with zucchini, tomatoes, peppers, olive oil

SALSA D'UMIDO DI RIGAGLIE   sauce with chicken livers and beef gravy

SALSA DELLA CASA   special house *or* restaurant sauce

SALSA DI CARNE   sauce with tomato, butter, Parmesan and brown meat sauce (same as SUGO or BOLOGNESE)

SALSA DI CARNE E FEGATINI   brown meat sauce and chicken livers

SALSA DI CIPOLLA   sauce of onions sautéed in butter and tomato paste

SALSA DI MAGRO   sauce of mushrooms, pesto, anchovy, olive oil, onion

SALSA DI MANZO E FUNGHI   meat sauce with mushrooms

SALSA DI PESCE   sauce of olive oil, anchovy, lemon, for fish

SALSA DI POMODORO   sauce of tomatoes, olive oil and herbs

SALSA DI POMODORO ALLA NAPOLETANA   tomato sauce with oil, garlic base

SALSA DI POMODORO FRESCO   fresh tomato sauce

SALSA FINTA   tomato sauce with onion, garlic, meat stock, oil, herbs

SALSA PER INSALATE AL VINO BIANCO   white wine salad sauce

SALSA PER VERDURE LESSATE   thin sauce of egg and lemon

SALSA PEVERADA   hot sauce of chicken liver, anchovy, sausage, wine, lemon

SALSA PICCANTE   spicy (sharp) sauce

SALSA POMMAROLA   tomato sauce for pasta

SALSA SEMPLICE AI CAPPERI   sauce of capers, lemon juice, oil, tabasco

SALSA VERDE   green pesto sauce

SALSA VERDE ALLA MILANESE   anchovy, parsley, oil, garlic sauce

SALSA VERDE ALLA PIEMONTESE   sauce of anchovies, egg yolk, parsley, garlic, capers and bread crumbs

SALSA VERDE PICCANTE   uncooked spicy green sauce

SALSETTA DI PEPERONI   uncooked sweet pepper sauce

SALSICCE   sausages eaten newly made and fried, or dry and seasoned

SALSICCE AL SUGO   fried pork sausages braised in meat sauce

SALSICCE AL VINO ROSSO E FUNGHI SECCHI   fried
sausages with red wine and dried wild mushrooms
SALSICCE ARROSTO   pork sausages grilled over open fire
SALSICCE COL CAVOLO NERO   sausages with red cabbage
SALSICCE CON CIPOLLE   sausages with smothered onions
SALSICCE CON MELANZANE   sausages with eggplants
SALSICCE CON UOVA   sausages with eggs
SALSICCE DI FEGATO   sausages of pigs' liver, with
garlic, salt and pepper, pinch of orange peel, eaten fried
after they have been dried
SALSICCE FRITTE   fried pork sausages
SALSICCIA   sausage (see SALSICCE)
SALTATE   sautéed
SALTIMBOCCA   slices of veal and prosciutto ham
sautéed in wine
SALTIMBOCCA ALLA GENOVESE   veal and ham rolls
sautéed in Marsala wine
SALTIMBOCCA ALLA ROMANA   veal cutlet flavored
with ham and sage, sautéed
SALTIMBOCCA ALLA SORRENTINA   thin veal slices
baked with ham and cheese slices and tomato sauce
SALUMI   sausages served sliced, cold
SALUMI NOSTRANI   local salami
SAN PIETRO   porgy type of fish
SAN PIETRO ALLA MUGNAIA   fish fillets floured, pan
fried in butter and lemon
SANATO   milk fed calf (veal)
SANGIOVESE   red table wine
SANGUE DI GIUDA   dark sparkling red wine, slightly sweet
SANTA GIUSTINA   red table wine
SANTA MADDALENA   light and fruity red wine
SARAGNO   porgy type of fish
SARAGO   ocean sunfish
SARDE   sardines
SARDE AL BECCAFICCU   stuffed baked sardines
SARDE AL FINOCCHIO   fresh sardines baked in tomato
wine sauce

SARDE AL VINO BIANCO   sardines baked with wine, anchovies

SARDE ALL'OLIO E ORIGANO   sardines baked in olive oil and oregano

SARDE ALLA BRACE   grilled sardines

SARDE IN CARPIONE   fried marinated sardines

SARDE IN TORTIERA   baked sardines with garlic, oil, lemon

SARDE RIPIENE   stuffed sardines

SARDELLE   sardines

SARDELLINE   young sardines

SARDINA   small sardine (also see SARDE)

SARDO   strong flavored sheep cheese

SARTICOLA   dry white wine

SARTÙ   rice casserole filled with chicken giblets, minced veal, tomato, mushrooms, buffalo cheese, cooked in oven

SARTÙ ALLA NAPOLETANA   baked rice mold with sausages, livers, peas, meat, cheese, bacon

SARTÙ DI RISO   bread crumb crust filled with rice, sauce, livers, meatballs, cheese

SASSELLA   robust, smooth red wine good with beef or game

SAVARIN   liquor-soaked cake ring filled with fruit and topped with whipped cream

SAVOIARDI   ladyfingers, cookies

SAVUTO   red, velvety wine with good bouquet

SCACCIATA   pizza dough sandwich enclosing cheese, anchovies, ham, onion, tomato, olives

SCALOGNO   shallot

SCALOPPA, SCALOPPINA   veal slice (see SCALOPPINE)

SCALOPPINE   thin veal slices

SCALOPPINE AI FUNGHI   pan-fried veal slices then grilled in mushroom cream sauce

SCALOPPINE AL BURRO   floured and pan-fried veal slices in butter

SCALOPPINE AL CARTOCCIO CON GLI ASPARAGI   veal slices and asparagus, Fontina cheese, Marsala sauce baked in foil pouch

SCALOPPINE AL FORMAGGIO   veal slices fried, covered with cheese and baked

SCALOPPINE AL LIMONE   veal slices marinated and sautéed in oil with lemon juice

SCALOPPINE AL MADERA   veal slices sautéed in butter and red wine

SCALOPPINE AL MARSALA   veal slices veal slices sautéed in Marsala wine

SCALOPPINE AL MARSALA ARRICCHITE   veal slices with Marsala wine and cream

SCALOPPINE AL POMODORO   veal slices sautéed in herb, tomato sauce

SCALOPPINE AL POMODORO E FUNGHI   veal slices sautéed in herb, mushroom, tomato sauce

SCALOPPINE AL VINO BIANCO   veal slices sautéed in butter and white wine

SCALOPPINE ALL'ARANCIO   veal slices sautéed in butter, oil and orange juice

SCALOPPINE ALLA BISMARK   veal slices fried and topped with fried egg

SCALOPPINE ALLA BOLOGNESE   veal slices breaded and fried with ham and cheese and meat sauce

SCALOPPINE ALLA BOSCAIOLA   veal slices sautéed, then broiled with onion, mushrooms and tomato

SCALOPPINE ALLA CACCIATORA   veal slices floured, pan fried in tomato, mushrooms, herb sauce

SCALOPPINE ALLA CAMPAGNOLA   veal slices sautéed then broiled with onion, mushrooms, tomato, carrot

SCALOPPINE ALLA CAPRICCIOSA   veal slices sautéed in mushroom sauce with ham, herbs, melted cheese

SCALOPPINE ALLA CONTADINA   veal slices sautéed in tomato sauce with onion, cheese, capers, olives

SCALOPPINE ALLA LOMBARDA   veal slices marinated and sautéed in oil with lemon juice and parsley

SCALOPPINE ALLA MILANESE   veal slices floured, breaded and fried with grated cheese

SCALOPPINE ALLA PANNA   veal slices sautéed in white cream sauce

SCALOPPINE ALLA PANNA E FUNGHI   veal slices sautéed in white cream sauce with mushrooms

SCALOPPINE ALLA PARMIGIANA   veal slices breaded, fried with grated cheese then baked with cheese on top

SCALOPPINE ALLA PIZZAIOLA   veal slices sautéed in garlic, tomato, oil and herb sauce

SCALOPPINE ALLA SORRENTINA   veal slices pan-fried then baked with mozzarella cheese and tomato sauce

SCALOPPINE ALLA VALDOSTANA   veal slices stuffed with Fontina cheese, breaded and fried

SCALOPPINE ALLA VIENNESE   veal slices breaded, topped with lemon and anchovies then fried

SCALOPPINE ALLA ZINGARA   veal slices sautéed in butter and red wine, mushrooms and herbs

SCALOPPINE AMMANTATE   veal slices with mozzarella

SCALOPPINE CON PISELLI   veal slices sautéed in butter and covered with peas

SCALOPPINE CREMATE   veal slices sautéed in white cream sauce with cognac

SCALOPPINE DI MAIALE AL MARSALA   pork fillet pan fried in wine

SCALOPPINE DI VITELLO   boneless thin slice of veal

SCALOPPINE PICCANTI   veal slices braised with butter and brandy, capers and anchovy

SCALOPPINE PICCATE   veal slices sautéed in butter and served with pan juices

SCAMORZA   aged mozzarella cheese

SCAMORZE RIVISONDOLI   soft cream cheese

SCAMORZINE   cheese from sheep's milk, sometimes roasted

SCAMPI   shrimp *or* prawns (also see GAMBERI)

SCAMPI ALL'AMERICANA   prawns sautéed in tomato sauce, wine, onion sauce

SCAMPI ALLA VENEZIANA   shrimp boiled and served cold with lemon juice

SCAMPI ARROSTO   shrimp marinated then baked in
tomato sauce

SCAMPI DORATI   breaded and deep-fried shrimp

SCAMPI E PEOCETI   shrimp cooked with capers,
mussels, butter, brandy, tomato, cream

SCAMPI FRITTI   breaded and deep-fried shrimp

SCANELLO   round steak

SCANELLO DI VITELLO   veal leg fillet braised in onion
and vinegar and sugar-glazed

SCAPECE   pickled, fried fish in white vinegar, seasoned
with saffron

SCAROLA   escarole lettuce

SCAVECCIO   eel in Tuscany

SCHIUDERE   to open

SCIROPPO   fruit syrup diluted with water

SCIUSCELLO   ricotta cheesecake with fruit, almonds,
brandy, chocolate, lemon peel

SCORFANO   Mediterranean scorpion fish

SCOTTADITO   veal cutlets

SCUNGILLI ALLA MARINARA   conch-like seafood
sautéed in tomatoes, wine, peppers

SCUOLA   school

SECCA   dried

SECCO   dry wine

SEDANI DI TREVI IN UMIDO   white celery sticks cooked
in tomato sauce

SEDANO   celery

SEDANO IN UMIDO   braised celery with tomatoes and onions

SEDIA   chair

SELLA DI DAINO   saddle of venison usually roasted

SELVAGGINA   game

SEMIFREDDO   ice cream cake

SEMIFREDDO ALLA CREMA   ice cream with almonds

SEMIFREDDO ALLO ZABAGLIONE   half frozen dessert
of cream, eggs, sugar, wine

SENAPE   mustard

SEPPIA   cuttlefish, squid

SEPPIA ALLA VENETA   squid marinated in garlic, oil, white wine and squid ink

SEPPIA IN UMIDO   stewed squid

SERVIZIO COMPRESO   includes service or tip

SERVIZIO NON COMPRESO   does not include service or tip

SFINCIUNI   stuffed pizza, sealed edges, sandwich form (see PIZZA)

SFIRENA   sea pike

SFOGIE   sole

SFOGLIA   homemade egg pasta

SFOGLIATELLE   cakes made of thin flakes of pastry wrapped around a filling of spiced cottage cheese and candied fruit

SFOGLIATELLE FROLLE   baked pastry filled with ricotta cheese, fruits, cinnamon

SFORMATO   baked mold

SFORMATO ALLA BESCIAMELLA   baked mold of egg whites, milk, cheese, meat sauce

SFORMATO DI BUCATINI   pasta boiled then baked with meat or cream sauce

SFORMATO DI CAPELLINI   mold of capellini with ham and mozzarella cheese

SFORMATO DI CARCIOFI   baked artichoke mold with bechamel sauce

SFORMATO DI FUNGHI   baked mushroom pudding

SFORMATO DI PATATE   potato pie with Parmesan cheese, ham and mozzarella cheese

SFORMATO DI TORTELLINI   baked pasta casserole

SFORMATO FREDDO DI TONNO E PATATE   cold tuna and potato mold

SGOMBRO   mackerel

SGOMBRO ALLA MARINARA   mackerel sautéed in tomatoes, wine, peppers

SGUAZZETO   braised lamb stew

SGUAZZETO ALLA BECHERA   stew made of various meats

SIDRO   cider

SIGNORE   women

SIGNORI   men

SILVANO   chocolate meringue *or* tart

SILVESTRO   herb and mint liqueur

SOAVE   dry white wine

SOAVE DI LEPRE   kid stewed in red wine

SOFFIONCINI IN BRODO   light dumplings in broth

SOFFRITTO   sautéed

SOGLIOLA   sole fish

SOGLIOLA AI FERRI   grilled sole

SOGLIOLA AL GRATIN   sole baked in cream sauce with mushrooms, shallots, garlic

SOGLIOLA ALL'ARLECCHINO   sole poached in cream sauce with onions, tomatoes, garlic and squash

SOGLIOLA ALLA MUGNAIA   sole floured and pan-fried in butter and oil served with lemon sauce

SOGLIOLA ALLA PARTENOPEA   sole poached in wine and served on pasta with cheese and white sauce

SOGLIOLA ARROSTO   sole baked in olive oil, herbs and white wine

SOGLIOLA DORATA   breaded and fried sole

SOGLIOLA FRITTA   breaded and deep-fried sole

SOGLIOLA MARGHERITA   sole poached in wine and herbs and served with hollandaise sauce

SOPA   soup (see ZUPPA, MINESTRA, MINESTRONE, CONSOMMÉ)

SOPPRESSATA   large sausages of a flattened oval shape, sometimes preserved in oil

SORBETTO   sherbet, flavored-water ice

SORRENTINA   casserole of potatoes with tomato sauce and grated cheese

SORSO DORATO   gold-colored wine, nutty and robust with special bouquet

SOTTACETI   pickled vegetables

SOTTACETO   pickled

SOTTOFILETTO   loin steak

SOTTOFILETTO FARCITO   loin steak stuffed with seasoned meat and roasted

SOTTONOCE DI VITELLO   veal leg fillet

SOUFFLÉ DI SPINACI E RICOTTA   spinach and cheese
   soufflé
SOUFFLÉ DI TAGLIATELLE   pasta soufflé
SPAGHETTI   spaghetti, long strings of pasta
SPAGHETTI AI CANESTRELLI   thin spaghetti with scallops
SPAGHETTI AI CARCIOFI   thin spaghetti with artichokes
SPAGHETTI AI FRUTTI DI MARE   spaghetti with sea food
SPAGHETTI AI TARTUFI NERI   spaghetti with flaked
   black truffles
SPAGHETTI AL CACIO E PEPE   spaghetti with strong
   goat cheese and pepper
SPAGHETTI AL GUANCIALE   spaghetti with bacon
SPAGHETTI AL POMODORO   spaghetti with tomato
   sauce and oil
SPAGHETTI AL POMODORO E BASILICO   spaghetti
   with fresh tomatoes and basil leaves
SPAGHETTI AL POMODORO E GRASSO DI PROSCIUTTO
   spaghetti with tomato and the fat of ham
SPAGHETTI AL POMODORO E ORIGANO   spaghetti
   with tomato and oregano
SPAGHETTI AL POMODORO E SCALOGNO   spaghetti
   with tomatoes and shallots
SPAGHETTI AL SUGO DI CIPOLLE   spaghetti with onion
   sauce
SPAGHETTI AL SUGO DI PESCE   spaghetti with fish-
   head sauce
SPAGHETTI AL TARTUFO NERO   spaghetti with black
   truffle
SPAGHETTI AL TONNO   spaghetti with tuna
SPAGHETTI AL TONNO E FUNGHI SECCHI   spaghetti
   with tuna and dried mushrooms
SPAGHETTI ALL'AGLIO E OLIO   spaghetti with olive oil,
   fried garlic and ginger
SPAGHETTI ALL'AGLIO, OLIO E ORIGANO   spaghetti
   with garlic, oil and oregano
SPAGHETTI ALL'AGLIO, OLIO E PEPERONCINO
   spaghetti with garlic, oil and hot peppers

SPAGHETTI ALL'AMATRICIANA   spaghetti with sauce of olive oil, bacon and tomato, seasoned with peppers or ginger, served with goat cheese

SPAGHETTI ALLA CAPRESE   spaghetti with sauce of tomato, anchovy, tuna, olives and cheese

SPAGHETTI ALLA CARBONARA   spaghetti with bacon, onion, wine, egg and cheese sauce

SPAGHETTI ALLA NURSINA   spaghetti with black truffles

SPAGHETTI ALLA PANNA ACIDA   spaghetti with sour cream

SPAGHETTI ALLA PUTTANESCA   spaghetti with sauce of tomato, garlic, anchovy, capers, cheese, olives

SPAGHETTI ALLA SICILIANA   spaghetti with eggplant and ricotta cheese

SPAGHETTI ALLA SIRACUSANA   thin spaghetti with eggplant, tomatoes, anchovies, olives

SPAGHETTI ALLE UOVA E FORMAGGIO   thin spaghetti with eggs and cheese

SPAGHETTI AROMATICI   spaghetti with anchovy sauce

SPAGHETTI COI WURSTEL   spaghetti with frankfurter type sausage

SPAGHETTI CON CIPOLLE   spaghetti with onions

SPAGHETTI CON CONDIMENTO VEGETALE CRUDO   spaghetti with raw tomatoes and basil

SPAGHETTI CON MELANZANE   spaghetti with eggplants, oil, garlic, cheese

SPAGHETTI CON MOZZARELLA   thin spaghetti with mozzarella cheese

SPAGHETTI CON OLIVE E CAPPERI   spaghetti with olives and capers

SPAGHETTI CON PEPERONI E MELANZANE   spaghetti with peppers and eggplant

SPAGHETTI CON PISELLI   spaghetti with peas

SPAGHETTI CON POLLO, MELANZANE E SALSA ALLA BOLOGNESE   spaghetti with chicken, eggplant and meat sauce

SPAGHETTI CON SALSA ALLA BOLOGNESE   spaghetti with meat and tomato sauce

SPAGHETTI CON VONGOLE   spaghetti with mussels
SPAGHETTI CON VONGOLE, POLPETTE E GAMBERETTI
   spaghetti with clams, squid, shrimp
SPAGHETTI ESTIVI FREDDI   cold spaghetti with
   spearmint, olives, anchovy, mushrooms, olive oil
SPAGHETTI VERDI   thin spaghetti made with spinach
SPAGHETTINI   thin spaghetti (see SPAGHETTI)
SPALLA   shoulder
SPALLA DI VITELLO AL FORNO   veal shoulder usually
   roasted
SPALLA DI VITELLO BRASATA   braised shoulder of veal
   with white wine
SPANNOCCHI   large prawns
SPARNOCCHIE   large shrimp-like shellfish
SPECIALITÀ   speciality
SPEZZATINO   meat *or* fowl stew
SPEZZATINO AL PROSCIUTTO   veal chunks braised in
   herbal tomato and wine sauce
SPEZZATINO ALLA CONTADINA   veal chunks braised
   with oil, onion, tomato, herbs, anchovy and cheese
SPEZZATINO ALLA PAESANA   veal chunks braised
   with oil, onion, tomato, mushrooms, herbs and cheese
SPEZZATINO D'AGNELLO O CAPRETTO   lamb or kid
   stew with Marsala wine
SPEZZATINO DI MAIALE AL POMODORO   pork
   stewed with tomatoes and onions
SPEZZATINO DI POLLO   small pieces of chicken sautéed
   in oil with pimentos, onion, mushrooms and tomatoes
SPEZZATINO DI POLLO PICCANTE   chicken fricassee
   with tomatoes, peppers and capers
SPEZZATINO DI STUFATO E PISELLI   beef stew with peas
SPEZZATO   veal chunks braised in herb, onion and wine
   sauce (also see SPEZZATINO)
SPEZZATO D'AGNELLO AL PEPERONE E PROSCIUTTO
   lamb stew with white wine, ham and pepper
SPEZZATO DI MUSCOLO   beef stewed slowly with
   tomatoes and onion

SPEZZATO DI TACCHINO   turkey braised with olives
SPEZZATO DI VITELLO   veal stew made in tomato,
wine, herb sauce
SPIEDI   roasted on a spit (see SPIEDINI)
SPIEDINI   pieces of meat grilled or roasted on a skewer
(usually basted)
SPIEDINI ALL'UCCELLETTO   skewered veal and sausage
with sage and white wine
SPIEDINI ALLA PISTOIESE   skewered little birds with
bread, bacon, sage, juniper berries, bay leaf
SPIEDINI DI AGNELLO   lamb brochette, grilled on skewers
SPIEDINI DI CAPRETTO   baby goat meat roasted on skewers
SPIEDINI DI MARE   fish and seafood skewered and roasted
SPIEDINI DI MOZZARELLA   bread and cheese pieces
baked and served with butter and anchovies
SPIEDINI DI PESCE   swordfish *or* tuna broiled on skewers
SPIEDINO DI CALAMARI   squid marinated then grilled
SPIEDINO DI SCAMPI   shrimp broiled on skewers
SPIGOLA   sea bass
SPIGOLA CON SALSA E CAPPERI   striped bass with
tomato caper sauce
SPINACI   spinach
SPINACI AL BURRO E PARMIGIANO   cooked spinach
with sauce of butter and grated cheese
SPINACI AL GRATIN   spinach with sauce of butter and
grated cheese
SPINACI ALLA GENOVESE COI PIGNOLI   spinach with
pine nuts, olive oil, anchovy paste and garlic
SPINACI ALLA PARMIGIANA   spinach with sauce of
butter and grated cheese
SPINACI ALLA PIEMONTESE   spinach sautéed with
anchovies, garlic
SPINACI COI FUNGHI   spinach and mushrooms
SPINACI E RISO IN BRODO   spinach and rice soup
SPOLETINA   truffles and anchovies added to tomato sauce
SPORCO   dirty
SPREMUTA   fresh fruit drink

SPREMUTA D'ARANCIA   orange-flavored drink

SPUGNOLA   morel mushroom

SPUMA GELATA ALLA CREMA   iced fruit vanilla mousse

SPUMANTE   sparkling wine

SPUMONE   ice cream with nuts and strawberries or raspberries

SPUMONI   multi-flavored ice cream dessert, usually with fruit pieces

SPUMONI AL CROCCANTE   candied, chopped toasted almond in and on ice-cream dessert

SPUNTATURA   short ribs of beef

SPUNTATURA DI MAIALE CON POLENTA   pork short ribs braised and served with cornmeal mush

SQUADRO   monk fish

STACCIATA UNTA   cake with sugar icing

STAGIONATA   long-aged meat

STAGIONE   in season

STARNA   gray partridge

STECCHINI ALLA BOLOGNESE   chicken livers, truffles, cheese, sweetbread, tongue on skewers, coated with a white wine sauce, egg and bread crumbs and fried in butter

STELLETTE   star-shaped pasta

STIMPIRATA DI SALMONE   salmon fried with olive oil, onions, celery, capers

STOCCAFISSO   dried cod

STOCCAFISSO ALL'ANCONETANA   dried unsalted cod, cooked with onion, tomato, garlic, oil, anchovies and milk

STOCCAFISSO IN UMIDO   dry salt cod stewed in tomatoes and herbs

STOCK   distilled wine brandy

STORIONE   sturgeon

STORIONE AFFUMICATO   smoked sturgeon fish

STORIONE ALLA MILANESE   sturgeon breaded and fried in butter and oil

STRACCHINO   creamy white soft cheese

STRACCIATELLA   thin batter of eggs, flour, grated Parmesan cheese, lemon rind, poured into boiling meat broth

STRACCIATELLA ALLA ROMANA   chicken broth with shirred egg, cheese and lemon juice

STRACOTTO   meat stew, slowly cooked for several hours

STRACOTTO ALLA TOSCANA   veal stew cooked in wine, herbs and tomato sauce

STRACOTTO DI BUE AL BAROLO   beef braised in red wine

STRACOTTO DI BUE CON PEPERONATA   beef braised with bell peppers

STRANGOLA PRETI   baked nut cake

STRASCINATI   shell-shaped fresh pasta with different sauces

STREGA   a strong herb liqueur

STRISCE   wide ribbon-style pasta

STRISCE E CECI   wide ribbon style pasta with chick-peas

STROZZAPRETI   spinach and cheese paste boiled, sliced and later added to soup

STRUFFOLI   pastries of sweet dough with a thin slice of onion, fried in olive oil

STRUFFOLI ALLA NAPOLETANA   fried pastry with honey, various fruits, ricotta cheese

STRUFFOLI DI NATALE   fried honey cookies

STUFATINO   meat stew

STUFATINO ALLA SICILIANA   beef stew with onions in thick sauce

STUFATINO D'AGNELLO ALL'ACETO   lamb stew with vinegar and green beans

STUFATINO DI MAIALE ALLA BOSCAIOLA   braised pork with wild mushrooms and juniper berries

STUFATINO DI MANZO COI PISELLI   beef stew with red wine and peas

STUFATINO DI VITELLO ALL'ANTICA   veal stew

STUFATO   stewing beef cooked slowly in sauce of tomatoes and other vegetables

STUZZICA APPETITO   antipasti of vegetables pickled in oil and vinegar

SU   up

SUBITO   right away

SUCCO   juice

SUCCO DI FRUTTA   thick fruit juice
SUCCO DI POMODORO   tomato juice
SUCCU TUNNU   soup with semolina and saffron dumplings
SUFFLÉ   soufflé, light frothy baked dish
SUGO   sauce *or* gravy (see SALSA)
SUGO DI ARANCIA   orange juice
SUGO DI CARNE   meat sauce
SUGO DI MARE   seafood sauce
SUGO DI RICOTTA   ricotta cheese sauce with ground
   meat, tomatoes, olive oil
SUPERIORE   higher alcohol content than required
SUPPLÌ   rice croquettes with cheese and meat sauce
SUPPLÌ AL RAGÙ   croquettes made of rice and meat
   sauce, dipped in bread crumbs and fried in olive oil
SUPPLÌ AL TELEFONO   rice croquettes with mozzarella
SUSINA   plum
SVIZZERINA DI VITELLO   grilled veal hamburger

T

TACCHINO   turkey
TACCHINO ALLA BOSCAIOLA   turkey breast in
   mushroom, tongue, ham and herb sauce
TACCHINO ALLA CANZANESE   turkey seasoned with
   bay leaf, rosemary, sage, pepper, served cold with gelatin
TACCHINO ALLA TETRAZZINI   cut up turkey with
   creamed mushroom sauce and pasta, covered with
   grated cheese and bread crumbs and baked
TACCHINO ARROSTO   roasted turkey
TACCHINO ARROSTO RIPIENO   roast stuffed turkey
TACCHINO ARROSTO RIPIENO DI CASTAGNE   roast
   turkey with chestnut stuffing
TACCHINO ARROSTO TARTUFATO   roasted turkey with
   Marsala, butter and truffles
TACCHINO BOLLITO   boiled turkey with vegetables and
   served cold
TACCHINO CON MAIONESE   cold turkey with mayonnaise

TACCHINO CON SALSA REALE   turkey breast in cream sauce with cognac

TACCHINO IN CARPIONE   turkey marinated in wine, herbs, oil and vinegar after cooking

TACCHINO NOSTRANO ARROSTO   turkey local grown and roasted

TACCHINO RIPIENO   stuffed turkey

TACCHINO RIPIENO ALLA LOMBARDA   turkey stuffed with veal, beef, sausage, apple, prunes, chestnuts, cheese and herbs

TACCHINO STUFATO AL VINO BIANCO   turkey stew with wine, mushrooms, vegetables and herbs

TAGLIATELLE   flat noodles

TAGLIATELLE AI QUATTRO FORMAGGI   white or green pasflat noodles ta with four cheeses

TAGLIATELLE ALLA BOLOGNESE   flat noodle pasta with tomato meat sauce

TAGLIATELLE ALLA GENOVESE   flat spinach noodles with mushroom sauce

TAGLIATELLE ALLA SALSA D'UOVO   flat noodle pasta with egg sauce

TAGLIATELLE VERDI ALLA GENOVESE   spinach pasta with sauce of basil, olive oil, garlic, cheese

TAGLIATELLE VERDI CON SALSA ALLA BOLOGNESE E CREMA   spinach pasta with sauce of tomato, meat, onion, olive oil

TAGLIERINI   narrow flat noodle made with egg dough

TAGLIOLINI   thin flat noodles

TAGLIOLINI ALL'OLIO, AGLIO E ROSMARINO   flat noodle with oil, garlic and rosemary

TAGLIOLINI ALLA BEBÉ   flat noodle with chicken, mushrooms and truffles

TAGLIOLINI BERNARDO   flat noodle with tuna

TALEGGIO   medium-hard mild cheese

TANTO   a lot

TAORMINA   sauce of bacon, black olives, anchovies, garlic and mushrooms

TARTARUGA   turtle

TARTINA   open-faced sandwich

TARTUFI   truffles

TARTUFI ALLA PIEMONTESE   truffles baked with
Parmesan

TARTUFI BIANCHI   white truffles

TARTUFI DI CIOCCOLATA   coffee-flavored chocolate
balls served cold

TARTUFI DI MARE   cockles *or* small clams with truffles

TARTUFI FRESCHI   fresh white truffles with butter

TARTUFI NERI   black truffles

TAURASI   full-bodied robust red wine good with meat,
game or rabbit

TAVERNA   small restaurant bar

TAVOLA   table

TAVOLA CALDA   quick-service snack bar

TEGAME   sautéed in butter or oil in small individual pan

TÈ   tea

TÈ AL LATTE   tea with milk

TÈ AL LIMONE   tea with lemon

TEGLIA   fried in a pan

TELEFONO   telephone

TELLINE   small shellfish

TENNERONI DI VITELLO CON PISELLI   veal braised in
wine with broth and peas

TERLANO   white, dry delicate wine from Venice, good
with soup, fish, eggs

TERMINARE   to end

TEROLDEGO   red wine, full, rich, good with game

TESTA DI VITELLO   calf's head

TESTARELLE D'ABBACCHIO   lambs' heads seasoned
with rosemary, basted with olive oil, browned in oven

TESTARELLE DI AGNELLO   roasted lambs' heads,
flavored with honey

TETTINI DI VITELLO ALLA PIZZAIOLA   veal slices
fried in garlic, herb oil and tomato sauce

TIMBALLO   baked pasta casserole with sauce

TIMBALLO DI FUNGHI   baked mold of mushrooms, bread crumbs, garlic, parsley, tomatoes, cheese

TIMBALLO DI INVERNO   pie filled with mozzarella, ham, pork, chicken livers, breast of chicken

TIMBALLO DI LASAGNE ALLA MODENESE   baked lasagna with meat and bechamel sauce

TIMBALLO DI LEGUMI   pie with thin layers of zucchini, ricotta, tomato, rice, vegetable puree

TIMBALLO DI MACCHERONI E POLLO   baked macaroni and chicken pie

TIMBALLO DI MELANZANE   baked eggplant ham and cheese pie

TIMBALLO DI RIGATONI RIPIENI   baked stuffed pasta casserole

TIMBALLO DI RISO   baked rice casserole

TIMBALLO DI SCAMORZA   baked potato and cheese pie

TIMBALLO DI SPAGHETTI E PESCE   baked spaghetti and fish pie

TIMBALLO DI TAGLIATELLE   baked or meat-stuffed pasta casserole

TIMBALLO DI ZUCCHINI   baked zucchini and egg loaf

TIMBALLO DI ZUCCHINI ALLA PIZZAIOLA   zucchini baked with tomato sauce, onion, cheese, anchovy

TIMO   thyme

TINCA CARPIONATA   fried fish marinated in wine, vinegar, sage, garlic and onion

TINCHE   fish, like bass

TINCHE MARINATE   bass marinated then pan-fried

TINCO   knuckle of veal, shin of beef

TIRARE   to pull

TOILETTE   lavatory

TOLETTA   toilet

TONNARELLI   square homemade noodles

TONNARELLI AI FUNGHI   square noodles with mushroom sauce

TONNARELLI AL ROSMARINO   square noodles with butter and rosemary

TONNATO   tuna sauce of garlic, oil, tomato, capers, anchovy

TONNO   tuna

TONNO ALL'AGRODOLCE ALLA TRAPANESE   sweet and sour tuna steaks sautéed in vinegar, wine and sugar

TONNO SOTT'OLIO   tuna fish in oil

TOPINAMBUR   Jerusalem artichokes

TOPINAMBUR AL POMODORO   Jerusalem artichoke smothered with tomato and onion

TOPINAMBUR FRITTI   fried, sliced Jerusalem artichoke

TORDI MATTI   veal pieces cooked on a skewer

TORDO   thrush

TORNEDÓ ALLA ROSSINI   fillet steak fried in butter with ham and mushrooms

TORRE QUARTO BIANCO   light, dry white wine, good with antipasto and seafood

TORRE QUARTO ROSSO   full, smooth red wine, good with meat or game

TORRESANI   small pigeons, domesticated

TORRONE   nougat candy

TORRONE AL CIOCCOLATO   chocolate nougat candy

TORRONE DI CREMONA   hard nougat candy made of egg white, honey, sugar, spices, toasted almonds and candied peel

TORRONE GELATO   iced nougat pudding

TORTA   pie, tart *or* cake

TORTA AL GIANDUIA   chocolate cake with jam, brandy, hazelnuts, honey, etc.

TORTA ALLE ALICI   baked anchovy pie

TORTA CASERECCIA DI POLENTA   cornmeal shortcake with dried fruit and pine nuts

TORTA DI CARCIOFI   artichoke pie in a flaky crust

TORTA DI FRUTTA   fruit flan

TORTA DI FRUTTA CON LA PANNA   fruit flan with cream

TORTA DI FRUTTA SECCA   baked fruit cake with nuts, figs, chocolate, eggs, candied fruit peel

TORTA DI MANDORLE   almond cake

TORTA DI MELE   apple pie *or* torte

TORTA DI MERINGA   fruit pie covered with whipped cream

TORTA DI NOCCIUOLE   hazelnut cake

TORTA DI NOCI   walnut cake

TORTA DI PERE ALLA PAESANA   plain cake with fresh pears

TORTA DI POLENTA E FONTINA   cornmeal and cheese pudding

TORTA DI PRUGNE   baked spongecake with wine, prunes, sugar, eggs

TORTA DI RICOTTA   ricotta cheesecake

TORTA DI RISO   rice cake

TORTA DI VERMICELLI   sweet noodle dessert with honey, raisins, powdered sugar, eggs, cinnamon

TORTA FRITTA   fritters

TORTA GELATA   ice cream cake

TORTA MILLE FOGLIE   thin cake layers separated with custard

TORTA PARADISO   spongecake

TORTA PASQUALINA   baked cheese and spinach pie

TORTA SUL TESTO   bread made on heated slab

TORTA TARANTINA DI PATATE   baked potato pie with cheese, oil, tomato, olives

TORTA ZUCCOTTO   liquor-soaked cake ring filled with fruit, ice cream, chocolate, whipped cream

TORTANO   baked savory cake made with pork renderings

TORTELLI   small fritters or fried cakes or stuffed pasta

TORTELLI ALLE ERBETTE   pasta stuffed with cheese, spinach, boiled

TORTELLI DI ZUCCA   ravioli made with pumpkin cheese stuffing

TORTELLINI   squares of dough stuffed with pork, turkey, veal, beef marrow, cheese

TORTELLINI ALLA BOLOGNESE   tortellini with tomato meat sauce

TORTELLINI ALLA MONTOVANA   tortellini stuffed with ham, veal, pork, chicken and Parmesan cheese, boiled

TORTELLINI ALLA PANNA   stuffed tortellini with cream sauce

TORTELLINI IN BRODO   tortellini stuffed with ham, turkey, cheese, boiled in soup

TORTELLINI VERDI   stuffed spinach tortellini
TORTELLONE   half-round stuffed tortellini
TORTIGLIONE   almond cake
TORTINA DI MARMELLATA   jam-filled tart
TORTINI AL CASTAGNACCIO   chestnut flour cake
TORTINO   tart filled with cheese and vegetables
TORTINO DI CARCIOFI   tart filled with slices of
   artichoke fried together with beaten eggs
TORTINO DI CRESPELLE   crepes stuffed with tomatoes,
   ham and cheese
TORTINO DI FUNGHI E PATATE   baked mushroom and
   potato pie
TORTINO DI MELANZANE E MOZZARELLA   pie with
   baked eggplant, mozzarella, eggs and tomatoes
TORTINO DI MOZZARELLA   cheese tart
TORTINO DI PATATE   potato and cheese tart
TORTINO DI VERDURE   vegetable casserole
TORTINO DI ZUCCHINE   baked zucchini mold with
   bechamel sauce
TORTIONATA ALLA LODIGIANA   almond cake
TOSCANA   tomatoes, celery and herbs
TOSTATO   toasted
TOSTO FRANCESE   French toast, mascarpone cheese,
   maple syrup
TOTANI   young squid
TOTANI E PATATE IN TEGAME ALLA GENOVESE   squid
   and potatoes, sautéed in olive oil, garlic, tomatoes and herbs
TOURNEDOS   beef *or* veal steak from tenderloin fillet
TOURNEDOS AL BAROLO   fillet steak fried in red wine
TOURNEDOS AL COGNAC   fillet steak fried in ham,
   mushrooms and cognac
TOURNEDOS AL MADERA   fillet steak fried in butter
   and Madera red wine
TOURNEDOS ALLA BISMARK   fillet steak fried and
   served with fried egg atop
TOURNEDOS ALLA BORDOLESE   fillet steak fried in
   butter, wine and marrow sauce

TOURNEDOS ALLA FINANZIERA   sweetbreads sautéed with marrow, wine and veal slices

TOVAGLIA   tablecloth

TRACCIOLE DI AGNELLO   lamb and vegetable chunks roasted on a skewer

TRAINIERA   sauce with olives, capers, garlic and ginger

TRAMEZZINO   small sandwich

TRAMINER   white wine

TRANCIA   slice

TRANCIA DI TORTA FARCITA   slice of fruit tart

TRANCIA DI VITELLO   roast veal slice

TRANCIA DI VITELLO AI FUNGHI   roast veal slice with mushrooms

TRASTEVERINA   tomato sauce with white wine, chopped bacon and chicken livers

TRATTORIA   small family-style restaurant

TREBBIANO   pleasant dry white wine good with pasta, fish and antipasti

TREBBIANO D'ABRUZZO   dark yellow dry wine

TRENETTE   flat ribbon-shaped noodles

TRENETTE AL PESTO   flat noodles with basil sauce

TRIESTINA   meat sauce with chopped ham, butter and cream

TRIGLIA   red mullet fish

TRIGLIA AL CARTOCCIO   mullet fish grilled in oiled paper

TRIGLIA ALL'ANCONETANA   mullet fish marinated, baked with ham

TRIGLIA ALLA CALABRESE   mullet fish baked with olive oil, lemon juice, oregano

TRIGLIA ALLA LIGURE   mullet fish sautéed in tomato, wine, anchovy

TRIGLIA ALLA LIVORNESE   mullet fish pan fried with tomato sauce, onion, garlic

TRIGLIA ALLA SICILIANA   mullet fish broiled in wine, meat gravy, orange and lemon juice

TRIPPA   stomach lining, tripe

TRIPPA AL SUGO   tripe sautéed in a meat mushroom sauce

TRIPPA ALLA BOLOGNESE   tripe braised in onion, garlic, lard, grated cheese and broiled

TRIPPA ALLA FIORENTINA   tripe stewed in meat sauce with tomatoes

TRIPPA ALLA GENOVESE   tripe cooked in a meat and tomato sauce, flavored with marjoram and served with grated cheese

TRIPPA ALLA LUCCHESE   tripe with onion, butter, cheese and cinnamon

TRIPPA ALLA MILANESE   tripe stewed with onions, leek, carrots, tomatoes, beans and spices

TRIPPA ALLA PARMIGIANA   tripe with herbs, vegetables, tomato sauce, Parmesan cheese

TRIPPA ALLA ROMANA   tripe in sweet and sour sauce with grated cheese

TRIPPA ALLA SENESE   tripe with local sausage and flavored with saffron

TRIPPA COI FAGIOLI   tripe and beans

TRIPPA CON OSTRICHE   tripe and oysters in a white wine sauce

TRIPPA MARCHIGIANA   tripe sautéed with onion, cabbage, potato, vegetables

TRITTATO   minced

TROTA   trout

TROTA AFFUMICATA   smoked trout

TROTA AL BURRO   pan-fried trout in butter

TROTA AL MARSALA   trout cooked in Marsala wine

TROTA AL POMODORO   trout casserole with tomatoes and garlic

TROTA ALLA BRACE   trout grilled or broiled with garlic oil

TROTA ALLA PIEMONTESE   trout pan fried in vinegar, oil and herbs

TROTA ALLE MANDORLE   stuffed trout, seasoned, baked in cream and topped with almonds

TROTA ARROSTO   trout marinated and baked in herb oil and white wine

TROTA BOLLITA   trout poached in white wine and herbs

TROTA IN BLU   trout boiled and served with mayonnaise

TROTA SALMONATA   salmon trout

TROTE ARROSTITE   spiced trout baked on an open fire or in the oven, sometimes steamed and served with oil, lemon or mayonnaise

TROTELLA   large lake trout (see TROTA)

TROTELLE AL POMODORO   trout with parsley, oil and tomato paste

TUBETTI   small tube-shaped pasta often used in salads

TURCINIELLI   macaroni in the form of little spirals, boiled and served with meat or tomato sauce and grated cheese

TURIDDU   biscuits made of flour, egg and almonds, powdered with sugar icing

TUTTO COMPRESO   everything included

U

UCCELLETTI   small birds

UCCELLETTI ALLA GOLOSA   gourmet veal dish with omelette, mozzarella, tomato sauce, wine

UCCELLETTI ALLA MAREMMANA   small birds cooked in oil with tomatoes, garlic, anchovy and olives, served on fried bread

UCCELLETTI DI CAMPAGNA   thin beef and ham slices rolled, skewered with bread slices and grilled

UMBRIA   sauce of anchovies, oil and garlic flavored with tomatoes and truffles

UMIDO DI GAMBERI E POMODORI PICCANTI   stewed shrimp with tomatoes and hot peppers

UMIDO DI PESCE   fish stew, with tomato, onion, garlic, oil, herbs

UOVA   eggs

UOVA AFFOGATE   poached eggs

UOVA AFFOGATE AL POMODORO   poached eggs in tomato sauce

UOVA AFFOGATE AL VINO   eggs poached in wine

UOVA AFFOGATE COL RISO   poached eggs served with
cheese and rice

UOVA AFFOGATE CON LE PUNTE DI ASPARAGI
poached eggs with asparagus tips

UOVA AGLI SPINACI   omelette with spinach

UOVA AL BURRO   eggs fried in butter

UOVA AL FORMAGGIO   eggs with cheese

UOVA AL FORNO   baked eggs

UOVA AL GROVIERA   eggs made with Swiss or Gruyère
cheese

UOVA AL GUSCIO   soft-boiled eggs

UOVA AL LARDO   fried eggs with bacon

UOVA AL POMODORO   omelette with tomatoes

UOVA AL PROSCIUTTO   omelette with ham

UOVA AL PROSCIUTTO E PANNA   fried eggs with ham
and Parmesan cheese

UOVA AL TEGAME   eggs cooked and served in
individual pan

UOVA ALL'AMERICANA   fried eggs with bacon and tomato

UOVA ALLA CACCIATORA   eggs poached in a tomato
sauce with herbs, onions and chopped chicken livers

UOVA ALLA CAMPAGNOLA   eggs with cooked
vegetables, cheese

UOVA ALLA CAPRICCIOSA   poached eggs in fried
bread with wine and bacon

UOVA ALLA CARDINALE   omelette with seafood,
mushrooms

UOVA ALLA COCOTTE   shirred eggs *or* coddled eggs

UOVA ALLA COQUE   boiled eggs

UOVA ALLA FIORENTINA   fried eggs, served on a bed
of spinach

UOVA ALLA MONACELLA   hard-boiled eggs stuffed
and coated with chocolate

UOVA ALLA PAESANA   omelette with vegetables and
diced ham or bacon

UOVA ALLA PORTOGHESE   omelette with tomato sauce
and paste

UOVA ALLA RUSSA   stuffed hard eggs with mayonnaise sauce

UOVA ALLA SARDA   hard-boiled eggs pan-fried then covered with bread crumbs, fried in garlic oil

UOVA ALLA SPAGNOLA   omelette with tomatoes, onions, peppers and garlic

UOVA ALLA TORINESE   eggs boiled, deviled, then deep fried

UOVA ALLA TRIPPA ALLA ROMANA   baked eggs cooked to look like tripe

UOVA ALLE ERBE   fried eggs cooked with herbs

UOVA BARROTTE   very soft-boiled eggs

UOVA BOLLITTE   boiled eggs

UOVA COI CARCIOFI   poached eggs with artichoke hearts

UOVA COI FEGATINI DI POLLO   eggs with sautéed chicken livers

UOVA COI FRUTTI DI MARE   eggs made with seafood

UOVA COI FUNGHI   eggs with mushrooms

UOVA CON ASPARAGI   egg omelette with asparagus

UOVA CON CONFETTURA   jam-filled omelette

UOVA CON MARMELLATA   eggs prepared with preserves

UOVA CON UVA PASSA AL GUANCIALE   eggs fried with raisins and bacon

UOVA E MOZZARELLA   mozzarella cheese sandwich, dipped in egg batter and deep fried

UOVA FARCITE   hard-cooked then stuffed eggs

UOVA FARCITE AL LIMONE   hard-boiled lemon-stuffed eggs

UOVA FARCITE AL PROSCIUTTO   hard-boiled, ham-stuffed eggs

UOVA FRITTE   fried eggs

UOVA FRITTE CON LA FONTINA   fried eggs on melted cheese toast with anchovies

UOVA FRITTE CON LA MOZZARELLA   fried eggs with cheese

UOVA IN FRITTATA   eggs in an omelette form

UOVA MOLLI   soft-boiled eggs

UOVA RIPIENE   stuffed hard-boiled eggs

UOVA SEMPLICI   plain omelette
UOVA SODE   hard-boiled eggs
UOVA STRACCIATE   scrambled eggs
UOVA STRAPAZZATE   scrambled eggs
UOVA STRAPAZZATE COI PEPERONI   scrambled eggs
   with peppers
UOVA, PANCETTA AFFUMICATA E SALSICCE   eggs,
   smoked bacon and sausage
UOVO   egg
UOVO IN CAMICIA   poached egg
USCITA   exit
UVA   grape
UVA PASSA   raisins
UVA PASSA E PROVOLA   raisins and cheese
UVA SPINA   gooseberries

V

VALDOSTANA   ham and Fontina cheese
VALIGETTA   stuffed braised *or* roasted veal breast
VALPOLICELLA   light red wine
VANIGLIA   vanilla
VARI   assorted (also VARIO)
VECCHIA ROMAGNA   wine distilled to brandy
VELLUTATA DI CARCIOFI   cream of artichoke thickened
   with egg yolk
VELLUTATA DI POLLO   cream of chicken thickened with
   egg yolk
VENTRESCA DI TONNO   belly of tuna fish often canned
   with oil
VENTRISCA   boiled pork belly served cold with white beans
VERDICCHIO   dry white wine, a favorite with seafood
VERDURE   green vegetables
VERDURE ALLA PARMIGIANA   vegetables cooked with
   butter, served with grated cheese
VERDURE COTTE   cooked green vegetables
VERDURE MARINATE   pickled green vegetables

VERDURE MISTE AL FORNO   mixed baked vegetables

VERMENTINO LIGURE   dry white wine, sometimes semi-sparkling

VERMICELLI   very thin long pasta strands

VERMICELLI AI CAPPERI   noodles with caper sauce of capers, anchovy, black olives, garlic, sharp cheese

VERMICELLI AI PEPERONI, OLIVE E CAPPERI   pasta noodles with peppers, olives and capers

VERMICELLI AL SALAME   pasta noodles with salami

VERMICELLI ALL'AGRO   pasta noodles with lemon and oil

VERMICELLI ALLA SICILIANA   pasta noodles served with eggplant, oil, garlic, cheese, olives, anchovies, capers

VERMICELLI CON VONGOLE   thin spaghetti, clams, spicy fresh tomato sauce, herbs

VERNACCIA DI SAN GIMINIANO   wine from Tuscany/Florence

VERZA   green cabbage

VERZADA   pork sausages sautéed in onion and cabbage

VETRO   glass

VIETATA L'ENTRATA   keep out, do not enter

VIETATO FUMARE   no smoking

VILLEROY   white sauce thickened with egg yolk, flavored with Parmesan, truffles, tongue, pieces of cooked ham

VIN SANTO   dessert wine

VINCISGRASSI   pastry filled with meatballs, ragout and bechamel sauce

VINO   wine

VINO APERTO   open wine

VINO BIANCO   white wine

VINO DA TAVOLA   table wine

VINO DEL PAESE   local wine

VINO REGIONALE   regional *or* local wine

VINO ROSATELLO   rosé wine

VINO ROSSO   red wine

VINO TIPICO   typical wine of the area

VISCIOLI   wild cherries

VITELLO   veal

VITELLO AI FUNGHI   veal cooked with mushrooms
VITELLO AL FORNO   veal roast
VITELLO AL UCCELLETTO   roast veal flavored with sage
VITELLO AL VINO ROSSO   veal stewed in red wine
VITELLO ALL'ASSISIANA   veal larded with ham and
   cooked with vegetables, herbs, white wine and milk
VITELLO ALLA MARENGO   veal simmered with wine,
   tomatoes, garlic, onions, mushrooms
VITELLO ALLE MELANZANE   pan-fried veal and
   eggplant slices
VITELLO ARROSTO   roast veal, usually leg
VITELLO ARROSTO AL SOAVE   roast veal in white wine
VITELLO ASCE AI FERRI   veal hamburger grilled
VITELLO BRASATO   veal roast marinated and braised in
   wine herb sauce
VITELLO IN GELATINA ALLA MILANESE   calf's foot
   cooked in wine, sliced, gelatine added, served cold
VITELLO MAGRO   veal loin slices
VITELLO TONNATO   thin veal slices served cold, after
   sautéed with tuna, anchovies, olive oil, wine
VITELLONE   young steer (best beef for steaks)
VOLERE   to desire
VONGOLA   small clam
VONGOLE   clam or mussel sauce, tomatoes, garlic and
   pimento

W

WURSTEL   boiled sausage
WURSTEL AL SUGO DI CARNE   sausage and brown
   sauce
WURSTEL COI CRAUTI   boiled sausage with sauerkraut

Z

ZABAGLIONE   dessert of egg yolks, sugar and Marsala
   wine, served warm

ZALETI   cake with white raisins, eggs, cornmeal, rum, sugar, pine nuts, lemon rind

ZAMPE DI MAIALE   pigs' feet boiled in broth

ZAMPONE DI MODENA   pig's foot stuffed with minced and spiced pork

ZEPPOLA   deep-fried fritter *or* doughnut

ZEPPOLE DI SAN GIUSEPPE   dessert fritters with cinnamon and sugar

ZIMINO   fish stew

ZITI   large macaroni

ZITI ALLA NAPOLETANA   macaroni with meat gravy

ZITONI   very long macaroni

ZUCCA   large yellow squash

ZUCCHERIERA   sugar bowl

ZUCCHERO   sugar

ZUCCHINE   Italian squash

ZUCCHINE ALL'AGRODOLCE   squash sautéed in a sweet and sour sauce

ZUCCHINE ALLA PANNA   squash in cream with rosemary

ZUCCHINE ALLA PARMIGIANA   squash sliced and sautéed in butter, garlic and lemon

ZUCCHINE ALLA SVELTA   shredded zucchini squash quick-fried in butter and lemon juice

ZUCCHINE COI PEPERONI   zucchini and peppers baked with anchovies, oil, tomatoes, cheese

ZUCCHINE CON PEPERONI AL FORNO   baked zucchini and peppers

ZUCCHINE FARCITE   squash stuffed with ham, mushrooms, herbs and cheese, baked

ZUCCHINE FRITTE   batter-dipped and deep-fried squash

ZUCCHINE GRATINATE   baked zucchini with tomato, herbs and cheese

ZUCCHINE IMBOTTITE DI CARNE   zucchini stuffed with meat

ZUCCHINE IN CARPIONE   marinated squash (usually cold)

ZUCCHINE IN SCAPECE   cold, fried zucchini squash with vinegar sauce

ZUCCHINE RIPIENE   stuffed zucchini

ZUCCHINE SALTATE ALL'ORIGANO   sautéed zucchini with oregano

ZUCCHINE TRIFOLATE CON LE CIPOLLE   sautéed zucchini with onions

ZUCCO   amber-yellow wine, pleasing bouquet, generous flavor

ZUCCOTTO   creamy icebox cake made with fruit and liquor

ZUPPA   soup, also see MINISTRINA, MINISTRONE, CONSOMMÉ

ZUPPA AI DUE COLORI   vanilla and chocolate pudding on spongecake

ZUPPA AL COLTIVATORE   thick vegetable soup with chopped bacon

ZUPPA ALL'EMILIANA   spongecake, custard, chocolate and cherry preserve

ZUPPA ALLA CERTOSINA   broth from fish, onion, olive oil, tomato, egg and cheese

ZUPPA ALLA CONTADINA   thick vegetable soup with garlic, wine and rice

ZUPPA ALLA MARINARA   stew of fish, with garlic, parsley and tomatoes, served with pieces of toasted, fried bread

ZUPPA ALLA PAESANA   peasant vegetable soup with anchovy, herbs and cheese

ZUPPA ALLA PAVESE CON L'UOVO   consommé in which floats an egg yolk, sprinkled with Parmesan cheese, on a little raft of toast

ZUPPA ALLA SARDA   soup of meat stock with eggs and cheese added then served over toast

ZUPPA CAODA   casserole made with pigeons, wine, cheese and baked

ZUPPA DEI POVERI ALLA RUGOLA   tart green salad and potato soup

ZUPPA DI ANGUILLE   eel soup with onions, vegetables, wine vinegar

ZUPPA DI BACCALÀ   soup with salt cod, wine, tomato, potato, herbs

ZUPPA DI CALAMARI E CARCIOFI   squid and artichoke soup

ZUPPA DI CASTAGNE   chestnut soup

ZUPPA DI CECI   chick-pea soup

ZUPPA DI CIPOLLE   onion soup

ZUPPA DI CODA DI BUE   oxtail soup

ZUPPA DI COZZE   mussel soup *or* chowder

ZUPPA DI DATTERI   fish soup

ZUPPA DI DATTERI ALLA VIAREGGINA   mussel soup heavily seasoned with olive oil, tomatoes, pepper and garlic

ZUPPA DI FAGIOLI   bean soup

ZUPPA DI FARINA ABBRUSTOLITA   light soup in which hard grain flour, slightly toasted, is cooked in place of the more usual greens or semolina

ZUPPA DI FINOCCHI SELVATICI   fennel casserole with sharp cheese, olive oil, toasted bread

ZUPPA DI FONTINA   bread and cheese soup

ZUPPA DI FRUTTI DI MARE   all shellfish soup

ZUPPA DI LATTUGHE RIPIENE   stuffed lettuce soup

ZUPPA DI ORTAGGI   vegetable soup of mostly greens

ZUPPA DI PESCE   fish stew

ZUPPA DI PESCE ALLA POZZUOLI   fish-stew soup

ZUPPA DI PESCE E GAMBERI   creamy fish soup with shrimps and saffron

ZUPPA DI PISELLI E VONGOLE   pea and clam soup

ZUPPA DI POLLO   chicken soup

ZUPPA DI RISO E CAVOLO STUFATO   rice and smothered cabbage soup

ZUPPA DI RISO, CAVOLO E RAPA   rice and kohlrabi cabbage soup

ZUPPA DI SEDANO   celery soup

ZUPPA DI TRIPPA   soup with strips of tripe, chopped potato and tomato, flavored with bacon, onion and celery

ZUPPA DI VERDURA   soup of vegetables and greens
ZUPPA DI VONGOLE   seafood stew with garlic, parsley,
    tomatoes served with pieces of toasted, fried bread
ZUPPA INGLESE   cake steeped in custard sauce and rum
    and cordials
ZUPPA PRIMAVERA   fresh spring vegetable soup
ZUPPA SANTA   puree of potato, sorrel and herbs